D0857375

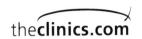

PEDIATRIC CLINICS
OF NORTH AMERICA

Pediatric Palliative Care

GUEST EDITORS
Tammy I. Kang, MD
David Munson, MD
Jeffrey C. Klick, MD

October 2007 • Volume 54 • Number 5

SAUNDERS

An Imprint of Elsevier, Inc.
PHILADELPHIA   LONDON   TORONTO   MONTREAL   SYDNEY   TOKYO

W.B. SAUNDERS COMPANY
A Division of Elsevier Inc.

1600 John F. Kennedy Boulevard • Suite 1800 • Philadelphia, Pennsylvania 19103

http://www.theclinics.com

THE PEDIATRIC CLINICS OF NORTH AMERICA
October 2007
Editor: Carla Holloway

Volume 54, Number 5
ISSN 0031-3955
ISBN-13: 978-1-4160-5107-7
ISBN-10: 1-4160-5107-4

The Pediatric Clinics of North America (ISSN 0031-3955) is published bi-monthly by Elsevier Inc. 360 Park Avenue South, New York, NY 10010-1710. Months of publication are February, April, June, August, October, and December. Business and Editorial Offices: 1600 John F. Kennedy Blvd., Suite 1800, Philadelphia, PA 19103-2899. Customer Service Office: 6277 Sea Harbor Drive, Orlando, FL 32887-4800. Periodicals postage paid at New York, NY and additional mailing offices. Subscription prices are $138.00 per year (US individuals), $281.00 per year (US institutions), $187.00 per year (Canadian individuals), $367.00 per year (Canadian institutions), $209.00 per year (international individuals), $367.00 per year (international institutions), $72.00 per year (US students), $110.00 per year (Canadian students), and $110.00 per year (foreign students). To receive students/resident rare, orders must be accompanied by name of affiliated institution, date of term, and the signature of program/residency coordinator on institution letterhead. Orders will be billed at individual rate until proof of status is received. Foreign air speed delivery is included in all Clinics subscription prices. All prices are subject to change without notice. POSTMASTER: Send address changes to *The Pediatric Clinics of North America*, Elsevier Periodicals Customer Service, 6277 Sea Harbor Drive, Orlando, FL 32887-4800. **Customer Service: 1-800-654-2452 (US). From outside of the US, call 1-407-345-4000**. E-mail: hhspcs@harcourt.com.

The Pediatric Clinics of North America is also published in Spanish by McGraw-Hill Inter-americana Editores S.A., Mexico City, Mexico; in Portuguese by Riechmann and Affonso Editores, Rua Comandante Coelho 1085, CEP 21250, Rio de Janeiro, Brazil; and in Greek by Althayia SA, Athens, Greece.

The Pediatric Clinics of North America is covered in *Index Medicus*, *Excerpta Medica*, *Current Contents*, *Current Contents/Clinical Medicine*, *Science Citation Index*, *ASCA*, *ISI/BIOMED*, and *BIOSIS*.

Printed in the United States of America.

GOAL STATEMENT

The goal of the *Pediatric Clinics of North America* is to keep practicing physicians and residents up to date with current clinical practice in pediatrics by providing timely articles reviewing the state-of-the-art in patient care.

ACCREDITATION

The *Pediatric Clinics of North America* is planned and implemented in accordance with the Essential Areas and Policies of the Accreditation Council for Continuing Medical Education (ACCME) through the joint sponsorship of the University Of Virginia School Of Medicine and Elsevier. The University Of Virginia School of Medicine is accredited by the ACCME to provide continuing medical education for physicians.

The University of Virginia School of Medicine designates this educational activity for a maximum of 15 *AMA PRA Category 1 Credits*™. Physicians should only claim credit commensurate with the extent of their participation in the activity.

The American Medical Association has determined that physicians not licensed in the US who participate in this CME activity are eligible for 15 *AMA PRA Category 1 Credits*™.

Credit can be earned by reading the text material, taking the CME examination online at: *http://www.theclinics.com/home/cme*, and completing the evaluation. After taking the test, you will be required to review any and all incorrect answers. Following completion of the test and evaluation, your credit will be awarded and you may print your certificate.

FACULTY DISCLOSURE/CONFLICT OF INTEREST

The University of Virginia School of Medicine, as an ACCME accredited provider, endorses and strives to comply with the Accreditation Council for Continuing Medical Education (ACCME) Standards of Commercial Support, Commonwealth of Virginia statutes, University of Virginia policies and procedures, and associated federal and private regulations and guidelines on the need for disclosure and monitoring of proprietary and financial interests that may affect the scientific integrity and balance of content delivered in continuing medical education activities under our auspices.

The University of Virginia School of Medicine requires that all CME activities accredited through this institution be developed independently and be scientifically rigorous, balanced and objective in the presentation/discussion of its content, theories and practices.

All authors/editors participating in an accredited CME activity are expected to disclose to the readers relevant financial relationships with commercial entities occurring within the past 12 months (such as grants or research support, employee, consultant, stock holder, member of speakers bureau, etc.). The University of Virginia School of Medicine will employ appropriate mechanisms to resolve potential conflicts of interest to maintain the standards of fair and balanced education to the reader. Questions about specific strategies can be directed to the Office of Continuing Medical Education, University of Virginia School of Medicine, Charlottesville, Virginia.

The authors/editors listed below have identified no financial or professional relationships for themselves or their spouse/partner:
Allison Ballantine, MD; Ivor Berkowitz, MBBCh; Jean M. Carroll, RN, BSN; Chris Feudtner, MD, PhD, MPH; Stephen J. Friedrichsdorf, MD; Carla Holloway (Acquisitions Editor); Tammy I. Kang, MD (Guest Editor); Leslie S. Kersun, MD, MSCE; Jeffrey C. Klick, MD (Guest Editor); Steven R. Leuthner, MD, MA; Daniel J. Licht, MD; Jennifer W. Mack, MD, MPH; Oscar H. Mayer, MD; Mary McSherry, ACSW, LSW; Wynne Morrison, MD; David Munson, MD (Guest Editor); Mary T. Rourke, PhD; Gina Santucci, MSN, APNP-BC; Renee A. Shelhaas, MD; Eyal Shemesh, MD; Christy Torkildson, RN, MSN, PHN; Christina K. Ullrich, MD; Jeannine S. Winsness, RN, MSN, CRNP; and, Courtney J. Wustoff, MD.

The authors/editors listed below identified the following professional or financial affiliations for themselves or their spouse/partner:
Kathy Kehoe, LCSW is employed by and on the Speaker's bureau for Samaritan Hospice.

Disclosure of Discussion of Non-FDA Approved Uses for Pharmaceutical and/or Medical Devices:
The University of Virginia School of Medicine, as an ACCME provider, requires that all authors identify and disclose any "off label" uses for pharmaceutical and medical device products. The University of Virginia School of Medicine recommends that each physician fully review all the available data on new products or procedures prior to clinical use.

TO ENROLL

To enroll in the Pediatric Clinics of North America Continuing Medical Education program, call customer service at 1-800-654-2452 or visit us online at *www.theclinics.com/home/cme*. The CME program is available to subscribers for an additional fee of $195.00.

GUEST EDITORS

TAMMY I. KANG, MD, Medical Director, The Pediatric Advanced Care Team; and Assistant Professor of Pediatrics, Division of Oncology, University of Pennsylvania School of Medicine The Children's Hospital of Philadelphia, Philadelphia, Pennsylvania

DAVID MUNSON, MD, Associate Medical Director, The Pediatric Advanced Care Team; and Assistant Professor of Clinical Pediatrics, Division of Neonatology, University of Pennsylvania School of Medicine, The Children's Hospital of Philadelphia, Philadelphia, Pennsylvania

JEFFREY C. KLICK, MD, Director of Education, The Pediatric Advanced Care Team, and Attending Physician, Division of General Pediatrics and The Pediatric Advanced Care Team, Children's Hospital of Pennsylvania; and Assistant Physician, Department of Pediatrics, University of Pennsylvania School of Medicine, Philadelphia, Pennsylvania

CONTRIBUTORS

ALLISON BALLANTINE, MD, Assistant Professor, Department of Pediatrics, University of Pennsylvania School of Medicine; and Attending Physician, Division of General Pediatrics and the Pediatric Advanced Care Team, The Children's Hospital of Philadelphia, Philadelphia, Pennsylvania

IVOR BERKOWITZ, MBBCh, Associate Professor, Division of Pediatric Anesthesiology and Critical Care Medicine, Johns Hopkins School of Medicine, Baltimore, Maryland

JEAN M. CARROLL, RN, BSN, Nurse Coordinator, The Pediatric Advanced Care Team, The Children's Hospital of Philadelphia, Philadelphia, Pennsylvania

CHRIS FEUDTNER, MD, PhD, MPH, Division of General Pediatrics and The Pediatric Advanced Care Team, Children's Hospital of Philadelphia; and the Leonard Davis Institute of Health Economics, University of Pennsylvania, Philadelphia, Pennsylvania

STEFAN J. FRIEDRICHSDORF, MD, Medical Director, Pain and Palliative Care, Children's Hospitals and Clinics of Minnesota, Minneapolis, Minnesota

TAMMY I. KANG, MD, Medical Director, The Pediatric Advanced Care Team; and Assistant Professor of Pediatrics, Division of Oncology, University of Pennsylvania School of Medicine The Children's Hospital of Philadelphia, Philadelphia, Pennsylvania

LESLIE S. KERSUN, MD, MSCE, Division of Oncology, The Children's Hospital of Philadelphia; and Assistant Professor of Pediatrics, Department of Pediatrics, The University of Pennsylvania School of Medicine, Philadelphia, Pennsylvania

KATHY KEHOE, LCSW, Bereavement Counselor, Marlton, New Jersey

JEFFREY C. KLICK, MD, Director of Education, The Pediatric Advanced Care Team, and Attending Physician, Division of General Pediatrics and The Pediatric Advanced Care Team, Children's Hospital of Pennsylvania; and Assistant Physician, Department of Pediatrics, University of Pennsylvania School of Medicine, Philadelphia, Pennsylvania

STEVEN R. LEUTHNER, MD, MA, Associate Professor of Pediatrics and Bioethics, The Medical College of Wisconsin, Wauwatosa; and Director, Fetal Concerns Program, Children's Hospital of Wisconsin, Milwaukee, Wisconsin

DANIEL J. LICHT, MD, Assistant Professor of Neurology and Pediatrics, Division of Child Neurology, The Children's Hospital of Philadelphia, Philadelphia, Pennsylvania

JENNIFER W. MACK, MD, MPH, Attending Physician in Pediatric Hematology/Oncology and Pediatric Palliative Care, Dana Farber Cancer Institute; Children's Hospital Boston, Department of Oncology; and Instructor in Pediatrics, Harvard Medical School, Boston, Massachusetts

OSCAR H. MAYER, MD, Assistant Professor of Clinical Pediatrics, Division of Pulmonology; and The Pediatric Advanced Care Team, The Children's Hospital of Philadelphia, Philadelphia, Pennsylvania

MARY McSHERRY, ACSW, LSW, The Pediatric Advanced Care Team, The Children's Hospital of Philadelphia, Philadelphia, Pennsylvania

WYNNE MORRISON, MD, Assistant Professor, Department of Anesthesiology and Critical Care, The Children's Hospital of Philadelphia, University of Pennsylvania School of Medicine, Philadelphia, Pennsylvania

DAVID MUNSON, MD, Associate Medical Director, The Pediatric Advanced Care Team; and Assistant Professor of Clinical Pediatrics, Division of Neonatology, University of Pennsylvania School of Medicine, The Children's Hospital of Philadelphia, Philadelphia, Pennsylvania

MARY T. ROURKE, PhD, Psychologist and Associate Director, The Behavioral Health Integrated Program, The Children's Hospital of Philadelphia, Philadelphia, Pennsylvania

GINA SANTUCCI, MSN, APNP-BC, The Pediatric Advanced Care Team, The Children's Hospital of Philadelphia, Philadelphia, Pennsylvania

RENÉE A. SHELLHAAS, MD, Epilepsy and Electrophysiology Fellow, Division of Child Neurology, The Children's Hospital of Philadelphia, Philadelphia, Pennsylvania

EYAL SHEMESH, MD, Director, Behavioral Health Integrated Program, Behavioral Health Center; and Department of Child and Adolescent Psychiatry, The Children's Hospital of Philadelphia, Philadelphia, Pennsylvania

CHRISTY TORKILDSON, RN, MSN, PHN, Doctoral Student, School of Nursing, University of California San Francisco, San Francisco; and National Director for Education, Research, and Professional Relations, George Mark Children's House, San Leandro, California

CHRISTINA K. ULLRICH, MD, Instructor in Pediatrics, Harvard Medical School; and Attending Physician in Pediatric Hematology/Oncology, Department of Pediatrics, Dana Farber Cancer Institute and Children's Hospital Boston, Boston, Massachusetts

JEANNINE S. WINSNESS, RN, MSN, CRNP, Pediatric Palliative Care Consultants, LLC, Wayne, Pennsylvania

COURTNEY J. WUSTHOFF, MD, Fellow of Child Neurology, Division of Child Neurology, The Children's Hospital of Philadelphia, Philadelphia, Pennsylvania

CONTENTS

In an ideal world, all of us—patients, parents, family members, nurses, physicians, social workers, therapists, pastoral care workers, and others—would always work together in a collaborative manner to provide the best care possible. This article bases the framework for pursuing this ideal upon studies of communication between patients, families, and clinicians, as well as more general works on communication, collaboration, decision making, mediation, and ethics, and is comprised of four parts: (1) what is meant by collaborative communication; (2) key concepts that influence how we frame the situations that children with life-threatening conditions confront and how these frameworks shape the care we provide; (3) general topics that are important to the task of collaborative communication, specifically how we use heuristics when we set about to solve complicated problems; and (4) three common tasks of collaborative communication, offering practical advice for patient care.

Quality end-of-life care includes the management of distressing symptoms; provisions of care, including the assessment and management of psychosocial and spiritual needs; and respite from diagnosis through death and bereavement. Meeting the palliative care goal of improved quality of life depends on medical and nursing practitioners understatnding and effectively assessing psychosocial symptoms.

care in children develop. Concomitantly, there arises the need to decide when it is appropriate to use these technologies. It is at this point that the skills of relationship building, listening, and empathic concern become indispensable.

FORTHCOMING ISSUES

RECENT ISSUES

Pediatr Clin N Am 54 (2007) xv–xvii

PEDIATRIC CLINICS

OF NORTH AMERICA

ELSEVIER
SAUNDERS

Preface

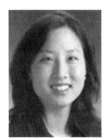 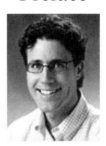 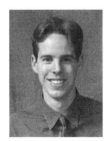

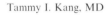

Tammy I. Kang, MD   David Munson, MD   Jeffrey C. Klick, MD

Guest Editors

Despite dramatic advances in the diagnosis and treatment of pediatric diseases, death during childhood remains a persistent reality—and a compelling clinical responsibility—for pediatric health care services. The past decade has seen an enormous shift in the attitudes, beliefs, and practices of pediatric palliative medicine. The concepts have been outlined and supported by national organizations, including the Institute of Medicine and the American Academy of Pediatrics.

In 2002, the Institute of Medicine issued a landmark report, *When Children Die*, that delineated the need for significant improvement in the palliative, end-of-life, and bereavement care received by this population [1]. In 2007, the American Boards of Medical Specialties—through a unique joint sponsorship by seven Boards (including Pediatrics, Internal Medicine, Family Medicine, Anesthesiology, Physical Medicine and Rehabilitation, Psychiatry and Neurology, and Surgery)—initiated a pathway that will establish a new subspecialty board of Hospice and Palliative Medicine.

However, this emphasis on the concepts of pediatric palliative care needs to be translated to bedside practice. We are often asked to describe pediatric palliative care to those unfamiliar with its goals and concepts. The World Health Organization and others offer a broad description of palliative care as "the active total care of patients whose disease is not responsive to curative treatment. Control of pain, of other symptoms, and of psychological, social, and spiritual problems is paramount. The goal of palliative care is achievement of the best quality of life for patients and their families." One of our courageous parents describes palliative care as "help with the

doi:10.1016/j.pcl.2007.08.003   *pediatric.theclinics.com*

'you never know.'" She echoes the feelings of many parents who say they "hope and pray that everything will be okay, but you never know. Palliative care helps me be the best Mom for him; to be emotionally and spiritually strong, to be a good parent, and to make the best decisions for him. Palliative care helps me to facilitate all of those things. Because when I'm falling apart, they are there to help put me back together."

We believe that palliative care can have different meanings for each child, each parent, and each sibling. For some children, aggressive pain and symptom management is a large focus of our team's involvement. For others, it is a focus on spiritual questions and struggles. One constant in all of our families is the need to maintain hope during seemingly hopeless moments. We constantly strive to develop ways to better communicate with families to help them through difficult transitions and discussions. As one of our nurses described: "We are constantly present." We are present for discussions that health care professionals historically avoided, we are present to aggressively treat physical pain and suffering, we are present at moments when parents are struggling with difficult decisions, we are present to celebrate moments with families when the disease unexpectedly improves, we are present through grief and bereavement.

Providing the highest quality care to dying patients—more generally, patients living with life-limiting or life-threatening conditions—and to their families is a vital, yet formidable, challenge. How do we, as health care professionals, translate the goals of palliative care into concrete practices for all those involved in caring for these children and their families? How do we incorporate the needs of individual children and their families into our daily practices?

In that vein, this issue of *Pediatric Clinics of North America* is dedicated to Pediatric Palliative Care in practice. We sought to provide the reader with a general overview of topics common to the care of children who have life-limiting illnesses and their families, as well as to provide information and practical advice for both the general practitioner and those who work in the field of palliative medicine. It is by no means intended to be all inclusive. As the field advances, the medical literature on these important topics continues to grow. Textbooks such as the *Oxford Text of Pediatric Palliative Care For Children* [2] can provide practitioners with more in-depth coverage of subjects integral to the practice of pediatric palliative care.

In general, Pediatric Palliative Care focuses on three prominent aspects that, although essential to approach in an interdisciplinary fashion blended together in a unified approach to care, can be discussed separately. First, and arguably most important, communication is the cornerstone of good pediatric palliative care. Understanding how disease processes and our innate abilities and liabilities affect that communication is essential to building a foundation of collaboration and a sense of teamwork with the family. Second, psychosocial aspects of pediatric palliative care are very important to the present and future well being of the child, family, and the practitioner. Focusing on the issues that affect the child's, families', and practitioners' physical and mental health must be a focus when caring for dying children. Finally, the aspect that is most easily translated into clinical practice is caring for the specific needs of the child in front of us. We provide tools for managing common symptoms, including pain, dyspnea, depression, agitation, anxiety, gastrointestinal complaints, spasticity, and seizures; provide insight into caring for children in unique circumstances, including fetal and neonatal care, chronic illness, and withdrawal of support; and provide practical advice in regards to "do not attempt resuscitation" discussions and orders as well as the practical aspects of caring for these children outside the hospital and in the community.

Regardless of your clinical focus or subspecialty, every practitioner will care for a child who is dying. We hope that minding the topics discussed in this issue will help to improve the quality of life for that child, their family, and even yourself.

Tammy I. Kang, MD
Pediatric Advanced Care Team
Division of Oncology
The Children's Hospital of Philadelphia
34 Street and Civic Center Boulevard
Philadelphia, PA 19104, USA

E-mail address: kang@email.chop.edu

David Munson, MD
Pediatric Advanced Care Team
Neonatology and Newborn Infant Center
The Children's Hospital of Philadelphia
34 Street and Civic Center Boulevard
Philadelphia, PA 19104, USA

E-mail address: munson@email.chop.edu

Jeffrey C. Klick, MD
Pediatric Advanced Care Team
Department of Pediatrics
The Children's Hospital of Philadelphia
34 Street and Civic Center Boulevard
Philadelphia, PA 19104, USA

E-mail address: klick@email.chop.edu

References

[1] Field M, Behrman R. When children die: improving palliative and end-of-life care for children and their families. Washington DC: The National Academies Press; 2003.
[2] Oxford Textbook of Palliative Care for Children. New York: Oxford University Press; 2006.

PEDIATRIC CLINICS
OF NORTH AMERICA

Pediatr Clin N Am 54 (2007) 583–607

Collaborative Communication in Pediatric Palliative Care: A Foundation for Problem-Solving and Decision-Making

Chris Feudtner, MD, PhD, MPH[a,b,*]

[a]*Division of General Pediatrics and the Pediatric Advanced Care Team, Children's Hospital of Philadelphia – North, 3535 Market Street, Room 1523, Philadelphia, PA 19104, USA*
[b]*Leonard Davis Institute of Health Economics, University of Pennsylvania, 3641 Locust Walk, Philadelphia, PA 19104, USA*

Let us communicate with each other clearly, compassionately, and collaboratively, as we strive to improve the quality of life for children including, when necessary, that part of life that is dying.

I offer us this goal at the outset, as it will guide our journey over the course of the following pages, and perhaps beyond. Throughout this article, I will address you, the reader, directly. I do so with respect, aiming to be as straightforward and clear as possible about the cognitive and emotional challenges of communicating in a collaborative manner. While I anticipate that most of you are clinicians, I will also attempt to make our discussion useful for those of you who are parents, or even patients. In an ideal world, all of us—patients, parents, family members, nurses, physicians, social workers, therapists, pastoral care workers, and others—would always work together in a collaborative manner to provide the best care possible to the patient: this article is committed to this ideal, and when I say "we" or "our" I respectfully mean to imply all of us. As much as possible, I base the frameworks and suggestions that I present in part upon studies of communication between patients, families, and clinicians [1–10], as well as more general works on communication, collaboration, decision-making, mediation, and ethics [11–19], all of which have been filtered through my own experiences as a physician, family member, and patient [20,21].

* Division of General Pediatrics and the Pediatric Advanced Care Team, Children's Hospital of Philadelphia – North, 3535 Market Street, Room 1523, Philadelphia, PA 19104.
 E-mail address: feudtner@email.chop.edu

0031-3955/07/$ - see front matter © 2007 Elsevier Inc. All rights reserved.
doi:10.1016/j.pcl.2007.07.008   *pediatric.theclinics.com*

This article unfolds in four parts. Part I explores what we mean by collaborative communication. Part II examines key concepts that influence how we frame the situations that children with life-threatening conditions confront, and how these frameworks shape the care we provide. Part III considers a few general topics that are important to the task of collaborative communication, specifically how we use little habits of thought—called heuristics—when we set about to solve complicated problems, how emotion affects the exchange of information between people, and how we can avoid certain pitfalls when engaging in difficult conversations. Part IV proceeds through three common tasks of collaborative communication, offering practical advice for patient care.

Part I: collaborative communication

What does the phrase "collaborative communication" aim to convey? The wide-ranging concept of communication indicates "the imparting or exchanging of information or news" [22]. Modifying this general concept is the idea that collaboration speaks to a particular type of communication, one that aims to be "produced or conducted by two or more parties working together" [22].

Collaborative communication encapsulates both the exchange of information and the nature of the collaborative relationship between the persons who are communicating. It recognizes the essential reciprocity and dynamic synergy of this pair of concepts, whereby better communication enhances collaboration, and more skillful collaboration can improve communication. Stated somewhat differently: collaborative communication emphasizes the relationships between people, viewing interpersonal communication and relationships as inexorably entwined [23].

Collaborative communication is distinguished by participants' desire to accomplish at least five important tasks:

1. Establishing a common goal or set of goals that guide our collaborative efforts.
2. Exhibiting mutual respect and compassion for each other.
3. Developing a sufficiently complete understanding of our differing perspectives.
4. Assuring maximum clarity and correctness of what we communicate to each other.
5. Managing intrapersonal and interpersonal processes that affect how we send, receive, and process information.

Part II: a general overview of pediatric palliative care

The challenges—and opportunities—of collaborative communication are best understood when situated in the broader context of palliative care, including the core tasks of palliative care, the ways in which the experiences of "dying" unfold for children with life-threatening conditions, and how our medical system distinguishes palliative care from other modes of care.

Palliative care

Over the past decade a consensus has emerged [24–27] that, in general, palliative care for adults involves eight interrelated core activities:

1. Provide effective pain and symptom management to help minimize suffering.
2. Attend to and minimize sources of emotional, social, and spiritual suffering.
3. Minimize the amount of time that patients spend with what they would deem to be an unacceptably poor quality of life before dying.
4. Communicate in a manner that prepares and empowers patients and families.
5. Enhance the patient's and family's ability to make what they feel are good decisions.
6. Assure that medical treatment is in accord with patient and family wishes.
7. Strive to strengthen important relationships between the patient and family and friends.
8. Provide loved ones with bereavement support and grief care.

In pediatric palliative care [28,29], we can organize this plethora of tasks into three domains, illustrated by Fig. 1.

1) Problem-solving and decision-making activities involve identifying and describing the problems or predicaments that confront the patient and those caring for the patient. They include clarifying the goals and hopes that motivate and guide care; and in light of these goals of care, evaluating the pros and cons of a variety of options, ranging from specific treatments to locations of care.
2) Interventions typically seek to improve the quality of life and minimize suffering for patients, family members, and clinical staff. They address the physical, mental, emotional, social, cultural, spiritual, and existential needs of the individual.
3) Logistical efforts aim to provide high-quality services in various settings, including the hospital and home; to coordinate these services; and to arrange appropriate payment.

Pathways of dying

Broadly speaking, the pathways of dying followed by infants, children, and adolescents who die in the United States display four different patterns, illustrated by Fig. 2.

For many children, death occurs suddenly, as in pattern *A*. These are the deaths due to traumatic injury (either unintentional, such as motor vehicle

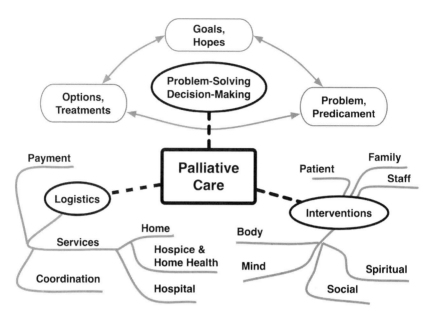

Fig. 1. Palliative care and its three core domains of tasks.

collisions, or intentional, such as homicide), precipitous premature birth, or occult conditions, such as cerebral aneurisms and cardiac arrhythmias. In these cases, pediatric palliative care focuses mostly on bereavement care for the family after the child's death, and support of the emergency responders and clinicians who cared for the patient.

The second pattern, pattern *B*, includes children who had been in good health until a disease or condition, such as a malignancy or a degenerative disorder, began to cause a steady decline in quality of life, predictably and inexorably. A major focus of palliative care for these children involves efforts to maximize a child's quality of life for as long as possible (as depicted in the figure by the arrow and the rightward shift of the alternative palliative care pathway, with higher quality of life levels but perhaps for a shorter length of time).

Pattern *B* also illustrates a peculiar aspect of the pathways to death, an aspect that may seem macabre but is important. In each of the patterns depicted in Fig. 2, the scale for quality of life ranges from 100 (maximum quality of life) to 0 (the quality of life associated with being dead). The scale then extends below 0 (a quality of life worse than being dead) as in patterns *B*, *C* and *D*. In common parlance, people will refer to certain circumstances as being "a fate worse than death." Researchers focused on developing concepts about quality of life have documented that conditions involving great suffering or profound impairment are viewed by many as being worse than death [30]. A core task of palliative care is to prevent a child's quality of life from descending into these states worse than death. In pattern *B*, the

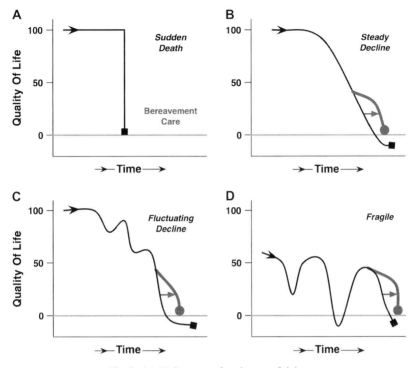

Fig. 2. (A–D) Patterns of pathways of dying.

alteration in the pathway brought about by palliative care therefore depicts not only maximization of quality of life, but also the minimization of time spent with the quality of life below 0.

Pattern C reflects, essentially, a variation on pattern B, whereby the pace of decline after the onset of the condition varies significantly, with episodes of worsening health interspersed among periods of relative recovery. Pattern C is the pathway for many children who die from a wide variety of medical conditions, ranging from malignancies that enter remission and then relapse, to cystic fibrosis with periodic exacerbations, to metabolic disorders that cause lasting injury with every episode of decompensation. Here again, palliative care aims to maximize quality of life by maximizing the "good" aspects of the child's life, for example by facilitating goals, such as residing at home and minimizing suffering through assiduous management of symptoms, and by preventing time spent with a quality of life worse than death.

A fourth group of children follow a different pathway, depicted as pattern D. These children have impairments of physiologic function that render them fragile and more vulnerable to recurrent health crises than other children are. These crises are often of sudden onset and precipitated by otherwise innocuous events, such as a common cold or a bout of emesis. This state of fragile health or extreme vulnerability to life-threatening illness is typically long-standing, with the quality of life less than ideal for months or years. Consequently—and very importantly—the pattern of fragile health comes to define the way of life for these children and their families, as they often live waiting for the next crises and setback. For a clinician or family member, determining when the child is dying can be difficult. Deciding when to redefine the goals of care from life extending to comfort seeking can be divisive within families, between families and clinicians, and among clinicians.

In large part, these difficulties of deciding when to redefine the goals of care arise as a result of difficulties of predicting what the child's health state will be in the future. As illustrated in Fig. 3, the difficulties of prognostication can be summarized by five major questions.

First, what was the child's health status and quality of life before this crisis? People are likely to have different answers to this question, based largely on their relationship to the patient, their degree of knowledge about the child over time, and their personal values and beliefs. These differences of perspective are worth exploring. For instance, if the clinicians have come to know the child chiefly when the child is critically ill and hospitalized, their perspective may be broadened if the family shares photographs of the child interacting with other family members, taken during a period of relative wellness.

Second, how likely is the child to survive the current crisis? Clinicians should be aware that parents may have witnessed the child survive severe crises in the past. They may then condition their assessment of the probability of survival on this past record of "beating the odds."

Third, if the child were to survive, what would the child have to endure on the path of recovery? For instance, in the best-case scenario, would a prolonged period of intubation and mechanical ventilation nevertheless be necessary?

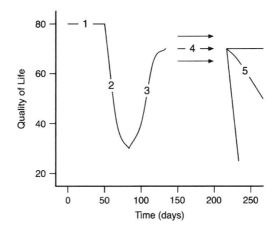

Fig. 3. Aspects of prognostic uncertainty for "fragile" children.

Fourth, after recover is complete and a new baseline of health and quality of life is established, what will this new baseline be? Not infrequently, the injury incurred during a health crisis can persist, diminishing the new baseline significantly from previous levels. Furthermore, the duration of time living at this new baseline is also uncertain. How long before the next crisis?

Fifth, how severe are future crises likely to be? Families will worry both in terms of the likelihood of dying and the degree of suffering that may be part of their child's future.

Conceptual models of care

Uncertainty is a fundamental aspect in all patterns of dying. To understand how to manage this irreducible element of uncertainty, we must understand how various conceptual models of care relate to each other. Fig. 4 illustrates three common models.

Until the past decade or so, largely because of the history of how hospice and palliative care arose in opposition to standard medical care, the reigning model was that typical medical care (labeled as "curative care," even though most diseases are managed rather than cured) and palliative care were mutually exclusive, incompatible domains of care. One had to pick one or the other, with a consequently abrupt transition from curative to palliative care—if the transition was ever made.

Beginning in the 1990s, a new conceptual model was presented, wherein the two modes of care could be provided simultaneously, with a gradual increase in palliative care over time as a proportion of all care and an offsetting diminishment of curative care [31]. Whether intended or not, this model still conceives curative and palliative care as in competition, with any effort devoted to one form of care coming at the expense of the other. Both of these first two models may hinder problem-solving and decision making by their dichotomization of care, foisting upon decision makers the seemingly unavoidable tradeoffs between the two modes (such as, "are we willing to forgo all forms of life-prolonging treatments in order to enroll in hospice?").

An alternative model categorizes all the interventions and acts of care based on their aims or objects: what does this act of care seek to accomplish? A single act of care can be motivated by one or several goals. Cure-seeking care aims to eradicate the underlying health problem. For example, penicillin can cure a bacterial pneumonia and chemotherapy can cure certain malignancies. This objective is often sufficient for most pediatric patients.

For many life-threatening conditions, however, cure is never a feasible goal. Instead, life-extending care seeks to enable the child to live with the condition longer, such as insulin therapy did for people with type 1 diabetes. Many of these interventions also enhance quality of life and are valued and used eagerly because of this effect.

Other interventions aim more specifically to improve quality of life and comfort maximizing care, such as the use of medications to reduce muscular

1. Incompatable Domains of Curative versus Palliative Care:

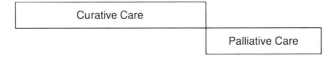

2. Competing Domains of Curative versus Palliative Care:

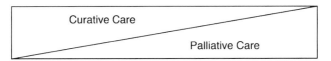

3. Complementary and Concurrent Components of Care:

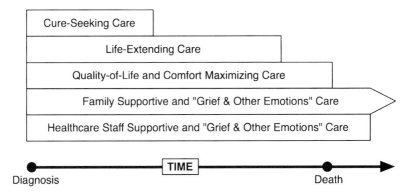

Fig. 4. Evolution of the relationships between conceptual models of care.

spasticity and its complications. Again, while the primary objective is to improve function, maximize quality of life, and minimize suffering, these interventions may also extend life.

For the practice of pediatrics, care important to the patient is not limited to just the patient but extends to the parents or other family members upon whom the patient depends for quality decision making and physical care. Family supportive care is an important mode of care that starts at diagnosis and extends beyond death, attending to the grief and other emotions of the parents and family members. While much of this care must be recognized and managed before the child's death, it extends past death in the form of bereavement care.

In parallel, a similar mode of care exists to support clinicians who in their humanity also grapple with a host of emotions in the care of children with life-limiting conditions. Health care staff supportive care, while not often delivered in a well-organized manner, aims to address the grief and other emotions associated with caring for these children.

This conceptualization of care, by avoiding the dichotomization of the modes of care and by organizing the acts of care based on goals, allows some of the problems arising from uncertainty to be managed in a more flexible manner.

Part III: the psychology of collaborative communication

Beyond working to understand how each of us view the concepts of pediatric palliative care, our ability to communicate collaboratively can be advanced if we also attend to our own habits of thought, emotions, and ways in which we handle interpersonal conflict. This section inspects this by exploring how our innate judgments and processes affect how we define situations and make decisions.

Depictions and detection

Over the past 30 years, the medical landscape of communication and decision-making has been shaped by the ideal of informed consent [32]. In the basic model of informed consent (as depicted in Fig. 5), a medical problem, such as a symptom or a disease, is evaluated by the physician. The physician then describes to the patient the range of reasonable treatment options and explains the pros and cons of each option, so that the patient can make an informed decision.

Often in pediatric palliative care, however, patients, parents, and clinicians have conceptualized the medical situation and predicaments quite differently (as in the difference between the viewpoints that "we can beat this"

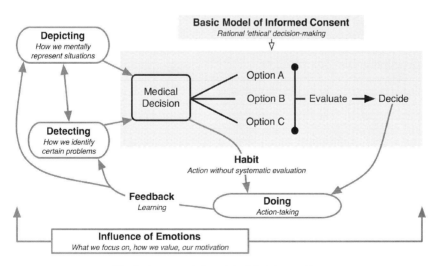

Fig. 5. An expanded model of decision making.

versus "there is no longer a realistic chance of cure"), leading us to differ regarding the way we think about various medical decisions and how we evaluate treatment options. Two psychologic processes, which we will call "depiction" and "detection," play large roles in creating these differences, as they help to define what constitutes the medical problem and thus determine how options are viewed and evaluated [33].

First, each of us creates, within our own minds, a depiction, or representation, of reality. As we interpret the meaning of symptoms, test results, behaviors, or events, we develop notions of what is going on and what it all means. These depictions reflect our individual temperaments, personal experiences, social circumstances, and cultural heritage and may be quite different than another person's interpretation. For example, a physician may consider the relapse of a malignant tumor in a patient as a challenge of medicine to rid the body of cancer, while a person of strong religious convictions may interpret the same event as a challenge of spiritual faith.

Second, based in part on how we have depicted a situation within ourselves, we focus on certain aspects of that situation while ignoring others. In the same way, the detection of problems warranting our attention will differ based on the individuals interpretation. Again, the same physician may detect as a problem the patient or family's steadfast belief in an extremely unlikely cure, while the patient and family may detect as their chief problem the challenge of maintaining their faith in an environment of disbelief.

Collaborative communication is fostered by acknowledging that "the problem" can differ from various points of view. Asking each other to share the sense of what is going on and what it means enables us to compare and contrast our depictions, and perhaps learn why we have focused on different problems.

Habits of thought and influence of emotions

Ideally, we make decisions on the basis of methodical consideration of all the advantages and disadvantages of the treatment options. However, collaborative communication must also be considered with our tendency to make decisions on the basis of quick assessments built upon habits or shortcuts of thought (what psychologists call "heuristics" [34,35]). While these habits may work well under most circumstances, they may also lead to systemic cognitive biases. Three of these heuristics are extremely pertinent to pediatric palliative care.

Availability and probability

Most of the time, we gauge how likely something is going to happen based on how easily we can imagine it happening, rather than as a quantified measure of probability. If we have witnessed a chain of events unfold before our eyes in the past and can readily imagine the same sequence happening again, we tend to believe that this is more likely to occur. Conversely, events that we have a hard time imagining we judge to be unlikely to occur. The memory of the experience is easily available to our imaginative mind.

This phenomenon may explain, in part, why parents who have watched their child recover "from death's door," defying prognoses offered by physicians, subjectively estimate the likelihood of recovery to be higher than what an objective assessment would estimate. It may also explain why physicians' prognoses are influenced by the outcomes of their most recent or most memorable patients (as exemplified when clinicians recall that they "once had a similar patient who recovered," and thus over-estimate the likelihood of recovery for the current patient).

To work with this innate habit of thought, collaborative communication sometimes involves helping each other envision possible events—desirable and undesirable—so that these events become mentally available, allowing a better assessment of the probability that these events may occur. The key issue is to recognize that a sequence of events that people cannot imagine will be judged as unlikely to occur, and a true assessment of the options must consider this bias.

Anchoring and evaluation

When it comes to evaluative judgments (that is, how we answer questions like "which is better, A or B?"), first impressions matter. For instance, if when presenting the pros and cons of various treatment options we decide to first talk about the risks, our subsequent thinking will be more dominated by concerns about risk than if we had started out by talking about possible treatment benefits. This phenomenon of how our thinking gets anchored to a particular concern, perspective, or fact is pervasive, subtle, and difficult to overcome.

One method that can shift the anchor is to draw attention to it and then try to take an alternative perspective. For example, if thoughts about risk have come to dominate a conversation, one might say: "I'm noticing that we are talking a lot about the bad things that could happen if we choose one of these treatments, and while this is important, why don't we try to focus just on the various good things that may happen and see how these treatments compare."

The second point of advice about anchoring is to make sure that the same anchoring bias is bestowed upon all treatment options. In other words, do not tolerate yourself or someone else presenting treatment A first in terms of benefits and then risks, and then presenting treatment B first in terms of risks and then benefits. Instead, be even-handed and present both in the same manner, devoting equal time and attention to each.

The affective heuristic and aversion

The prospect of a child suffering or dying often evokes deeply disturbing images that generate strongly unpleasant feelings. Consequently, many people develop an aversion to contemplating the possibility of suffering, death, or even certain treatment options that seek to minimize suffering but not prevent death. People often use these aversions associated with the disturbing images as a guide or shortcut to figure out the best course of action. Usually they pick the course of action that minimizes the negative images and feelings.

One example of this mode of thinking was expressed by a father who had dialed 9-1-1 when his child, who was at home with hospice care for an intractable tumor, became somnolent. The father said, "I couldn't image just sitting there doing nothing and watching my child die." After empathetically wishing that neither he nor his child had to go through any of this, the conversation gently turned to imaging what could be done while sitting at the child's bedside, perhaps holding a hand and talking with his child, or climbing into bed and rocking his child. In effect, this approach helped to create and explore new images with perhaps different feelings, still sad, but hopefully not as scary. The challenge presented when working with the affective heuristic, points more broadly to the influence that emotion has on individuals and groups when they try to work together to solve problems and make decisions.

Emotional intelligence

To handle emotions well, people engaged in collaborative communication use emotional intelligence, which is "the ability to process emotion-laden information competently, to use it to guide cognitive activities like problem solving, and to focus energy on required behaviors." [36] This vital ability can be broken down into four specific aptitudes, as illustrated in Fig. 6.

1) Emotional perception and expression: your ability to perceive emotions in others and to effectively express your emotions to others, creating a two-way flow of emotional communication.
2) Emotional understanding: when perceiving or feeling an emotion within yourself, to be able to interpret it correctly (for instance, when feeling sad, recognizing the emotion as sadness and not misinterpreting it as anger or irritation).
3) Emotional facilitation of thought and action: your ability to use emotion to improve your ability to think more clearly or perform behaviors with greater skill (in other words, the ability to "psych yourself up" or "calm down" to perform a specific task).
4) Emotional management: the ability to manage or influence your own emotions and the emotions of others when working together.

This model can help when coaching either yourself or others on how to handle emotionally challenging situations. You might ask, "which of these aptitudes do I need to focus on to best help myself or another person through a difficult situation?" While many educational or training programs (which have been introduced in a wide variety of settings from elementary

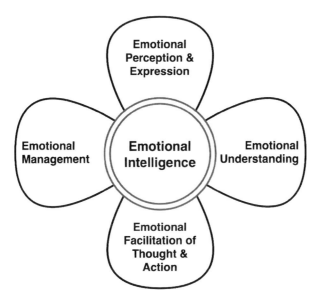

Fig. 6. Emotional intelligence and its four core aptitudes.

schools to corporate businesses) claim to improve emotional intelligence, none can be specifically recommended because lack of rigorous evaluations.

Managing conflict

Sometimes in the course of providing clinical care—despite our best efforts to clarify goals, understand each other's perspectives, and manage our emotions—conflicts arise. These conflicts may be between parents and physicians, or between family members, or among various clinicians on the health care team, or almost any other combination of individuals who care about and for the patient. Often in these situations, what is most palpable is the feeling of discord, disagreement, or disgruntlement. Typically, the actual heart of the conflict remains unspoken, and this root source may be unclear or unknown to one or even both parties. Regrettably, we often try to communicate while avoiding the source of conflict, under the assumption that the conflict is either unsolvable or could be solved only if "they" would be reasonable. To proceed in collaborative communication, the conflict must be addressed and managed.

A useful strategy to address conflict and have more productive "difficult conversations" is to fundamentally shift our thinking about interpersonal conflict and how we deal with it [11,20]. Fig. 7 illustrates some details of this shift.

Difficult conversations are usually viewed as involving the delivery or receipt of accusations, debating who is right and who is wrong. Participants often settle for simple notions of what caused the conflict and what needs to

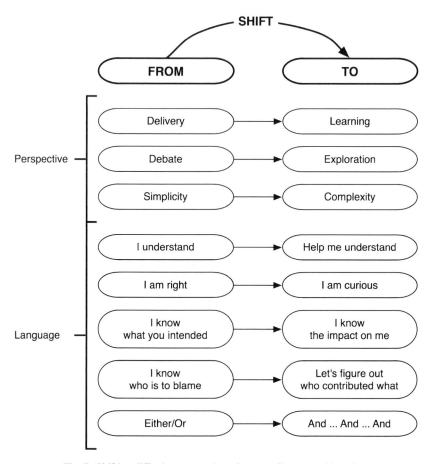

Fig. 7. Shifting difficult conversations from conflict toward learning.

be done to resolve it. We must recognize, however, that we usually do not know the intentions that motivated other people's actions; instead, we infer these intentions (often inaccurately) from the impact that the actions had on us: we think (without really thinking about it) that "I feel hurt; therefore you meant to hurt me."

Productive conversations about difficult issues focus on learning more about the perspectives of both parties, exploring what may be a complex web of actions that contributed to the conflict. This shift in approach is mirrored by a shift in perspective from the certainty of one's understanding and rightness to a more curious posture, seeking not to blame but striving to understand everyone's contributions. People engaging in collaborative communication should avoid the assumption that other people wanted to have a certain effect on them and, rather, talk openly about the impact that specific behaviors or actions did have.

Participants in collaborative communication should also attend to what they think the conflict says about themselves and their sense of personal identity: that is, whether they feel insecure or threatened, devalued or disappointed, incompetent or insensitive. Because we all make mistakes, sometimes acting in a manner that contributes to conflict with a mixture of motives that guides our behavior, some of these self-reflections may have a kernel of truth.

A way to acknowledge these reflections, while also endorsing the encompassing truth that our intentions are good, is to use the simple word "and" repeatedly and avoid the word "but." For example, "I hear you that when I had to cancel our last meeting on short notice that you felt upset AND that you felt that I did not value your time AND I want to apologize AND I want to assure you that I did not want to upset you AND that I do value your time AND I want to thank you for coming back in today to talk about your child AND I hope we can make some good progress today in our plans." Using "and" while avoiding "but" shifts the tone of the language from argument to mutual exploration.

Part IV: three common tasks in pediatric palliative care

While the work of pediatric palliative care involves a myriad of tasks that require our best efforts at collaborative communication, the remainder of this article focuses on three common tasks: communicating bad news, reframing and reanchoring situations, and conducting family meetings.

Communicating bad news

Clinicians who have the duty to communicate bad news to patients or family members might improve their performance of this task by following some guidelines that have been developed, based on interviews with patients and family members as well as expert experience and opinion [37–41]. Fig. 8 illustrated these guidelines. First, the overall task of communicating bad news can be usefully subdivided into three phases: preparation, delivery, and follow-up.

The first phase, preparation, is essential. Taking the time to formulate a plan of how to deliver the news can dramatically improve how well the information is conveyed. Key parts of preparation include:

- Rehearsing what to say and how to say it. This should include visualizing how to get the right people to the proper setting and then how to deliver the news.
- Considering where to deliver the news. Should the setting be a private conference room or at the bedside? Who should be present at the meeting? Should the talk be with just the patient? Should it include a parent alone or wait for both parents to be available? Will it be helpful to include the nurse or social worker?

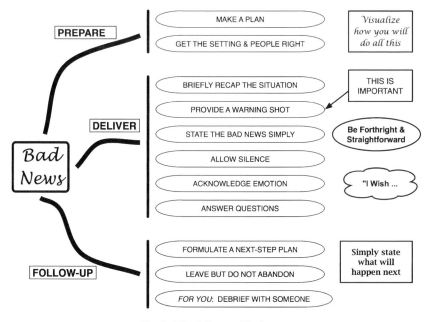

Fig. 8. The delivery of bad news.

- Investigating if the patient or family is of a particular culture that handles the communication of bad news in a particular way. Then make plans to work with their cultural values and expectations.
- Visualizing how to get the right people to the proper setting and then how the delivery of the news will unfold. This may take a small amount of time, but will yield many benefits in clinical practice.

The second phase involves the actual delivery of the news. Starting by briefly recapping the clinical situation provides some necessary context for receiving and interpreting the news. Even the most complex episode of hospital care can, for the purpose of providing a conversational context for some upcoming bad news, be condensed and conveyed in a minute or two.

At this point in the discussion, provide the patient or family with a "warning shot," meaning a phrase that alerts them to the fact the news to follow is not good; for instance, one might say that "The results of the test are now back, and I am afraid that the news is not good." A pause should follow. According to patients and family members, this pause before the actual statement of the news provides a moment to brace themselves for the news, so that they are not caught off guard.

When communicating the news, state the facts simply and in plain language, such as "the cancer has spread." Then be quiet. The core aspect of the news is often conveyed in a sentence, perhaps two or three. Avoid the temptation to continue to talk after this core news has been spoken. Instead, allow silence. Persons receiving bad news often are flooded with emotion and become disengaged from the conversation for a period of time. Although allowing silence may at first feel awkward, most people appreciate the silence as a sign of respect and empathy. Continuing to talk can be interpreted as unfeeling. The duration of silence can vary from one conversation to the next, and no reliable rules guide when to resume speaking other than remaining fully engaged and responsive to the reactions of the people in the room.

One way to resume speaking is to acknowledge your own emotion with an "I wish" statement, such as "I wish this news was different" or "I wish that the cancer had not spread." Be careful to avoid making statements that attempt to relate yourself to another person's emotions, such as "I can't image how you feel." Instead, acknowledge their emotions with simple observational statements, such as "I can see that you are very upset" or "I hear how angry you are."

If the patient or family members ask questions, provide forthright and straightforward answers. Realize that much of the information may need to be repeated later, as strong emotions can impair the subsequent recall of information. If no questions are asked, even after you have solicited them ("I don't know if you want to ask any questions at this point; if you are, I can answer them; if not, you can ask them later"), then move on to the next phase.

Phase three involves making plans for the next steps in care and communication. While the family may need time to digest the bad news, they will need clear information on what the next step of care includes. This often includes reframing the situation, reanchoring the framework of understanding, or readdressing the goals of care for the child (methods that will be discussed shortly).

Before ending the meeting, the patient and family will need to know when they can next expect more information or a future opportunity to ask questions. This may be a meeting with you or with someone else, such as a new specialist or another trusted physician. Tell them what to expect at that meeting, for example "I am going to leave now and will be back in an hour [or whenever; just be specific]. We'll review what we just talked about and I'll answer questions. We'll then start to map out how we want to move forward." By spelling out how you will be returning you will be much less likely to give the impression that you are abandoning them.

The final step regards self-care, so I will speak about it more personally. I find telling another person bad news to be a remarkably stressful task. Having a plan has made it less stressful for me over the years, but it is still challenging, intellectually and emotionally. Sometimes I can deliver bad news and keep moving to the next clinical task; other times I am blown away, either because I did not do as good a job as I had intended, or because the reaction of the patient or family to the news really affected me. Following these kinds of encounters, I have found it helpful to acknowledge my own emotions—sadness, anger, fear, guilt—to myself and to a trusted colleague, often within minutes of the conversation. If I wait, I rarely do this self-care debriefing, and it becomes less effective. Again, a minute or two is all this usually takes, but it is personally priceless time.

Reframing and reanchoring situations

One of the most common events in collaborative communication involves framing a situation [13,42]. We do this every time we start a conversation, as we quickly answer a series of questions: What are we talking about? What problem or opportunity concerns us? What are we trying to achieve? What is the pertinent context of our discussion? What are the key facts that we should all know?

We have already seen how these questions can be addressed when the conversation is about bad news. While many of those tactics can be used for a wide range of conversational subjects, several inter-related issues that more decisively frame clinical situations warrant special attention here.

Goals of care and the range of hopes

First, excellent pediatric palliative care requires that the goals of care be conceived through a process that is compassionate and holistically comprehensive. Quite often, however, the goals of care are obscure because they are never discussed explicitly, clearly, openly.

Typically, when a child first presents with signs of a medical problem, the primary goal is to rid them of the problem, often through a cure. This xcommon goal is usually left unstated as it is assumed by the patient, family members, and clinicians alike. However, when more prognostic information about the medical problem becomes available, and the prognosis shifts to a problem that will be life-long and potentially life-shortening, the situation needs to be reframed and reanchored.

Indeed, a change in clinical status usually causes people to reframe their understanding of a situation, altering how they depict it to themselves and others, and shifting their focus regarding what problems they detect. Alongside this process of reframing, family members may also reconsider what had been their previous goals, potentially reanchoring their evaluations of treatment options with a new set of priorities.

A question that can facilitate this process is to inquire: "Given what we now know about what your child is up against, it would help me if I could hear from you what you are hoping for, what you are worried about and, what you want to see happen." Expect, that the first response will be for a miracle, such as for the problem to go away. This is a normal and completely understandable desire and does not indicate that the family is not realistic. After the hope for a miracle is voiced, be patient and gently ask about what other hopes they have. Often, after a pause, a variety of hopes may be expressed: hopes about going home, about not having death occur too soon, about not suffering or having any further invasive interventions, or about being reunited with loved ones. These hopes can then be translated into goals and become the starting point for a conversation about how the different modes of care can support these goals of care.

Second, once these goals are clarified and articulated clearly, they must be disseminated throughout the health care team. While they should be documented in the medical record with sufficient detail that any reader would know what the goals are, the health care team should work together so that the spirit, as well as the letter, of the goals of care are understood by everyone. Often this requires face-to-face conversations.

Third, any agreements about the limits of care—usually documented as a Do-Not-Attempt-Resuscitation (DNAR) or Allow-Natural-Death order on the patient's chart—must be incontrovertibly clear to everyone involved making these sorts of treatment decisions for the child. Standardized forms for documenting these orders should be simple and clear, yet sufficiently detailed so that the limits of care can be drawn at a variety of important gradations across the spectrum of treatments, for example from no cardioversion to no medications to support blood pressure, or from no tracheal intubation to no supplemental oxygen. This information must be readily transferable with the patient across settings of care, from an intensive care unit to a general ward and from the hospital to the home. Finally, the DNAR order must not lead to a "do nothing" mentality. Instead, by specifying a limit to the invasiveness of care while affirming the goals of care, it should result in a "totally committed" attitude about caring for the child. The health care team should work in concert to assure that this attitude prevails.

Conducting family meetings

Finding consensus in a plan of action

Family meetings, when clinicians and family members join together to engage in a dialogue and devise a plan of action, are a mainstay of pediatric hospital-based clinical practice. Often the focus of these meetings is determining a consensus of care and can help everyone take stock of the situation and come up with a plan. Surprisingly little is known about how these meetings are run or how to run them better. The advice offered below (and summarized in Fig. 9) is based mostly on recommendations that are based on the care of adult patients in intensive care units [43–47], and my own experiences.

Because most meetings of this sort do not include the child patient, I will refer to meeting with the family (as opposed to meeting with the patient). The assumption that children do not attend these meetings, however, should be examined case-by-case, as some older children, adolescents, and young adults may very much want to be and should be included in these discussions. Sometimes families request a meeting. However, often a member of

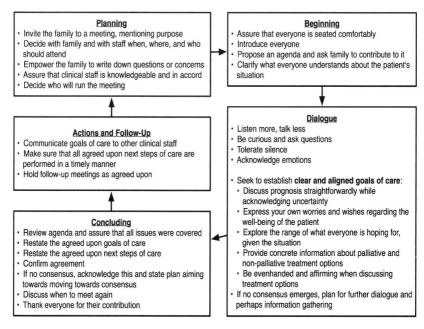

Fig. 9. Guidance on conducting family meetings.

the health care team, recognizing a need for reframing or reanchoring communication, proposes a meeting to the family.

Planning

Just as planning is a crucial activity for the delivery of bad news, it is equally important for family meetings. In this setting, it is also helpful for the family to be prepared as well.

First, schedule the meeting so that all the people the patient or family think should be present can attend, and make plans so that a private room with adequate space and chairs is reserved. Encourage the family members to prepare themselves for the meeting by writing down any questions, concerns, or ideas that they have so that all of these points can be addressed at the meeting. At the same time, make sure that the participating clinicians are all prepared, having reviewed all available information about the patient's condition. Decide who among the clinicians will be responsible for running the meeting.

Furthermore, work so that any disagreements between clinicians are identified, addressed and, if possible, resolved before the meeting. If disagreements cannot be resolved, then develop a plan about how the disagreement will be described to the family, and what plan of action will be used to resolve this disagreement, such as ordering an additional confirmatory test, initiating an empirical trial of therapy, or seeking the opinion of the family.

In general, attempting to hide conflicts from families is a dubious and often counter-productive strategy. It is far better to be candid and decide how to manage them.

Beginning

At the scheduled time and place, assure that everyone in attendance is seated comfortably. Have everyone introduce themselves regarding their role in the care of the child. At this stage, the point is to generate an agenda for the meeting and not to discuss each issue as it is mentioned. The clinician running the meeting should propose an agenda and invite the family's input. For example: "Thanks for coming in this morning. For the next 30 minutes, from my point of view, I think we want to talk about how the patient is doing [using the child's name], what we think might happen in the next few days, and then make some plans together about how to best care for your child. I also want to know what you want to talk about at this meeting." Make sure to write down whatever questions, concerns, or ideas that the family mentions, encouraging them to keep getting all these issues "out on the table" at the start of the meeting. Once all the issues are written down, promise the family that by the end of the meeting you will have discussed each of them.

Having formulated the agenda, provide a brief summary of the clinical status of the patient. For instance, suggest that everyone alloy you to provide a brief 1 or 2 minute overview of the child's main health problems and the child's current clinical status. When the summery is complete, solicit questions: "Is there anything about that overview that is new information to anyone, or that you don't agree with?" If there are no questions to clarify, move on to the dialogue.

Dialogue

How to manage the ensuing dialogue can be divided into advice regarding process and suggestions regarding how to establish clear and aligned goals of care. First, monitor how much the clinicians (including whoever is leading the meeting) are speaking. Try to achieve a balance whereby the family is speaking as much as the clinicians and thus the clinicians are doing more listening. Be inquisitive about what the family is thinking and feeling by intently listening to their thoughts, by asking questions, and by respectfully listening to the answers. Allow for periods of silence. Instead of filling the void with your own voice, enable the family to share their thoughts. If emotions are evident, acknowledging and affirming them can be very helpful in creating a supportive, collaborative exchange.

Second, the clarification and alignment of care goals can be fostered by maintaining an empathetic but forthright tone. Present information about the patient's prognosis, acknowledging any degree of uncertainty in a straightforward manner. Empathy can be expressed by voicing your worries about what might happen to the patient or your wishes regarding how the situation might be different.

Ask the family members to discuss what they are hoping for (as outlined in the previous section). Listing each of the hopes can be transformative. Translate these hopes into a spectrum of possible goals of care for the patient, establishing a concrete framework for evaluating information and making decisions about both palliative and nonpalliative care options.

These care options should then be presented in an even-handed manner, seeking to minimize the influence of the biases that heuristic short cuts of thinking can create. Help the family to visualize what the different courses of treatment could look like, present the benefits and risks in the same order, suggest focusing explicitly on a set of concerns that previously have taken a back seat, and spend roughly equal time discussing each option with similar amounts of detail. If true, let the family know that loving, devoted families choose treatment option A (such as remaining on high-intensity life support) while other loving, devoted families choose treatment option B (such as gathering the family together and holding the child while the life-extending interventions are replaced by comfort-seeking interventions), and that they will be supported with either choice.

At some point in this discussion, a consensus will likely emerge about what the most important goals of care are and how to best pursue them. If consensus is not forthcoming, and the various family members or clinicians are not close to agreement about how to proceed, the leader should shift the discussion to focus on how the conversation can continue and what new information might be gathered to help reach agreement.

Concluding

Once a consensus has emerged, move onward by reviewing the meeting agenda and assuring that all the items were covered adequately, all questions answered and concerns addressed, and a plan of care established. Restate the goals of care and the plan of care. Confirm that everyone agrees.

If a consensus did not emerge, note this fact and the plan for further dialogue in a nonjudgmental manner; for example: "Well, today we have talked about many important things and have learned a lot. We still differ in our views about what is the best way to take care of this child, and we have agreed to continue to meet and talk about how to come to an agreement." Discuss when the next scheduled meeting should take place. Lastly, thank everyone for their time and effort, and end the meeting.

Actions and follow-up

The diagram regarding family meeting guidance presents a cyclic pattern, where the planning and conduct of one meeting is linked to subsequent meetings by a phase of action and follow-up that is critical. Meetings are most productive when they guide patient care and positively influence the family's experience. The consensus goals of care must be disseminated outward from the meeting so that all clinicians are aware of them. If no consensus emerged, then this information too must be disseminated along with the plan regarding how the family-clinical team is working toward consensus. Implement the next steps of care in a timely manner and then abide by the agreed upon schedule for future meetings.

Summary

Collaborative communication builds the foundation upon which pediatric palliative care of the highest possible quality can be created. While I hope that the material we have covered and the advice offered is helpful to all of us as we strive to work together better, there is still much to learn about how to improve our communication skills. Let us commit to advancing this area of medical care—through personal reflection and practice as well as rigorous research—so that in the future patients, families, and clinicians can all benefit.

References

[1] Meyer EC, Ritholz MD, Burns JP, et al. Improving the quality of end-of-life care in the pediatric intensive care unit: parents' priorities and recommendations. Pediatrics 2006;117(3): 649–57.
[2] Hays RM, Valentine J, Haynes G, et al. The Seattle Pediatric Palliative Care Project: effects on family satisfaction and health-related quality of life. J Palliat Med 2006;9(3):716–28.
[3] Back AL, Arnold RM. Dealing with conflict in caring for the seriously ill: "it was just out of the question". JAMA 2005;293(11):1374–81.
[4] Katz J. The silent world of doctor and patient. Johns Hopkins Paperbacks edition. Baltimore (MD): Johns Hopkins University Press; 2002.
[5] Steinhauser KE, Christakis NA, Clipp EC, et al. Factors considered important at the end of life by patients, family, physicians, and other care providers. JAMA 2000;284(19):2476–82.
[6] Homer CJ, Marino B, Cleary PD, et al. Quality of care at a children's hospital: the parent's perspective. Arch Pediatr Adolesc Med 1999;153(11):1123–9.
[7] Curtis JR, Patrick DL, Caldwell E, et al. The quality of patient-doctor communication about end-of-life care: a study of patients with advanced AIDS and their primary care clinicians. AIDS 1999;13(9):1123–31.
[8] Tulsky JA, Fischer GS, Rose MR, et al. Opening the black box: how do physicians communicate about advance directives? Ann Intern Med 1998;129(6):441–9.
[9] Braddock CH, Fihn SD, Levinson W, et al. How doctors and patients discuss routine clinical decisions. Informed decision making in the outpatient setting [see comments]. J Gen Intern Med 1997;12(6):339–45.
[10] Hays RM, Haynes G, Geyer JR, et al. Communication at the end of life. In: Carter BS, Levetown M, editors. Palliative care for infants, children, and adolescents: a practical handbook. Baltimore (MD): Johns Hopkins University Press; 2004. p. 112–40.
[11] Stone D, Patton B, Heen S. Difficult conversations: how to discuss what matters most. New York: Viking; 1999.
[12] Keeney RL. Value-focused thinking: a path to creative decision making. Cambridge (MA): Harvard University Press; 1992.
[13] Hammond JS, Keeney RL, Raiffa H. Smart choices: a practical guide to making better decisions. Boston: Harvard Business School Press; 1999.
[14] Fisher R, Ury W. Getting to yes: negotiating agreement without giving in. Boston: Houghton Mifflin; 1981.

[15] Ury W. Getting past no: negotiating with difficult people. New York: Bantam Books; 1991.

[16] Ury W. The power of a positive no: how to say no and still get to yes. New York: Bantam Books; 2007.

[17] Beauchamp TL, Childress JF. Principles of biomedical ethics. 5th edition. New York: Oxford University Press; 2001.

[18] Strong C, Feudtner C, Carter BS, et al. Goals, values, and conflict resolution. In: Carter BS, Levetown M, editors. Palliative care for infants, children, and adolescents: a practical handbook. Baltimore (MD): Johns Hopkins University Press; 2004. p. 23–43.

[19] Dubler NN, Liebman CB. Bioethics mediation: a guide to shaping shared solutions. New York: United Hospital Fund of New York; 2004.

[20] Feudtner C. Tolerance and integrity. Arch Pediatr Adolesc Med 2005;159(1):8–9.

[21] Feudtner C. A piece of my mind: dare we go gently. JAMA 2000;284(13):1621–2.

[22] McKean E. The new Oxford American dictionary. 2nd edition. New York: Oxford University Press; 2005.

[23] Habermas J. The theory of communicative action. Boston: Beacon Press; 1984.

[24] Field MJ, Cassel CK, Institute of Medicine (US). Committee on Care at the End of Life. Approaching death: improving care at the end of life. Washington, DC: National Academy Press; 1997.

[25] Ferrell B, Connor SR, Cordes A, et al. The national agenda for quality palliative care: the National Consensus Project and the National Quality Forum. J Pain Symptom Manage 2007;33(6):737–44.

[26] National Consensus Project for Quality Palliative Care. Clinical practice guidelines for quality palliative care, executive summary. J Palliat Med 2004;7(5):611–27.

[27] Mularski RA, Curtis JR, Billings JA, et al. Proposed quality measures for palliative care in the critically ill: a consensus from the Robert Wood Johnson Foundation Critical Care Workgroup. Crit Care Med 2006;34(11 Suppl):S404–11.

[28] Field MJ, Behrman RE, Institute of Medicine (US). Committee on Palliative and End-of-Life Care for Children and Their Families. When children die: improving palliative and end-of-life care for children and their families. Washington, DC: National Academy Press; 2003.

[29] Himelstein BP, Hilden JM, Boldt AM, et al. Pediatric palliative care. N Engl J Med 2004; 350(17):1752–62.

[30] Patrick DL, Starks HE, Cain KC, et al. Measuring preferences for health states worse than death. Med Decis Making 1994;14(1):9–18.

[31] Lynn J. An 88-year-old woman facing the end of life. JAMA 1997;277(20):1633–40.

[32] Faden RR, Beauchamp TL, King NMP. A history and theory of informed consent. New York: Oxford University Press; 1986.

[33] Klein GA. Sources of power: how people make decisions. Cambridge (MA): MIT Press; 1998.

[34] Kahneman D, Slovic P, Tversky A. Judgment under uncertainty: heuristics and biases. Cambridge (UK): Cambridge University Press; 1982.

[35] Kahneman D, Frederick S. Representativeness revisited: attribute substitution in intuitive judgment. In: Gilovich T, Griffin DW, Kahneman D, editors. Heuristics and biases: the psychology of intuitive judgement. Cambridge (UK): Cambridge University Press; 2002. p. 49–81.

[36] Salovey P, Mayer JD, Caruso D. The positive psychology of emotional intelligence. In: Snyder CR, Lopez SJ, editors. Handbook of positive psychology. New York: Oxford University Press; 2005. p. 159–71.

[37] Buckman R, Kason Y. How to break bad news: a guide for health care professionals. Baltimore (MD): Johns Hopkins University Press; 1992.

[38] Quill TE, Arnold RM, Platt F. "I wish things were different": expressing wishes in response to loss, futility, and unrealistic hopes. Ann Intern Med 2001;135(7):551–5.

[39] Friedrichsen MJ, Strang PM, Carlsson ME. Receiving bad news: experiences of family members. J Palliat Care 2001;17(4):241–7.

[40] Contro N, Larson J, Scofield S, et al. Family perspectives on the quality of pediatric palliative care. Arch Pediatr Adolesc Med 2002;156(1):14–9.

[41] Contro NA, Larson J, Scofield S, et al. Hospital staff and family perspectives regarding quality of pediatric palliative care. Pediatrics 2004;114(5):1248–52.

[42] Kahneman D, Tversky A. Choices, values, and frames. New York: Cambridge University Press; 2000.

[43] West HF, Engelberg RA, Wenrich MD, et al. Expressions of nonabandonment during the intensive care unit family conference. J Palliat Med 2005;8(4):797–807.

[44] Curtis JR, Engelberg RA, Wenrich MD, et al. Missed opportunities during family conferences about end-of-life care in the intensive care unit. Am J Respir Crit Care Med 2005; 171(8):844–9.

[45] Boyle DK, Miller PA, Forbes-Thompson SA. Communication and end-of-life care in the intensive care unit: patient, family, and clinician outcomes. Crit Care Nurs Q 2005;28(4): 302–16.

[46] Boyle D, Dwinnell B, Platt F. Invite, listen, and summarize: a patient-centered communication technique. Acad Med 2005;80(1):29–32.

[47] Lautrette A, Ciroldi M, Ksibi H, et al. End-of-life family conferences: rooted in the evidence. Crit Care Med 2006;34(11 Suppl):S364–72.

ELSEVIER
SAUNDERS

PEDIATRIC CLINICS
OF NORTH AMERICA

Pediatr Clin N Am 54 (2007) 609–629

Psychosocial and Spiritual Needs of Children Living with a Life-Limiting Illness

Mary McSherry, ACSW, LSW[a], Kathy Kehoe, LCSW[c],
Jean M. Carroll, RN, BSN[a], Tammy I. Kang, MD[a],
Mary T. Rourke, PhD[b],*

[a]The Pediatric Advanced Care Team, The Children's Hospital of Philadelphia,
34th and Civic Center Blvd, Philadelphia, PA 19104, USA
[b]The Behavioral Health Integrated Program, The Children's Hospital of Philadelphia,
34th and Civic Center Boulevard, Philadelphia, PA 19104, USA
[c]Marlton, NJ, USA

Pediatric palliative care has been defined as an active and total approach to care that embraces physical, emotional, social, and spiritual elements. Its focus is to enhance quality of life for the child while supporting the family. Quality end-of-life care includes the management of distressing symptoms; provision of care, including the assessment and management of psychosocial and spiritual needs; and respite from diagnosis through death and bereavement [1]. Providing this care requires an interdisciplinary team approach that involves the child and family and a multitude of health care professionals. Although most pediatric palliative care teams employ psychosocial and chaplaincy professionals to assist in their mission, the general practitioner is also an integral part of providing this support. Meeting the palliative care goal of improved quality of life depends on medical and nursing practitioners understanding and effectively assessing psychosocial symptoms. This focus is necessary to help children and their families process the death and dying experience and to help health care teams adequately advocate for the needs of children within the treatment team and hospital and hospice contexts.

Consistent with this mission, the past decade has brought greater attention to the needs of children facing life-limiting illnesses and their families.

* Corresponding author.
E-mail address: rourke@email.chop.edu (M.T. Rourke).

0031-3955/07/$ - see front matter © 2007 Elsevier Inc. All rights reserved.
doi:10.1016/j.pcl.2007.08.002 *pediatric.theclinics.com*

Several national and international organizations, including the Institute of Medicine, The American Academy of Pediatrics, and the National Association of Social Workers, have developed guidelines to emphasize the need for comprehensive, multidisciplinary, compassionate care that spans home and hospital. These organizations have sought to address not only physical needs, but also the emotional, psychologic, and spiritual dimensions of pediatric palliative care [1–6].

Despite this agreement, however, there are limited empirical data demonstrating the specific needs of children receiving pediatric palliative care and their families, and even scarcer evidence on the most effective ways in which to provide the best possible care.

The goal of this article is to address this issue directly by reviewing the limited data available and integrating them with relevant theoretic conceptualizations and our multidisciplinary team's clinical experiences. The ultimate objective is to provide a general outline of how medical teams can understand, assess, and respond to the psychosocial needs of children and families receiving palliative care.

Overview of psychosocial pediatric palliative care literature

Awareness of what is known about long-term outcomes of parents after the death of a child and parents' perspectives regarding their psychosocial, emotional, and spiritual needs is essential in designing an appropriate psychosocial plan for an individual family. Research exploring how the death of a child affects family members physically and emotionally has shown that these affects can be profound and long lasting [7–13].

Parental impact

As might be expected, bereaved parents seem to be at risk for psychologic distress, particularly in the first years after the death of a child. In a cohort of 1,082,503 people identified from national registers in Denmark, parents who lost a child had an increased risk for a first psychiatric hospitalization for any disorder, compared with those parents who did not lose a child. Bereaved mothers had a higher relative risk for being hospitalized for any psychiatric disorder than bereaved fathers. This risk was highest during the first year after the death of the child but remained elevated 5 years or more after the death [8,9]. Similarly, in a population-based, nationwide study in Sweden, Kreicbergs and colleagues [14–16] found higher-than-average levels of distress in bereaved parents compared with a nonbereaved group, and found specifically that bereaved mothers and parents who lose a child 9 years or older have an increased risk for long-term psychologic distress. In this study, psychologic morbidity in bereaved parents decreased to levels similar to those among nonbereaved parents 7 to 9 years after the loss. Although no specific diagnoses have been identified by the limited literature in this area, parents may be most susceptible to posttraumatic responses, including high levels of worry, hypervigilance, arousal, and numbing/detachment or avoidance [17].

It is unclear what other factors may predict significant parental distress after a child's death. In the Kreicbergs and colleagues study, interviews with 449 bereaved parents suggested that the child's physical pain and circumstances at the moment of death contributed to parents' long-term distress [18]. In addition, there are some small studies that have postulated that a child's death at home as opposed to death in the hospital may result in improved parental adjustment [19–21]. The need to build evidence-based practice is crucial to better understanding how to minimize parental risk for long-term effects.

There are a few studies that document parental preferences regarding the palliative care experience. In a survey done by Mack and colleagues, parents associated quality end-of-life care with physicians (1) giving clear information about what to expect in the end-of-life period, (2) communicating with care and sensitivity, (3) communicating directly with the child when appropriate, and (4) preparing the parent for circumstances surrounding the child's death [22]. A survey of 56 parents whose children died in a pediatric intensive care unit identified similar priorities for pediatric end-of-life care: (1) honest and complete information, (2) ready access to staff, (3) communication and care coordination, (4) emotional expression and support by staff, (5) preservation of the integrity of the parent–child relationship, and (6) faith [20]. These studies are helpful guides to designing care, but there are no studies to date that document specific relationships between these practices or principles and psychosocial outcomes.

Sibling impact

Healthy children have been found to be greatly impacted by the death of a sibling, in the short and long term. In the 1950s and 1960s, studies indicated that siblings of a child who dies are at risk for developing adjustment difficulties, having feelings of guilt, becoming withdrawn, and having acting-out behaviors [23]. In a study of siblings of childhood cancer survivors, siblings showed clinical levels of posttraumatic stress at even higher rates than the survivors themselves [24]; these traumatic reactions are likely to exist and perhaps even be exacerbated in siblings of children who did not survive. Studies of sibling adjustment to serious illness have indicated that parental coping, marital stresses, financial resources, degree of disruption to family life, and parent–sibling communication are all important factors in determining a sibling's adjustment [25]. As with the literature on bereaved parents, there are few indicators regarding what factors place surviving siblings most at risk. One study does suggest advantages to a home (versus hospital) death. Lauer and colleagues [26–28] found that most siblings who had a sibling die at home were prepared for the death, received support, and reported closer family relations thereafter. Conversely, children whose sibling died in the hospital were more likely to describe themselves as unprepared for the death, isolated, and lacking personal involvement in the death.

The lack of information on sibling reactions leads to a paucity of knowledge on how interventions for siblings should be structured. It is clear from research and from clinical experience, however, that outreach to siblings in most institutions is currently inadequate. In a longitudinal study of families with a child diagnosed with cancer, for example, it was found that the sibling's emotional support needs were met at a lower level than for other family members [29]. Contro and colleagues [29] interviewed bereaved parents who stated that sibling support was lacking specifically in relation to accessibility of support groups, bereavement follow-up, and attention from medical teams. There are a multitude of interventions, such as the use of art, play, and music therapy, to aid in addressing the needs of siblings [30–34]. More research is needed, however, to better define these interventions and to demonstrate their effectiveness.

Defining psychosocial assessment in pediatric palliative care

It is rarely the case in pediatric palliative care that the experience of psychosocial distress in a child or family is immediately understood in a way that defines treatment. In contrast to non–medically ill children, children receiving palliative care most often report distress that is linked to various illness-related factors [23]. Identifying the factors responsible for distress is necessary to design an appropriate intervention. Successfully integrating psychosocial care into pediatric palliative care therefore includes a careful assessment of the following factors:

  The patient's and family's developmental level and ability to complete appropriate developmental tasks
  The child's experience of pain and discomfort and the family's ability to tolerate the child's discomfort
  The experience of emotional symptoms by the child and family members
  The effectiveness of complex communication channels within the family, within the medical team, and between the family and the team
  Practical factors affecting the family, including financial status, living situation, and social support
  Religious or spiritual/existential background, preferences, related beliefs, rituals, and practices of the patient and family.

Currently, there is no validated psychosocial assessment tool available to assess these domains. Most psychosocial professionals agree that careful assessment is a multidimensional activity that occurs across several interactions and includes gathering information through open-ended questions to children and to parents, observing the patient's behavior and responses in a variety of situations, and observing family behaviors and family members' reactions to the child and to medical events. The most effective assessment is not conducted by one team member but rather is the result of information gathered by all team members and assembled in a team-wide discussion of a family's care plan. Finally, assessment depends on the establishment of a respectful relationship between the assessor and the family and patient. Such a relationship requires resisting the temptation to give advice; accepting the family as they are, without judgment about how "appropriate" their reactions are; identifying and respecting a family's strengths to accomplish the difficult tasks ahead; curiously asking open-ended questions that provide unstructured and helpful information to round out a team's understanding; and giving clear, concrete, and honest feedback and reactions to a family. These characteristics, along with honestly and genuinely being "in the moment" with children and families, have been theoretically linked to successful psychologic encounters [35,36].

A consideration of each of the areas to be assessed follows. In addition, examples of how to use open-ended questions and child and parent observation to guide assessment within each area can be found in Table 1.

The patient's and family's developmental level and ability to complete appropriate developmental tasks

Children's understanding of their medical illness and of death and dying vary according to their level of cognitive and social development, and these developmental differences lead to different psychosocial concerns [22]. In general, until mid to late adolescence, children do not have the same existential reactions to life-limiting illness that adults may have. They are more likely to grieve intermittently, in between doing other things, and their grief may be focused on things they are missing (eg, "I miss my Little League team." "I really wish I could go to camp." "Usually my sister is here in the room when Dad reads my good-night story." "I was supposed to go to Disney World on my Make-a-Wish trip this week."). In contrast to adults, children's understanding of palliative care is much more likely to be focused on immediate, concrete realities, such as pain and discomfort. They may, for example, be focused on their pain or their significant dislike of being in the hospital or unable to go outside and play.

Developmental understandings of death, related to cognitive development, may result in expected emotional and behavioral reactions. Very young children may become fearful of separations and are unlikely to understand the concept of death and its finality [37]. Children at this age may be afraid of the permanent separation from their parents, and may therefore resist any temporary separation at all from caregivers.

By the elementary school age years, children might still have an imcomplete understanding of death [37]. For example, some children, after being

Table 1
Examples of open-ended questions and behaviors to observe when assessing psychosocial concerns and strengths in children receiving palliative care and their families

Area being assessed	Open-ended questions	Patient behaviors to observe	Parent behaviors to observe
Developmental appropriateness and understanding	Tell me about what is happening with your treatment. What questions do you have that you have been too shy/too scared to ask? Why do you think this is happening to you? (Same questions can be asked of parents.)	Indications of fearing sleep (will not go to sleep, resists sedative medication) Indications of fear of separation Degree to which patient can enjoy some developmentally appropriate activities (artwork, talking to peers, planning fun activities)	Coddling an older child Apparent discord between treatment of child and child's developmental level Ability to let child explore some developmentally appropriate activities Ability to effectively soothe/nurture or comfort the child.
Beliefs about pain	What do you think is happening now that is making you hurt? How worried do you get when you feel pain? What do you worry about? What do you like (or not like) about using your pain meds? What concerns do you have about using your patient controlled analgesia? (Same questions can be asked of parents.)	Use of a range of physical behaviors to demonstrate different levels of pain. Behavioral manifestations of anxiety with increased pain. Over- or underuse of pain medications.	Degree of own distress or focus on child's daily pain experience Ability to comfort and reassure the child Ability to distract the child from pain and engage in other activities.
Emotional issues	How are you feeling? What are the things you are sad about? What are you missing because you are sick? What are you worried about?	Sadness, apathy Lethargy Unwillingness to engage in activities or conversation (must rule out physical causes for these symptoms).	Hypervigilance over child's pain, labs, or physical condition Signs of anxiety or excess sadness Avoidance of discussing important issues or of seeing the child or physician Asking same questions over and over again of the medical team.

Communication	Sometimes it's hard to talk about some medical things. Who can you talk to about the hardest things? What things would you like to talk or hear about, but haven't been able to find someone to listen or talk to? What opportunities are people offering you to talk, and how does it work if you tell them you don't feel like talking?	Patient asking questions about death, dying, prognosis, or related issues. Patient becoming annoyed when people "push" him or her to talk.	Reluctance to talk to child or to be alone with him/her. Eager insistence that child needs to talk despite child indicating need not to talk. Expressing anger or exaggerated conflicts regarding the medical care.
Practical issues	To parents: How have the extra medical expenses and any lost income you may have experienced affected your family? How do you get to the hospital for visits? What meals do you eat when here? Who cares for members of the family still at home? Who lives at home? Who cares for your child when he/she is not in the hospital? What space is available in your home for hospital equipment? What would it be like for your family to have home care nursing in the house?	Missed appointments Frequently bouncing back to the hospital after discharge Desire to want to stay in the hospital despite being medically cleared to go home Strong desire to have no medical intervention (including equipment or home care staff) at home.	Same as child observations

(continued on next page)

Table 1 (*continued*)

Area being assessed	Open-ended questions	Patient behaviors to observe	Parent behaviors to observe
Spiritual needs	What religious group, if any, do you belong to? What help would you like in thinking about religious or spiritual issues? What does your family believe about what happens after death? What traditions or rituals does your family practice when someone is sick or dying? What support from the hospital would be most helpful to you?	Confusion or distress regarding afterlife issues Worries about what kind of service to have Unusual behaviors that may be explained or understood as cultural rituals around illness or death	Same as child observations.

The questions and areas of observation here are examples to guide and illustrate an assessment, and are not meant to represent an exhaustive assessment tool. The text of this article should supplement this outline, and information should be adapted to meet a patient's specific clinical situation. Most questions for the child can also be rephrased and asked of the parents to gain helpful information. In addition, the questions and areas of observation often overlap and tap more than one area. They were arbitrarily placed in one category here to conserve space.

told that dying is like going to sleep, may become afraid to go to sleep and may fight sleep or medicines that make them feel sleepy. During these years, children may have rule-based understandings of death and an afterlife, and may be afraid that they will not go to heaven because they have been bad. They may believe that something that they did caused their illness, or they may feel guilt at what they are putting their families through.

By adolescence, children may have a more adultlike understanding of death [25,37], and may feel more overtly sad at anticipated losses, such as not going to the prom or to college, or not getting to see a sibling grow. Although they understand the finality and irreversibility of death, adolescents—even in the midst of experiencing a life-limiting illness—may manage by distancing themselves from the reality. Even though they may at times be able to acknowledge and have meaningful discussions about the reality of their impending death, they may want to continue planning for a future as they normally would have planned, and may become annoyed when parents and medical team members accuse them of not "getting it." At all ages, children may fear the unknown, including what death will feel like (eg, "Will it hurt?" "Will I be very cold?"), where they will go ("Do you think there is a heaven?" "Will there be a Gap store there?"), and who will take care of their families ("I am the one who watches my brother after school!" "I think my mom will be too sad after I die.").

Although practiced pediatricians and pediatric health care providers can easily estimate the developmental and cognitive level of most healthy children, several factors make this assessment difficult in children who have serious illnesses. First, seriously ill children often are not able to participate in the age-appropriate activities that spur further development, which may cause them to experience distress or to look younger than their age-mates. For example, adolescents receiving palliative care may have fewer peer and social experiences than is typical due to prolonged illnesses and missed school or social activities. Older adolescents may therefore can look like much younger teens, and may not have the social skills or independence of their peers or siblings. Second, distress and pain often cause behavioral regression, causing children to look and behave like much younger children. Preschoolers and early school-aged children may become unable to articulate their concerns, and may regress to whining and crying when upset. Older children may be unable to explain that they are worried or sad, or that something hurts, and may also cry. Children may lose milestones that they have achieved (eg, toileting, self-care, or feeding skills), or may need to be held, helped to sleep, or reassured in ways not typical based on their age or even their past experiences. This change in behavior is not always isolated to the child. Parents are likely to alter their caretaking style and may begin feeding or bathing formerly independent children, or cooing and speaking in babyish terms to a teenager.

There are two additional factors that are important to factor into a consideration of development. First, just as children have developmental paths, so do families. The tasks of a family with very young children are different from those of a family with school-aged children, which are different again from families of adolescents [38]. Serious illness, and end-of-life care in particular, often requires families to reorganize in ways that directly oppose their family's stage. This asynchrony can cause distress in any member of the family, and factoring this systemic issue into a thorough assessment is important.

Second, one major difference that exists between adult and pediatric palliative care is the reality that children, despite serious and life-limiting illnesses, will often continue to progress through normal developmental stages. This may mean that a child's understanding of her illness will change over time, and the issues causing her distress will change over time. Parents and medical team members may not be prepared for changes or growth in cognition and emotion, and may continue to interact with a child at an earlier developmental level. Assessing the developmental fit between the child and those working with him is therefore an important aim, as is ongoing reassessment of a child's and family's status and needs. This growth during illness also becomes evident in children's ability to plan for the future even while they are facing the end of their lives. Talking about getting a driver's license, going to a best friend's sleepover next year, or what might happen at Christmas time, for example, may perplex or concern family or team members, who might in turn believe that the child does not understand that he is going to die. This orientation in children, however, may be adaptive; thinking about these issues is developmentally appropriate and allows children to remain engaged with life in potentially joyful ways. As long as children are able in some way to acknowledge the current reality, their focus on future milestones that they may not live to see is not currently considered detrimental, and may even be a source of coping and strength [36]. Children and families may take solace in being able to plan developmentally appropriate or fun events at an otherwise difficult time. Thwarting this planning may evoke even more distress.

Case example

Kayla was a 14-year-old girl in her last week of life. The team believed that Kayla had a realistic understanding of her prognosis until she began to choose her courses for her next semester at school. On hearing these plans, Kayla's parents and the team members became concerned and sent a psychologist in to meet with Kayla to be sure that she "gets it" and to help reorient her to "what she needs to do before she dies." After a few questions about Kayla's understanding of the medical issues and her thinking about courses for next semester, Kayla—with some exasperation—responded by saying, "Look, you can tell everyone that I know that I'm never going to take these courses. But planning them is just what I'm supposed to be doing right now!"

Interventions to manage developmental issues

There are various ways in which developmental issues can impact the pediatric palliative care process. The first step in configuring an appropriate intervention is to be sure that a thorough assessment of the situation accurately identifies the developmental issue. The assessment then dictates the intervention. For a child who is distressed because of the lack of appropriate developmental experiences, creatively arranging appropriate developmental activities may help. For example, introducing peers (in person, through mail, or by way of technology) may help. Child life specialists are expert at designing such interventions and can provide helpful consultation around these issues. In cases in which there is a mismatch between a child's growing developmental needs and a family's interactional style with the child, a family meeting that gently addresses these issues and suggests alternate possibilities to a family may be helpful. For the family thrust into a way of operating that is inconsistent with the family's developmental level, helping the family to identify the mismatch and then to identify ways in which to integrate pieces of both sets of tasks may be helpful. Again, ongoing collaboration with social workers, psychologists, and child life specialists can help in constructing interventions in all of these situations.

The child's experience of pain and discomfort and the family's ability to tolerate the child's discomfort

The experience of pain is part of most end-of-life experiences, and pediatric palliative care teams are often called upon in the treatment of pain. A thorough consideration of the medical management of pain issues is handled elsewhere in this issue.

An important psychosocial component of pain assessment and management that should complement medical management includes a consideration of the child's and family's ability to tolerate pain and discomfort. Most often this requires an assessment of what the pain means to the child and family.

Case example

Louis was a 9-year-old at the end of a several-year-long battle with cancer. While receiving pediatric palliative care, he was fortunate enough to experience several long periods of time during which he maintained a good quality of life and attended school, rode bikes with friends, and participated in many developmentally appropriate activities. Each time Louis experienced even minor pain, however, he immediately became confined to bed, cried often, and flinched when anyone touched him. His parents, who usually worked hard to allow Louis to experience a "normal life," supported his behavior during these pain episodes and hovered over him worriedly. Because pain at any level resulted in the same kind of reaction, it became difficult for the team to address the pain because they could not discriminate pain intensity. Collaboration with the multidisciplinary team indicated that the experience of even a minor twinge triggered all of Louis' fears that he was dying at that moment; his subsequent behavior, then, reflected not just his pain but also his intense anxiety about dying. For his parents, the pain also triggered their beliefs that "the end is near," according to Louis' mother. "Each time he feels any pain at all and I see him like this, I think, 'OK, here we are, we're not going home with him this time.'" Once this cycle was identified, the team began each investigation of the pain recognizing the source of pain in many children is not just physical, by addressing what Louis and his parents believed about the pain and, when possible, reassured them that the pain was just part of the process and would be addressed. The team also had a clear conversation with Louis' parents, opening channels of communication about whether "this was it" around each pain admission. Once this was acknowledged, it was easier for the team to calm Louis after each new pain episode, and to get a more accurate read on the level of pain experienced.

A second psychosocial factor than can complicate pain management is a family's concern to use adequate levels of opioid medications [39]. Parents often express concerns that their child will become addicted to opioids, and therefore resist their use directly with the medical team, or indirectly by instructing the child not to "push the button" too often. For parents and for some children, use of opioids may signal or remind them of the life-limiting nature of the disease. Refusing the use of these medications can therefore be a sign of denial of the reality of disease progression.

Interventions to manage psychosocial aspects of pain

Assessing a child's and family's beliefs about the experience of pain and what it means, and the meaning of changes in pain medication, is an important part of pain interventions. Medicating pain is only one component of intervention, and should always be accompanied by behavioral pain management strategies, including attention to the beliefs that children and family have about what the pain means. Communication within the multidisciplinary team is crucial in integrating information from all sources in order to provide the most accurate and complete assessment. In addition, addressing family concerns openly, with clarity, is crucial. This form of communication should happen regularly, with enough time for family members to express their concerns and for team members to address them.

The experience of emotional symptoms by the child and family members

Emotional symptoms at the end of life are expected and can be related to various developmental and contextual issues. Although a small proportion of children may report classic psychopathology, it is believed that these illnesses occur at rates comparable to those in the general population and are not necessarily related to the experience of having a life-limiting condition. It is more common that children report expected symptoms of emotional distress related to their experience [40].

Many of the common emotional responses to the life-limiting illness experience are affected by a child's developmental level. Most commonly, children report anxiety over the unknown and sadness over losses. The specific form of worry and sadness, however, and whether it is experienced sporadically or continuously are likely to vary by age. Younger children may have a series of sad moments about missed opportunities or being in the hospital, interspersed with moments of developmentally appropriate behavior. Older children or adolescents may have a more continuous sadness over losses.

Clinical experience suggests that children's losses about three issues cause the most distress: loss of control over their bodies and what is happening at any given moment, loss of a personal identity (eg, soccer player, cheerleader, social leader, class clown), and loss of interpersonal relationships (eg, best friends, friendship groupings) [41]. Identifying the degree to which each of these issues affects a child (and his family members) is important.

Assessing the emotional state in family members is also critical; parents' and siblings' emotional responses can affect the patient directly, and can shape how the family is able to respond to and support the child. Siblings can experience some of the same losses that the patient experiences; loss of control and predictability over their schedules and what is happening in the family, loss of a personal identity (eg, becoming the child whose sibling is dying), and loss of interpersonal relationships (because of being actively excluded or because of changes in routine that remove siblings from their normal social opportunities) are common. Sadness, guilt, and worry can accompany these changes for siblings.

Interventions to manage emotional issues

A thorough assessment with input from all members of the multidisciplinary team is crucial in the development of a plan of care. For significant emotional symptoms (eg, extreme sadness, intense worry and agitation), psychopharmacologic approaches can be helpful and are discussed elsewhere in this issue.

Identifying and addressing developmental challenges can be one component of an intervention for emotional distress. Cognitive–behavioral techniques, a set of therapeutic interventions that promote healthy thoughts and beliefs to facilitate coping with pain and discomfort, are also promising approaches, and can be implemented by a psychologist or trained counselor. Supportive counseling can also be helpful for parents and siblings, as can family therapy, to help distressed families reorganize during and, when appropriate, after the death of a child. Therapy to address or remediate long-standing dysfunction in individuals or families is usually not indicated during this time of crisis. In cases in which an individual or family has a long history of difficulty, addressing the problem as it interferes with or impinges on the child's medical care is advised.

The effectiveness of complex communication channels within the family, within the medical team, and between the family and the team

One question that often arises in the care of seriously ill children is how much information should be shared with them about their illness, prognosis, and possible death. Many who care for dying children believe that giving children the opportunity to openly discuss death, grief, and illness allows them to explore their fears, ask questions, and as a result, minimize their confusion and fears. In one study, 100% of Swedish parents who discussed death with their children later reported satisfaction with that decision, whereas a small percentage of those who chose not to have the discussion were dissatisfied with their decision [41]. These beliefs are generally based on small case scenarios or professional experiences, however, and the study of parents reflects only one sample within a particular culture.

There is no one agreed-upon way in which to have conversations about death and dying with children, although it is clear that a child's developmental and cognitive ability and family influences, such as culture, religious or spiritual beliefs, or individual communication preferences, must be considered. It is helpful to conceptualize these "conversations" with children as a series of discussions that take place over a period of time and over multiple interactions with more than one person. Children express their emotions in various ways, and so many discussions can be encouraged through play, art, music, and writing, and through simple conversation.

As children become comfortable speaking about their illness and possible death, the multidisciplinary team members can anticipate questions from the child. When children feel safe, they confide in and ask questions of those people with whom they feel most comfortable. Even before the prognosis has been provided by a team member, children may ask questions like, "If I take my medicine, will I get better?" or "The medicine isn't working anymore, is it?" Children may ask directly, "Am I going to die?" Team members need to be prepared for these questions, but should not respond to them quickly or automatically. Because they have a different frame of reference, children can often be asking something different than what their question means to an adult.

Case example

Jesse was a 7-year-old in the hospital for pain, who was fully expected to live at least another several months. In the middle of the night, he asked his nurse if he was going to die. His nurse, who had a good rapport with Jesse and knew that his parents had discussed this possibility with him, responded that, yes, he was going to die. Despite her gentle words and approach, and her spending a good deal of time with Jesse, he became extremely agitated and upset. The next day, after Jesse remained inconsolable, his mother was able to discern that Jessie's question to the nurse had not been, "Am I going to die from my disease?" but rather, "Does this pain mean that I am dying right now, tonight?"

To avoid responding to questions that children did not ask, it is good practice to clarify the question that a child is asking before responding. When asked, "Am I going to die?" for example, a good first response might be, "I want to answer your question as honestly as I can, so let me first ask you a few things. Tell me why you are asking. What do you think?" By gathering more information about what caused the child to ask the question, the question itself can be defined and the response and ensuing conversation will be most helpful. Conversations that focus on a child's concerns and fears (many of which would never have been guessed by family or team members) can reduce feelings of isolation, guilt, and anxiety. Because children have a tendency to express themselves in different ways, caretakers should pay attention to the verbal and nonverbal communications from the patient.

Facilitating communication between parents and their children is also a critical aspect of pediatric palliative care. Parents are often hesitant to have these difficult conversations with their children, and may rely on the health care team to provide guidance and support. By assessing the degree to which parents are talking with their children and the degree to which children feel comfortable raising questions with their parents, teams can provide advice and direction to parents. There may be times when the parents would prefer to have the physician or other health care provider present during discussions for support and medical expertise. Again, discussions between parents and children about medical issues should happen continuously, not just in one "discussion," and can take the form of talking, drawing, playing, or writing, among other modalities.

It is important to realize that communication with children about death can occur in all health care settings. In particular, children and families referred to hospice programs have access to a multidisciplinary team of providers who can help facilitate these conversations. In hospice work, there are often opportunities to talk with children about death and dying. It is often assumed that children are unaware of the severity of their illness and impending death. Children know much more than is often perceived and are very skilled at hearing their parents' unspoken feelings [42]. Frequent questions and comments from parents and other adult caregivers include: "What should we say? How much should we tell them? Do you really think they know they are dying?"

An intervention sometimes used to enlighten parents and loved ones about children's perception often surprises them about just know much children are aware about themselves and their families. With parental permission, children are spoken with in general terms about death and dying to assess their thoughts and feelings. Parents are requested to remain out of sight but within hearing distance of the conversation. The discussion can begin with the sharing of a pet fish dying, and the child is asked if they have ever experienced such a loss. Often, very openly and willingly, children share stories of their losses. Often, what children do not know about death is filled in with imaginary details or secondary information they may have seen or heard on television, in school, or from peers. This type of intervention not only reinforces how much children know or think they know about death, but offers wonderful opportunities to dispel frightening images and present a more comforting reality.

Ongoing and effective communication between the family and the medical team is also a critical component of palliative care, and disruptions in this process can compromise the care delivered. To promote the most effective communication as possible, regular times for communication should be structured into routine provision of care. Parents should know when and how to contact providers with any questions, and providers should use clear and concrete language whenever appropriate. It is important to remember that parents may be experiencing trauma symptoms and high anxiety during conversations, which may reduce their ability to take in (and then accurately recall) information. Reducing stimulation and distractions during conversations can maximize comfort. Conversations should, for example, occur with everyone sitting down in a space where interruptions are limited. Conversations about difficult issues are hindered if multiple providers are in the room with the parents at the same time; being careful to have only those individuals who need to be present for a conversation in the room increases the likelihood that real issues and concerns are addressed. Providers should be clear about how much time they have to talk (eg, "I have 5 minutes right now to talk, but if we need more time, we can schedule something for later in the day."). Stopping periodically to listen to parents' concerns and understandings of information just provided to them can also provide a check on whether parents understood what the provider intended to communicate.

Interventions to manage communication and conflicts between the family and the team

Good communication is on ongoing process that requires attention; it does not occur automatically. Following the guidelines above can promote effective communication, but there are occasions when conflicts arise and complicate the rapport between a family and the medical team. Conflicts are best resolved when they are addressed directly, without accusation, in a comfortable environment. Parents (who should be encouraged to bring a support person) should sit down, present their issues, and calmly discuss their options as they move forward. It is rare that a pediatric palliative care conflict cannot be worked out through discussion. In those cases, adding a neutral third party (perhaps a psychosocial professional or hospital mediator) to the conversation may promote positive movement.

Practical factors affecting the family, including financial status, living situation, and social support

General factors in a child's and family's life can have a direct influence on physical and psychologic symptoms and treatment. For example, a single-parent family with several children and little extra money living in a chaotic environment without access to regular transportation is going to face several obstacles in meeting their child's medical needs. A careful assessment of family constellation, financial resources and constraints, living situation, access to social support, transportation, and ability to manage the many practical demands of palliative care treatment is essential. Once such an assessment identifies barriers, hospital and community resources can be identified to help a family. Social workers are best equipped to facilitate this form of assessment for a team, and to match families with appropriate resources.

Religious or spiritual/existential background, preferences, related beliefs, rituals, and practices of the patient and family

Integral to providing comprehensive pediatric palliative care is an understanding of a family's spiritual needs and how the individual family's beliefs influence the decisions they make. The need to incorporate religion and spirituality into the medical care of children and families is important because most of the United States population considers themselves to be religious or spiritual [43,44]. Although spirituality is tied closely to religion and more formal religious affiliations, it should not be confused with religious affiliation [45]. In the context of caring for seriously ill and dying children and their families, it is vital that the definition of spirituality remain broad and include a focus on the individual's views on life, search for meaning and purpose, and self-awareness.

Several survey studies reveal that parents of children who have serious illnesses believe that their religious or spiritual beliefs were important factors in their coping efforts and decision-making [29,46–48]. Additionally, in a qualitative study, parents of children in the pediatric intensive care unit identified four spiritual/religious themes: (1) faith, (2) access to clergy, (3) care from clergy, and (4) belief in the transcendent quality of the parent–child relationship that endures beyond death. A total of 73% of the families interviewed found spiritual interventions helpful during times of crisis or at their child's end of life [48].

Although parents may have a clear view of their religious or spiritual beliefs and use these beliefs in difficult situations, a child will likely be more confused. Parents may look to pastoral care providers to help answer difficult spiritual questions, but a child is likely ask these questions of parents, friends, other family members, or members of the health care team. In a survey of pastoral care providers at children's hospitals in the United States, respondents believed that most children had spiritual care needs that were only partially being addressed. The barriers to providing spiritual care for children included: (1) inadequate staffing, (2) lack of training of health care providers, and (3) late consultation with the pastoral care service [45].

All members of the health care team can play a role in providing children and families with the opportunity to discuss spiritual and religious beliefs. Although doing a spiritual assessment is a requirement of hospital accreditation standards, most health care providers feel ill prepared to conduct such an assessment. It is important that the team be open to spiritually focused discussions and readily access available resources, such as hospital or community-based pastoral care services, to support children and families.

Managing spiritual concerns in pediatric palliative care

Committee members of the Children's International Project on Children's Palliative/Hospice Services identified several aspects relevant to spirituality in pediatric palliative care and developed guidelines for clinicians working in this specialty [2].

These guidelines included:

The interdisciplinary team should include professionals with skill in assessing and responding to common spiritual and existential issues of patients who have life-threatening illnesses and conditions and their families.

Regular, ongoing exploration of spiritual and existential concerns should occur and be documented (including but not limited to developmentally appropriate considerations of life review, assessment of hopes and fears, meaning, purpose, beliefs about afterlife, guilt, forgiveness, and life completion tasks). Use of a standardized instrument can facilitate this exploration.

The team should identify religious or spiritual/existential background, preferences, and related beliefs, rituals, and practices of the patient and family.

Pastoral care and other palliative care professionals should facilitate contacts, as desired by the family, with spiritual/religious communities, groups, or individuals. Patients should have access to clergy in their own religious traditions.

Professional and institutional use of religious symbols must be sensitive to cultural and religious diversity.

The patient and family should be encouraged to display their own religious/spiritual symbols.

The palliative care service should facilitate religious or spiritual rituals as desired by patient and family, especially at the time of death.

Periodic reevaluation of spiritual/existential interventions and patient and family preferences should occur and be documented.

Assessing and providing spiritual care to children who have life-limiting illnesses and their families is an area that deserves continued exploration and attention. Educating health care providers on the importance of being open to discussing spiritual issues and making appropriate resources available to families is vital. Although seemingly not a traditional part of health care delivery, meeting a child's and family's spiritual needs and facilitating a family's involvement in traditions that are comforting or help to make meaning of the distressing experience are an integral part of providing comprehensive high-quality palliative care.

Summary

Helping children to die well and assisting families in coping with this devastating experience is the responsibility of health care professionals. Accomplishing this mission depends on the accurate identification of the psychosocial and spiritual needs of dying children and their family members. Attention to practical concerns, family reactions, developmental issues, communication, and spiritual needs can address many of these concerns. A carefully orchestrated team that communicates well within the team and with the family is essential for the accomplishment of these tasks. Attending to the relationship built between providers and their child patients is also critical. Frequently children astound professionals and loved ones by demonstrating an inner wisdom well beyond their biologic years. Remaining open and teachable to the wisdom children offer enables professionals to support them through this experience with humanity, honesty, and integrity. We know that every child and family has a unique experience on the end-of-life journey. From each experience, practitioners learn lessons about the psychosocial and spiritual needs at the end of life that offer insights when caring for future families.

References

[1] American Academy of Pediatrics. Committee on Bioethics and Committee on Hospital Care. Palliative care for children. Pediatrics 2000;106:351.
[2] Clinical Practice Guidelines for Quality Palliative Care. In: National consensus project for quality palliative care. Brooklyn 2004.
[3] The pediatrician and childhood bereavement. American Academy of Pediatrics. Committee on psychosocial aspects of child and family health. Pediatrics 2000;105:445–8.
[4] Field M, Behrman R. When children die: improving palliative and end-of-life care for children and their families. Washington DC: The National Academies Press; 2003.
[5] Jones BL. Companionship, control, and compassion: a social work perspective on the needs of children with cancer and their families at the end of life. J Palliat Med 2006;9:774–88.
[6] Masera G, Spinetta JJ, Jankovic M, et al. Guidelines for assistance to terminally ill children with cancer: a report of the SIOP Working Committee on psychosocial issues in pediatric oncology. Med Pediatr Oncol 1999;32:44–8.

[7] Goodenough B, Drew D, Higgins S, et al. Bereavement outcomes for parents who lose a child to cancer: are place of death and sex of parent associated with differences in psychological functioning? Psychooncology 2004;13:779–91.

[8] Li J, Laursen TM, Precht DH, et al. Hospitalization for mental illness among parents after the death of a child. N Engl J Med 2005;352:1190–6.

[9] Li J, Precht DH, Mortensen PB, et al. Mortality in parents after death of a child in Denmark: a nationwide follow-up study. Lancet 2003;361:363–7.

[10] Payne JS, Paulson MA. Psychosocial adjustment of families following the death of a child. In: Shulman JL, editor. The child with cancer: clinical approaches to psychosocial care-research in psychosocial aspects. Springfield (IL): Charles C Thomas; 1980.

[11] Spinetta JJ. Impact of cancer on the family. Front Radiat Ther Oncol 1981;16:167–76.

[12] Spinetta JJ, Swarner JA, Sheposh JP. Effective parental coping following the death of a child from cancer. J Pediatr Psychol 1981;6:251–63.

[13] Whittam EH. Terminal care of the dying child. Psychosocial implications of care. Cancer 1993;71:3450–62.

[14] Kreicbergs U, Valdimarsdottir U, Onelov E, et al. Care-related distress: a nationwide study of parents who lost their child to cancer. J Clin Oncol 2005;23:9162–71.

[15] Kreicbergs U, Valdimarsdottir U, Onelov E, et al. Anxiety and depression in parents 4-9 years after the loss of a child owing to a malignancy: a population-based follow-up. Psychol Med 2004;34:1431–41.

[16] Kreicbergs U, Valdimarsdottir U, Steineck G, et al. A population-based nationwide study of parents' perceptions of a questionnaire on their child's death due to cancer. Lancet 2004;364:787–9.

[17] Block SD. Perspectives on care at the close of life. Psychological considerations, growth, and transcendence at the end of life: the art of the possible. JAMA 2001;285:2898–905.

[18] Mack JW, Hilden JM, Watterson J, et al. Parent and physician perspectives on quality of care at the end of life in children with cancer. J Clin Oncol 2005;23:9155–61.

[19] Binger CM, Ablin AR, Feuerstein RC, et al. Childhood leukemia. Emotional impact on patient and family. N Engl J Med 1969;280:414–8.

[20] Cain AC, Fast I, Erickson ME. Children's disturbed reactions to the death of a sibling. Am J Orthopsychiatry 1964;34:741–52.

[21] Cobb B. Psychological impact of long illness and death of a child on the family circle. J Pediatr 1956;49:746–51.

[22] Alderfer MA, Labay LE, Kazak AE. Brief report: does posttraumatic stress apply to siblings of childhood cancer survivors? J Pediatr Psychol 2003;28:281–6.

[23] Brown MR, Sourkes B. Psychotherapy in pediatric palliative care. Child Adolesc Psychiatr Clin N Am 2006;15:585–96.

[24] Micucci J. The adolescent in family therapy: breaking the cycle of conflict and control. New York: Guilford Press; 2000.

[25] Poltorak DY, Glazer JP. The development of children's understanding of death: cognitive and psychodynamic considerations. Child Adolesc Psychiatr Clin N Am 2006;15:567.

[26] Lauer ME, Mulhern RK, Bohne JB, et al. Children's perceptions of their sibling's death at home or hospital: the precursors of differential adjustment. Can Nurse 1985;8:21–7.

[27] Lauer ME, Mulhern RK, Schell MJ, et al. Long-term follow-up of parental adjustment following a child's death at home or hospital. Cancer 1989;63:988–94.

[28] Lauer ME, Mulhern RK, Wallskog JM, et al. A comparison study of parental adaptation following a child's death at home or in the hospital. Pediatrics 1983;71:107–12.

[29] Contro N, Larson J, Scofield S, et al. Family perspectives on the quality of pediatric palliative care. Arch Pediatr Adolesc Med 2002;156:14–9.

[30] Duncan J, Joselow M, Hilden JM. Program interventions for children at the end of life and their siblings. Child Adolesc Psychiatr Clin N Am 2006;15:739–58.

[31] Giovanola J. Sibling involvement at the end of life. J Pediatr Oncol Nurs 2005;22:222–6.

[32] Pratt RR. Art, dance, and music therapy. Phys Med Rehabil Clin N Am 2004;15:827–41.

[33] Rollins JA. Childhood cancer: siblings draw and tell. Pediatr Nurs 1990;16:21–7.

[34] Wilson JM. Child life services. Pediatrics 2006;118:1757–63.

[35] Kazak AE, Noll R. Child death from pediatric illness: conceptualizing interventions from a family systems and public health perspective. Prof Psychol 2004;35:219.

[36] Stuber ML, Shemesh E. Post-traumatic stress response to life-threatening illnesses in children and their parents. Child Adolesc Psychiatr Clin N Am 2006;15:597–609.

[37] Frager G. Children's concept of death. In: Joishy SK, editor. Palliative Medicine Secrets. Philadelphia: Hanley & Belfus; 1999.

[38] Carter B, BcGoldrick M. The expanded family life cycle: individual, family and social perspectives. Boston: Allyn & Bacon; 1999.

[39] Stoddard FJ, Usher CT, Abrams AN. Psychopharmacology in pediatric critical care. Child Adolesc Psychiatr Clin N Am 2006;15:611–55.

[40] Poltorak DY, Benore E. Cognitive-behavioral interventions for physical symptom management in pediatric palliative medicine. Child Adolesc Psychiatr Clin N Am 2006;15:683–91.

[41] Kreicbergs U, Valdimarsdottir U, Onelov E, et al. Talking about death with children who have severe malignant disease. N Engl J Med 2004;351:1175–86.

[42] Gottlieb D. Voices of conflict; voices of healing. Lincoln (NE): People with Disabilities Press; 2001.

[43] Levin JS, Larson DB, Puchalski CM. Religion and spirituality in medicine: research and education. JAMA 1997;278:792–3.

[44] Maugans TA, Wadland WC. Religion and family medicine: a survey of physicians and patients. J Fam Pract 1991;32:210–3.

[45] Feudtner C, Haney J, Dimmers MA. Spiritual care needs of hospitalized children and their families: a national survey of pastoral care providers' perceptions. Pediatrics 2003;111: e67–72.

[46] Davies B, Brenner P, Orloff S, et al. Addressing spirituality in pediatric hospice and palliative care. J Palliat Care 2002;18:59–67.

[47] Dell'Orfano S. The meaning of spiritual care in a pediatric setting. J Pediatr Nurs 2002;17: 380–5.

[48] Robinson MR, Thiel MM, Backus MM, et al. Matters of spirituality at the end of life in the pediatric intensive care unit. Pediatrics 2006;118:e719–29.

ELSEVIER
SAUNDERS

PEDIATRIC CLINICS

OF NORTH AMERICA

Pediatr Clin N Am 54 (2007) 631–644

Compassion Fatigue in Pediatric Palliative Care Providers

Mary T. Rourke, PhD

The Behavioral Health Integrated Program, The Children's Hospital of Philadelphia,
9th Floor Main Hospital, Room 9S35, 34th and Civic Center Boulevard,
Philadelphia, PA 19104, USA

Few people would deny that the death of a child is traumatic for most families. It is less common, however, for people to recognize that a child's death can also be traumatic for the health care professionals who care for the child. Further, the cumulative impact on health care professionals of routinely experiencing children's deaths may be significant.

Despite these issues, there is little research that examines the common experiences of health care professionals who routinely provide pediatric palliative or end-of-life care. This article proposes a general framework, borrowed in part from the study of trauma workers in other professions, through which we can understand the experience of health care professionals who provide pediatric palliative care. It focuses on ways in which predictable and common reactions of palliative care team members might be clarified and, in turn, well managed. These reactions are illustrated by clinical vignettes, which are based on composite case examples and clinical experience.

Common psychologic reactions to trauma

Many labels have been applied interchangeably to describe the kinds of psychologic consequences experienced by professionals working with people in the wake of traumatic events, including secondary traumatic stress (STS), vicarious traumatization, and compassion fatigue [1–3]. Secondary traumatic stress, one of the more commonly used labels, has been defined as "...the natural consequent behaviors and emotions resulting from knowing about a traumatizing event experienced by a significant other—the stress

---

E-mail address: rourke@email.chop.edu

0031-3955/07/$ - see front matter © 2007 Elsevier Inc. All rights reserved.
doi:10.1016/j.pcl.2007.07.004   *pediatric.theclinics.com*

resulting from helping or wanting to help a traumatized or suffering person" [2]. Specific secondary traumatic stress reactions are known only through theoretic assumption and anecdotal reports. No definitive empiric findings illustrate the specific manifestations of these reactions. It makes sense, however, that stress resulting from witnessing the trauma of others would parallel the stress the victims themselves experience after a trauma. Most conceptualizations of STS include aspects common in posttraumatic stress reactions, including re-experiencing (intrusive thoughts, nightmares, vivid distressing imagery), avoidance or emotional numbing, and high physiologic arousal [4]. The most common articulations of STS suggest a constellation of these trauma reactions across three domains: psychologic, cognitive, and interpersonal (Box 1). These reactions are considered common and even expected for professionals who help others by providing care and empathy. For this reason, Figley [2] advocates the term compassion fatigue to reflect the inevitable experience of the emotional exhaustion that comes from continuous compassion directed toward those in crisis. The term compassion fatigue is used in the remainder of this article.

Compassion fatigue must be distinguished from the concept of burnout. Burnout refers to the global long-term consequences of working in a stressful caregiving environment and includes the experience of emotional exhaustion and a depleted sense of personal accomplishment and achievement [2,5]. Burnout is believed to be the end result of a gradual process of wearing down, whereas compassion fatigue may represent a more immediate, specific, trauma-related reaction [2].

Pediatric palliative care professionals as trauma workers

It may seem odd to consider pediatric palliative care professionals, who by definition aim to provide a less distressing end-of-life experience for children and their families, as "trauma workers." Evidence shows, however, that children and families going through serious pediatric illness and injury are experiencing trauma and do report significant posttraumatic stress [6]. Although these data were collected on children who were still living, one can surmise that family members of those children who did not survive also experience their child's illness as a trauma. In most cases, the death of a child after a serious illness or injury is the culmination of a trauma that began at diagnosis. Day-to-day aspects of palliative treatment may be experienced as traumatic by children or their families, including the experience of a child's pain that is not responsive to treatment. For some families, waiting for scans, making treatment decisions (eg, withdrawal of curative care, "Do Not Resuscitate" orders), and fearing death may in and of themselves be traumatic.

Within this context, palliative care workers may indeed be doing something akin to trauma work. Just as EMTs and other trauma personnel enter the scene after a catastrophic event, responding to the most serious

---

Box 1. Common symptoms of compassion fatigue across three domains

Psychologic
Strong emotions (sadness, anger, guilt, worry)
Intrusive thoughts or images/nightmares
Feeling numb or frozen
Avoiding the patient/family or situation
Somatic complaints (gastrointestinal distress, headaches, fatigue)
Anxiety or agitation
Compulsive or addictive behaviors (drinking, smoking, shopping sprees)
Feeling isolated or personally responsible, with no back-up

Cognitive
Mistrust of others (family, patient, other staff)
Increased personal vulnerability or lack of safety
Belief that others aren't competent to handle the problem
Increased or decreased sense of power or control
Increased cynicism
Increased sense of personal responsibility or blame
Belief that others don't understand the work that you do

Interpersonal
Withdrawal from the larger treatment team
Withdrawal from personal relationships (because people "don't understand")
Difficulty trusting others personally and professionally
Overidentifying with the distress of others leading to skewed boundaries in relationships
Detachment from emotional situations or experiences (including the patient/family)
Becoming easily irritated with others

Data from Refs. [1,2,11]

---

injuries and providing a sense of safety and support, palliative care teams enter the scene of a family's personal crisis, attending to the serious issues of symptom management and providing safety by ensuring the comfort of the dying child. Just as trauma workers at a catastrophic event must navigate the confusion and intense emotional devastation of those who have just endured the event, so must palliative care teams do their difficult work in the face of the intense emotions and confusion of the family members. Many of the family members may demand time and attention that is

simultaneously required to be directed toward helping the child die peacefully and without pain or distress. Finally, just as trauma workers at the
scene of a natural disaster must work in intense chaos, with no clearly evident or accessible organizational structure on the scene, palliative care teams
often operate outside the routines of hospital care. Many of their tasks are
performed in collaboration with hospices or in the homes of dying patients,
removed from the hospital's organizational resources.

The routine practice of presiding over the death of children can lead
easily to the experience of compassion fatigue. Repeated exposure to dying
children can erode the myth of safety that guides most people through life,
revealing a harsh and frightening reality. Further, health care providers at
the end of life are both witnesses to and participants in a child's and family's
trauma. Physicians or nurses are often required to provide treatments that
are necessarily painful or upsetting and may be unable to provide full relief
from pain. As a result, their complex role in a family's trauma can be
distressing.

The intense relationships that often occur between palliative care providers
and patients and their families can themselves be sources of compassion
fatigue. Palliative care providers often encounter situations that echo losses
in their own lives and reactivate their personal pain and grief, even if only temporarily. During these times, health care providers may actually be responding
emotionally as much to their own personal grief as to the present reality of the
patient and family for whom they are caring [2]. In addition, parents may also
be reacting with strong emotions that are more closely linked psychologically
to their own traumatic experience than to the objective aspects of the situations. These reactions can seem inappropriate, offensive, and often exasperat-
ing to health care providers. Traumatized parents may, for example, "check
out" and be emotionally unavailable to their children or to the medical
team, or they may accuse the medical team of not working hard enough on
their child's behalf. In cases like these, most parents are reacting out of their
own fear or trauma. These reactions can nonetheless lead team members to
feel abused, angry, powerless, or resentful.

Only one unpublished study examines traumatic stress in pediatric health
care providers at a tertiary care medical center. Early data analyses, which
are continuing, do suggest that doctors, nurses, allied health care workers,
and psychosocial staff are at risk for high levels of compassion fatigue. Overall, the combined sample's average level of compassion fatigue exceeded that
of trauma workers and a larger sample of nonpediatric health care workers
(P.M. Robins, L. Meltzer, and N. Zelikovsky, unpublished data, 2007).

Who is most at risk for compassion fatigue?

Compassion fatigue is an occupational hazard for those who work with
people in trauma. It is critical to recognize that if a team is doing its job

correctly and engaging in caring and supportive ways with families around the death of a child, all members of the team are susceptible at some time or another to experiencing the natural consequences of such care [7,8]. The effects of compassion fatigue, however, may endure or worsen over time, developing into serious reactions that compromise a health care provider's ability to interact in positive and helpful ways with patients and families [9,10].

No published data to date suggest specific factors that may predispose pediatric health care practitioners to develop compassion fatigue. In a sample of adult cancer nurses, however, unusually high levels of job stress (poor physician/nurse communication, heavy workload) were associated with high levels of exhaustion and depersonalization [10]. For trauma workers who responded to an earthquake-related disaster, exposure to repeated traumas, poor psychologic adjustment, lack of professional experience, low sense of control, and lack of social support predicted higher levels of traumatic distress [3]. One recently completed study of compassion fatigue in pediatric health care professionals suggests that weak personal coping skills, high levels of distress, and high levels of empathy, along with being a physician (versus a nurse or psychosocial professional), were most predictive of compassion fatigue (P.M. Robins, L. Meltzer, and N. Zelikovsky, unpublished data, 2007).

Strategies for preventing and ameliorating compassion fatigue

Compassion fatigue cannot be completely eradicated in those who provide pediatric palliative care. It is important to prevent a normal response of compassion fatigue from developing in strongly negative and destructive ways, however [7]. Multiple recommendations for protecting professionals from the cumulative and complicated effects of compassion fatigue include three tiers of strategies: personal strategies, professional strategies, and organizational strategies [2,7,11,12,13].

Personal strategies

Most of the strategies believed to be most helpful personally reflect the same kind of good self-care that health care providers recommend to patients [10]. In a moving discussion of the challenges of their work, a group of oncologists emphasize that doing their job well requires a commitment to ensuring their own personal well-being [12]. Along the same lines, suggestions for developing a good self-care plan that can minimize the impact of compassion fatigue include:

- Getting appropriate amounts of sleep, good nutrition, and regular exercise.
- Building relaxation and a moderate pace into most days, including the regular use of tools such as meditation, deep breathing, visual imagery, and massage [7].

Engaging regularly in a non–work-related activity to rejuvenate and restore energy, commitment, and focus [7,12,13].

Maintaining a good balance between work, family, and non-obligatory events to defuse the tension and monotony that come from an intense caseload [7,12,13].

Finding and allowing adequate personal time to grieve the inevitable losses that come with losing a patient [12].

Developing a specific set of coping skills, including assertiveness, stress management, organization, time management, communication, and cognitive restructuring, to ease the challenges of day-to-day issues [7,10].

Relying on psychotherapy, particularly for caregivers who are experiencing very strong emotional reactions to their work, who are strongly reminded of their own personal losses frequently, or who have no clear confidante in their daily lives [5,13].

Attending to one's spiritual needs and existential understanding to build a personal meaning system through which daily professional experiences can be understood [13].

Professional strategies

Perhaps the most helpful professional strategy for containing and managing compassion fatigue is recognizing and accepting the realities of working in pediatric palliative care: some children will die from their disease or injury, and health care providers are limited in their ability to relieve a patient's and family's suffering [7]. Having acknowledged that reality, health care providers can find it easier to identify the many ways in which they can help.

Other professional strategies include:

Engaging in peer consultation, which is most helpful if it occurs regularly and predictably in a safe, confidential, and nonjudgmental environment [13].

Being clear and consistent with oneself and others about boundaries and personal limit-setting [7,13]

Diversifying one's workload, so that not all professional time involves providing care to the most distressed patients. This strategy should include mixing more and less acute cases; having clear limits around time on service (for all professionals on the team, not only the physicians), adding research, teaching, or other activities to round out clinical service, and having coverage schedules that accommodate work-life balance for providers as much as possible [7,11,13].

Identifying the one or two scenarios that are most difficult and exhausting for a professional, and identifying and reviewing potential responses to use when these situations arise [12].

Finding and focusing on the positive features of one's own and one's patients' experiences.

Connecting regularly with a respectful team of professionals that meets regularly and shares a common goal or mission [13].

Organizational strategies

The organization within which any palliative care provider works sets the stage for how stressful the work is, and for how effectively the provider is able to defuse that stress. It is essential that the larger organization recognize that pediatric death occurs in large enough numbers to warrant the resources necessary to do the job well. The organization needs to provide structures for addressing compassion fatigue. Accomplishing these tasks may take time and public advocacy. On a more concrete level, organizations can be the focus for important interventions to prevent or reduce compassion fatigue [14]. Some strategies that may move organizations closer to these goals include:

Breaking the "culture of silence" that can sometimes exist around the experience of compassion fatigue (P.M. Robins, L. Meltzer, and N. Zelikovsky, unpublished data, 2007). From the training of health care providers and continuing through regular continuing education channels, it is critical to recognize that compassion fatigue is an expected occupational hazard, not a weakness [1,10,12,13].

Providing physical settings that are comforting or soothing and offering meeting spaces that are appropriately furnished and private. In nonpatient areas, allowing for personal items that anchor clinicians to their lives outside of work [13].

Providing adequate resources for the job, including regular and supportive supervision, continuing education opportunities, days off without undue hassle, appropriate benefits, and an overall positive work climate [1,13].

Developing an atmosphere of respect for the work [1,13]. Organizations tend to be governed by principles of power, and those who are traumatized, such as dying children, their families, and care providers, often lack institutional power. Commonly, institutions lack respect for the role of working with dying children and their families. Teams and organizations can respond by aligning the work of a palliative care group or provider with a larger, more organizationally powerful division or department. They may also enhance respect by framing the mission of palliative care as one that supports the overall mission of the larger institution.

Developing a working support team. When working with situations that can provoke compassion fatigue, a connected, supportive team is critical. Through the process of regular case discussion, in which all team members, regardless of role, are encouraged to contribute, teams can recognize compassion fatigue, discuss its implications, and collaboratively formulate a team approach to manage repercussions [8]. The team should provide a forum for active listening and limited criticism [12].

These strategies are an amalgam of recommendations from the medical and mental health literature and draw heavily on the child abuse literature. No studies document the effectiveness of these specific strategies in preventing compassion fatigue, although there are indications that they may relate to overall physician well-being. Oncologists who report high levels of psychosocial well-being, for example, also report using more of the strategies suggested above than those who report lower levels. Specifically, having a positive outlook; developing a specific approach to deal with end-of-life issues; participating in regular hobbies, activities, and exercise; and incorporating work–life balance into one's life were all related to higher levels of well-being among oncologists [15].

Clinical examples of relational complications of compassion fatigue

Because the palliative care workers who experience symptoms of compassion fatigue are often taking care of patients and families and interacting with colleagues at the same time, the risks for complications in these relationships is high [1,2,8]. Below are three common examples of relational complications attributable to compassion fatigue, along with suggestions for how to address them.

Splitting

Splitting is a relationship pattern common to people who have experienced trauma, and usually involves perceiving one person or subgroup of people as entirely good and helpful, and an opposing person or subgroup as entirely bad and extremely unhelpful [8]. In the following example, a physician providing care to a dying patient has been demonstrating several signs of compassion fatigue, including exhaustion, cynicism, and a subtle distrust of other members of the team. She recognizes that her decisions about her personal boundaries, such as how much personal information and contact information to share with families, have shifted recently also. The family, in the midst of their own traumatic reaction, is also experiencing a high level of anxiety and distrust of almost everyone on the team.

> Dr. Smith has been on-service with the palliative care team for the past 10 days and has been meeting daily with the family. Jaden, the patient, is a 6-year-old who is actively dying after being treated for histiocytosis for 3 years. Dr. Smith is the physician who introduced the family to the palliative care team and its approach. She has shared with the family that she also has a 6-year-old son, and she has interacted with Jaden over the past week about Ninja turtles, his favorite TV shows, and how much his 8-year-old brother bugs him. The family has felt somewhat relieved by

Dr. Smith's care, and has been able to make some difficult decisions this week regarding Jaden's DNR status. They attribute their and Jaden's increased comfort and their decisions to Dr. Smith's exceptional skill. Over the course of the past several days, the palliative care team's nurse practitioner has attempted to work with Jaden and the family. On each occasion, the family questioned his judgment and appealed to Dr. Smith for a final decision, saying, "She just knows us and Jaden better." In private, they confided to Dr. Smith that until now, they have felt that they felt "used" by the large teaching hospital treating Jaden, and that they believed that only Dr. Smith cared enough about them and their child to provide the best care. Dr. Smith, feeling cynical about increased administrative pressures and lack of support by the administration, responded with a half-hearted defense of the hospital. She then increased her focus on the family. She informed the rest of the team that she would be the primary team representative to work with the family, and wanted to be kept apprised of Jaden's care even after she rotated off service. Once the new physician rotated on service and introduced himself to the family and Jaden, the family immediately called Dr. Smith to complain. They gently but firmly insisted that the new physician did not understand their concerns and was not good at reading Jaden's signals. Dr. Smith explained that there was no way around having this new physician care for the family, but she then gave the family her direct pager number and suggested that they call her with any questions about Jaden's care. The family did just that several times over the ensuing week, much to the distress of the on-service palliative care team, all of whom felt undermined and angry at Dr. Smith's "arrogance."

In this example, Dr. Smith was already feeling depleted by the ongoing demands of her work, and possibly by the similarities between her son and this actively dying patient. The family, understandably distressed, has the common reaction of assuming that Dr. Smith is all good, and anyone else on her team must not be nearly as good, and may even be incompetent to care for their child. Dr. Smith's halfhearted verbal support of her team is undone by allowing the family to call her for advice when another clinician is supposed to be providing care. Although this permission allows the family to stay connected to someone familiar on the team, it distances them from of the rest of the team and complicates Jaden's care. The team then exacerbates the splitting by interpreting Dr. Smith's behavior as arrogance, rather than the response of someone who is experiencing understandable effects of compassion fatigue and needs to be connected to a supportive group.

Managing splitting on a team

Splitting is a group phenomenon, and must be managed at the team level. The interventions discussed earlier regarding appropriate organizational environments for teams involved in trauma-related work are relevant. Teams must have regular meetings at which they build group identity, making it easier for members who begin to feel isolated to ally primarily with the team. These meetings must be safe places to openly discuss incipient attempts to split the team or form alliances, and to discover potential solutions [10]. Team members should acknowledge the risk for this type of splitting, and should protect themselves by agreeing on how they will respond to it. Acknowledging to families that different levels of comfort with different care providers are normal and helping to support a family's connection to a new provider are critical. Team members should resist ongoing independent conversations with the family. Finally, when splitting does occur, team members not involved should resist the temptation to take sides, because doing so can only deepen the conflicts. Instead, supporting team members on both sides can help resolve the problem.

The savior versus the helper

Another common pattern of relationship between physicians and patients that relates to compassion fatigue is the challenge of maintaining the role of helper and avoiding the role of savior [12]. The following example illustrates this difficulty:

> Dr. Jones has been an attending physician who was providing end-of-life care to Jesse, a 16-year-old who is in her last weeks of life after a several-year struggle with acute lymphocytic leukemia. Dr. Jones met Jesse when she was initially diagnosed during his fellowship years, and has been her primary oncologist through multiple relapses, a bone marrow transplant, and the transition to palliative care. This week, Jesse's mother has become increasingly insistent that "no stone be left unturned," and has begged Dr. Jones in multiple phone calls and e-mails that he "not give up on us, not let us down." Her most recent e-mail to Dr. Jones had, as its subject line, "If anyone can help us, you can." In addition, Jesse's parents have begun researching experimental treatments that "just might pull Jesse out of this nosedive." They call and e-mail Dr. Jones multiple times each day, and request numerous meetings with the team to review the treatments and plans to manage Jesse's symptoms. Her parents ask the same questions repeatedly, seemingly without having heard answers given during previous meetings.
>
> Dr. Jones' own level of anxiety and frustration has increased considerably as the family's campaign has increased. Although he was at first able to respond carefully and clearly about the limits of curative medicine in Jesse's case, he has slowly begun exploring the other "options" suggested by the family. He has allowed the family to delay discussion of DNR until "we know what we're doing," despite that he had a clear plan outlined to help manage Jesse's symptoms. Dr. Jones has found himself struggling with guilt, knowing that he would be forced to let this family down in the end. In addition, Dr. Jones himself has been responding to so many issues with this family that he has had less and less time available for other patients, further increasing his guilt and anxiety.
>
> Jesse's family clearly continued their respect for Dr. Jones, praising him often to the nursing staff, and even writing a letter commending his work to

the hospital administration. Their continuing close attachment to Dr. Jones led them to sense his anxiety, however. At one point, Jesse's mother pulled aside the team social worker and asked, "Is Dr. Jones OK? He seems so upset." Despite the social worker's assurances that Dr. Jones was doing just fine, the next day, Jesse's parents presented Dr. Jones with a "care package" including tickets for the local college's basketball game.

In this example, Dr. Jones began in the role of helper, with several factors setting him up for a meaningful and positive end-of-life experience with the family: he knew them well, had their respect, and had a good end-of-life care plan in mind. The family's distress, however, led him to accept, however passively, their request that he rescue them. He may, in fact, have been affected by his own anticipatory grief. By responding to their pleas, Dr. Jones set himself up as responsible for producing a miracle, and would no doubt confront a strong sense of guilt for his inability to actually produce that miracle [12]. As his attempts to manage the family's anxious pleas increased, and the demands on him intensified, Dr. Jones was also limited in his ability to seek support from colleagues. His engagement in a clinical impossibility became his own personal mission. His collusion with the family's crusade opened up the possibility that Jesse would endure more painful treatment, rather than comfort and freedom from symptoms, in her last days [12]. Further, Jesse's parents sensed Dr. Jones' distress, which placed them in the role of caring for the physician, a complication that frequently arises in trauma work. Giving gifts is an obvious example of care-taking that can include more subtle manifestations, such as patients' and families' reluctance to share information or concerns for fear of upsetting the physician [1].

Managing the savior versus the helper dichotomy

The most important rule of thumb when attempting to remain a "helper" is to use frequent, clear communication. Articulating a clear plan with the patient and family that explicitly acknowledges the goals of care and revisiting the plan with the family regularly may reduce the anxiety that prompts families to ask for inappropriate help [8]. As part of that plan, the clinician should have a prepared response for the likely family press for more treatment. Even after a family has acknowledged a transition to palliative care, the realization than their child is actively dying is likely to reactivate a sense of crisis and push them to search, once again, for a rescue. After the clinician has listened carefully to a family's concerns and empathically acknowledged their distress, letting them know that they have been heard and understood, then he or she can calmly reiterate the decision-making process they have agreed on and the potential consequences of changing course. These steps often redirect families to the most sensible care plan, keeping the physician and family, and not the trauma reactions of both, in charge of the plan. As always, it is critical that a team be available to back up the primary clinician connected with the family [8]. Inclusion of other team members in the regular planning conversations with the family reduces the likelihood that the physician will be drawn into an isolated role of rescuer with a family he or she knows well.

Becoming detached

Compassion fatigue can result not only in becoming overinvolved in a patient's care at the end of life but also in detachment. Sometimes physicians and others involved in a patient's care gradually or abruptly withdraw as the emotional intensity increases. A clinical vignette illustrates this form of compassion fatigue:

> Dr. Marsh was the attending physician on the palliative care service while she was 24 weeks pregnant. On her first day on service, Dr. Marsh met the mother of a 7-month-old baby who was receiving palliative care since being diagnosed with a severe neurologic disorder at birth. As she reviewed the active patients with the team, one of the other physicians offered to cover this case, suggesting that her pregnancy might make this case difficult for her. Dr. Marsh considered the offer, but didn't believe that this case would be an overly emotional one for her. After meeting the mother and examining the baby, she adjusted the baby's care plan, asked the mother if she had any concerns, and moved on to her next patient.
>
> During her week on service, the baby's condition deteriorated, requiring Dr. Marsh to have several difficult conversations with the baby's parents. As the care team became increasingly distressed over the baby's condition and the mother's anguished response, they paged Dr. Marsh more frequently. She started to become irritated by the requests for her attention, feeling that nothing unexpected was occurring and the care plan in place was adequately addressing the issues. She found the team meetings with the baby's parents to be overly long and repetitive, and began feeling excessively tired during them. Twice, at the last minute, she found reasons to delay these meetings by several hours. By the end of the week, the baby's parents complained about Dr. Marsh's unavailability to the team nurse, claiming that she barely examined the baby, was not responsive to their requests for information, and seemed cold.

Dr. Marsh is clearly attempting to avoid the distress she might feel if she allowed herself to engage with a family more personally around their trauma. Although examples of detachment are rarely this obvious, attempts to avoid connection are common among physicians who care for dying children. For instance, a clinician might put an especially distressing family last on his or her list of patients to see for the night, leaving less time to spend with them. He or she might shut off emotionally when dealing with a particular family, or might feel intense irritation, or exhaustion, when working with them [1].

Managing detachment

Perhaps the biggest risk factor for detachment is working alone or not being part of a supportive and collaborative team when providing end-of-life care. Being part of a team that meets regularly and discusses the details of patient care is critical. If such a team is not available, care providers can seek supervision or collegial support from peers or others familiar with a patient or family, such as social workers, nurses, and physicians from other specialties who have treated the patient. Discussions of patient care should include considerations of how the work is affecting individual caregivers, and is most effective with a minimum of criticism and high levels of support [7,8].

Compassion satisfaction

Compassion satisfaction is a term for the personal and professional sense of fulfillment that can accompany the difficult work of providing compassionate care to those in crisis. It includes feeling pleasure in helping others and believing that one's work is important and meaningful (P.M. Robins, L. Meltzer, and N. Zelikovsky, unpublished data, 2007) [2,16]. Those who provide palliative care find varying degrees of benefit or reward in the work.

At the same time, compassion satisfaction may be related to compassion fatigue in important ways. In a study of child protective workers, compassion satisfaction seemed to protect professionals from experiencing compassion fatigue [17]. No studies of compassion fatigue and compassion satisfaction in pediatric health care providers are yet available, but the preliminary analyses in the unpublished study cited earlier in this article indicate that compassion satisfaction is evident in pediatric health care providers and may be related to these care providers often having reasonable clinical loads, children of their own, and many years of professional experience. The connections between compassion satisfaction and compassion fatigue may be important for future investigation (P.M. Robins, L. Meltzer, and N. Zelikovsky, unpublished data, 2007).

Summary

The experience of compassion fatigue is an expected and common response to the professional task of routinely caring for children at the end of life. Symptoms of compassion fatigue often mimic trauma reactions. They have the potential to create personal distress for health care providers and to complicate the relationships between these providers and the children and families for whom they provide care. Implementing strategies that span personal, professional, and organizational domains can help protect health care providers from the damaging effects of compassion fatigue. Providing pediatric palliative care within a constructive and supportive team can help caregivers deal with the relational challenges of compassion fatigue. Finally, any consideration of the toll of providing pediatric palliative care must be balanced with a consideration of the parallel experience of compassion satisfaction. Preliminary work suggests that compassion satisfaction emerges particularly in those who have years of experience and a strong balance in their professional and personal lives and that compassion satisfaction itself may protect health care providers from compassion fatigue.

References

[1] Collins S, Long A. Working with psychological effects of trauma: consequences for mental health workers—a literature review. J Psychiatr Ment Health Nurs 2003;10:417–24.

[2] Figley C. Compassion fatigue as secondary traumatic stress disorder: an overview. In: Figley C, editor. Compassion fatigue: coping with secondary traumatic stress disorder. New York: Brunner/Mazel; 1995. p. 1–20.

[3] Weiss DS, Marmar CR, Metzler TJ, et al. Predicting symptomatic distress in emergency service personnel. J Consult Clin Psychol 1995;63(3):361–8.

[4] American Psychiatric Association. Dianostic and statistical manual of mental disorders. 4th edition. Arlington (VA): American Psychiatric Association Publishing; 1994.

[5] Maslach C, Jackson S, Leiter P. Maslach Burnout inventory. 3rd edition. New York: Consulting Psychologists Press Inc.; 1996.

[6] Kazak AE, Rourke MT, Alderfer MA, et al. Evidence-based assessment, intervention and psychosocial care in pediatric oncology: a blueprint for comprehensive services across treatment. J Pediatr Psychol, in press.

[7] Yassen J. Preventing secondary traumatic stress disorder. In: Figley C, editor. Compassion fatigue: coping with secondary traumatic stress disorder. New York: Brunner/Mazel; 1995. p. 178–208.

[8] Munroe J, Shay J, Fisher L, et al. Preventing compassion fatigue: a team treatment model. In: Figley C, editor. Compassion fatigue: secondary traumatic stress disorders in those who treat the traumatized. New York: Brunnel/Mazel; 1995. p. 209–31.

[9] Shanafelt T, Chung H, White H, et al. Shaping your career to maximize personal satisfaction in the practice of oncology. J Clin Oncol 2006;24(24):4020–6.

[10] Firth-Cozens J. Intervention to improve physicians' well-being and patient care. Soc Sci Med 2001;52:215–22.

[11] Dutton MA, Rubinstein FL. Working with people with PTSD: research implications. In: Figley C, editor. Compassion fatigue: coping with secondary traumatic stress disorder. New York: Brunner/Mazel; 1995. p. 82–100.

[12] Shanafelt T, Adjei A, Meyskens FL. When your favorite patient relapses: physician grief and well-being in the practice of oncology. J Clin Oncol 2003;21(13):2616–9.

[13] Pearlman LA, Saakvitne KW. Treating therapists with vicarious traumatization and secondary traumatic stress disorders. In: Figley C, editor. Compassion fatigue: secondary traumatic stress disorders in those who treat the traumatized. New York: Brunnel/Mazel; 1995. p. 150–77.

[14] Barnard D, Street A, Love AW. Relationships between stressors, work supports, and burnout among cancer nurses. Cancer Nurs 2006;29(4):338–45.

[15] Shanafelt T, Novotny P, Johnson M, et al. The well-being and personal wellness promotion strategies of medical oncologists in the North Central Cancer Treatment Group. Oncology 2005;68:23–32.

[16] DePanfilis D. Compassion fatigue, burnout, and compassion satisfaction: implications for retention of workers. Child Abuse Negl 2006;30:1067–9.

[17] Conrad D, Kellar-Guenther Y. Compassion fatigue, burnout, and compassion satisfaction among Colorado child protection workers. Child Abuse Negl 2006;30:1071–80.

ELSEVIER
SAUNDERS

PEDIATRIC CLINICS
OF NORTH AMERICA

Pediatr Clin N Am 54 (2007) 645–672

The Management of Pain in Children with Life-limiting Illnesses

Stefan J. Friedrichsdorf, MD[a],
Tammy I. Kang, MD[b,c],*

[a]Pain and Palliative Care, Children's Hospitals and Clinics of Minnesota,
2525 Chicago Avenue South, Minneapolis, MN 55404, USA
[b]Division of Oncology, Children's Hospital of Philadelphia, 34th and Civic Center Boulevard,
4314 Wood Building, Philadelphia, PA 19104, USA
[c]The Pediatric Advanced Care Team, Children's Hospital of Philadelphia,
Philadelphia, PA 19104, USA

Despite increasing awareness about causes and treatment of pain in children, at the beginning of the 21st century most children with advanced illness still experience pain. Multiple studies have shown that children have suboptimal pain control in the last days of life [1–6]. Although there are discrepancies in the percentage of time and the degree to which it occurs, there is clear room for improvement in the management of pain in children with life-limiting illnesses. The treatment of pain not only affects the child, but can also have a significant impact on the family [2,7,8].

Pain can be somatic, visceral, or neuropathic in nature and can be disease-related, treatment-related, or caused by spiritual or psychologic distress. The key to effective pain control is obtaining a detailed assessment, developing a child-specific treatment plan, and frequently re-evaluating to determine efficacy.

This article focuses on topics common to practitioners caring for children with life-limiting illnesses. These topics include a review of myths and obstacles to achieving adequate pain control, a review of the pathophysiology of pain, an overview of the use of opioids in children, an approach to the management of neuropathic pain, and a brief discussion of nonpharmacologic pain management strategies. As pediatric palliative medicine providers, the authors have found these topics to encompass the most common situations encountered. Clearly, there are many other aspects important to the

---

* Corresponding author. Division of Oncology, Children's Hospital of Philadelphia, 34th and Civic Center Boulevard, 4314 Wood Building, Philadelphia, PA 19104.

E-mail address: kang@email.chop.edu (T.I. Kang).

0031-3955/07/$ - see front matter © 2007 Elsevier Inc. All rights reserved.
doi:10.1016/j.pcl.2007.07.007
pediatric.theclinics.com

management of pain in this patient population, including assessment and management of emotion and spiritual pain, and the use of more advanced pain regimens, including regional anesthesia techniques.

Myths and obstacles to good pain control

No parent or health care provider wishes a child to suffer pain unnecessarily. The pain suffered by children during their illness, regardless of the cause, is a significant source of distress for parents. Why then does there seem to be reluctance to manage pain aggressively? The barriers that health care professionals encounter from both family members and colleagues in aggressively managing pain needs to be highlighted.

For many parents, the words "morphine" or "methadone" conjure up societal, cultural, and familial beliefs that they may or may not discuss with their child's health care team. In qualitative surveys, concerns parents have voiced regarding their reluctance to use opioids for pain control have included [1,3,9,10]:

- Fear of giving up
- Misconceptions of opioids as "too strong for children"
- Fear of side effects
- Worry their child will become "addicted" to pain medications
- Cultural or religious beliefs

In addition to parental hesitation, health care providers have also expressed reluctance to manage pain with opioids. Reasons cited have included [11,12]:

- Lack of sufficient education regarding managing pain
- Misconceptions about frequency and severity of side effects, such as respiratory depression
- Worries that opioids will shorten life expectancy
- Concerns that escalating opioid doses will increase the likelihood of tolerance, and thus make pain control more difficult as the disease progresses

Pathophysiology in brief

To better understand pediatric pain management strategies, it is important to have a basic understanding of the pathophysiology of pain. In general, pain can be broadly divided into categories based on likely pathophysiology. The main categories managed in pediatric palliative care include nocioceptive, visceral, and neuropathic pain.

Nocioceptive pain is used to describe pain that is related to the degree of receptor stimulation by processes causing tissue injury. Peripheral nociceptors are activated by noxious stimuli, which causes impulses to be transmitted to the spinal cord and higher centers within the central nervous system

[13]. Peripheral nociceptors have various response characteristics and can be found in skin, muscle, joints, and some visceral tissues. Nocioception consists of four processes: transduction, transmission, perception, and modulation.

Transduction

The nociceptive process begins with transduction (depolarization) at the peripheral nociceptors in response to noxious stimuli.

Transmission

Transmission is the process by which these stimuli proceed along primary afferent axons via myelinated A-D fibers and nonmylelinted C fibers to the spinal cord, and then on to higher centers in the brain.

Perception

Perception refers to the process when impulses reach higher centers and the individual recognizes pain.

Modulation

A very complex system exists to modulate and inhibit pain perception. This involves mediation by the binding of endogenous opioid compounds to subsets of receptors: mu, delta, and kappa. These endorphins are widely distributed and tied to systems regulating pain and stress. In addition, other neurotransmitters, such as serotonin and norepinephrine, also play a role in the endogenous pain modulating system through structures such as descending inhibiting pathways.

Nocioceptive pain can be further classified as somatic or visceral. Somatic pain is characterized by being well localized and described as aching, squeezing, stabbing, or throbbing. Bone pain caused by cancer metastasis is an example of somatic pain. Pain arising from stimulation of afferent receptors in the viscera is referred to as "visceral" pain. Visceral pain is not evoked from all organs and is not always associated with direct visceral injury. It is characterized as diffuse and poorly localized, and described by patients as dull, crampy, or achy.

Management strategies

The cornerstone to effective pain management in palliative care patients is a repetitive approach involving a detailed assessment of the pain, a patient-specific multimodial treatment plan, and regular, frequent reevaluation. Clinicians managing pain in children benefit from a consistent approach and a set of tools that they use often and can modify based on individual clinical situations. One commonly used approach comes from the World Health Organization (WHO). To address some of the confusion surrounding pain treatment for children, and encourage the use of opioids when necessary, the WHO developed a simple stepwise approach to the management of pain in children with cancer, called the "WHO three-step analgesic ladder" [14–16]. Under the assumption that pain would increase as the child's disease progresses, the goal was to give providers steps to follow to escalate treatment, using progressively stronger analgesics. The first step for the treatment of mild pain uses nonopioid analgesics, such as acetaminophen or nonsteroidal anti-inflammatory drugs (NSAIDs), with our without adjuvant pain medications. For more moderate pain, or pain not relieved with the previous medications, weak opioids, such as codeine or tramadol, are added. For severe pain, strong opioids, such as morphine, oxycodone, hydromorphone, or fentanyl are used. Limitations to the initial WHO approach include its lack of utility in neuropathic pain syndromes, its emphasis on the use of opioids to control pain, and the absence of supportive, behavioral, and cognitive methods for alleviating pain. For this reason, the authors use a slightly modified form of the ladder to eliminate this confusion, as shown in Fig. 1.

In addition to the stepwise approach to medications, the WHO pain management guidelines for children with cancer and children receiving palliative care consists of four concepts: "by the ladder," "by the clock," "by the mouth," and "by the child." The basic premise is that treatment should be escalated according to the WHO three-step analgesic ladder approach outlined above, be administered on a scheduled basis to provide stable blood concentrations with rescue doses as needed, be given by the most appropriate route (which is usually the least invasive most convenient route, such as oral, sublingual, transmucosal, transdermal, or rectal), and be tailored to the individual child's circumstance, needs, and response to treatment.

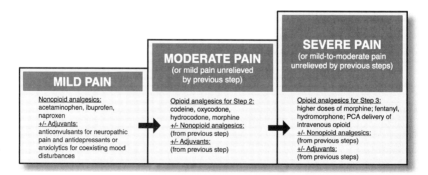

Fig. 1. Three-step analgesic ladder. Based on the World Health Organization "three step ladder" approach to cancer pain management. PCA, patient-controlled analgesia.

Pain assessment in children

The first step in aggressive pain management, regardless of whether the practioner chooses to use the guidelines above, is an accurate age appropriate assessment of the child's pain. This involves obtaining a thorough evaluation, including a detailed assessment and physical exam. Components in a detailed pain assessment are listed in Table 1.

Most hospitals have standard pain assessment tools that are incorporated into daily practice. Behavioral scores for infants, young children, and children who are cognitively impaired are available [17–22]. Examples are listed in Tables 2–4. For older children, self-report scores, such as faces, numerical rating, or visual analog scales are widely used (Fig. 2). When using these scales, it is important to recognize their limitations to interpret their results. Behavioral scales can often incorporate fear or anxiety and make the result difficult to interpret. Self-report scores can be used too literally, where a child's pain is considered severe only if the number reported is greater than a four or five. For some patients, lower numbers may signify severe pain. The authors have found the use of standardized pain assessments extremely valuable in assessing the efficacy of a pain intervention and in heightening the awareness of the health care team in the importance of measuring pain. Lastly, for most children, especially those with life-limiting illnesses, pain is multidimensional. The assessment of emotional,

Table 1
Components of pain assessment in children

Assessment	Components
History of primary illness	Primary disease
	Other potential causes of pain (ie, treatment related, procedures)
Detailed description of pain	Location
	Intensity
	Duration
	Exacerbating factors
	Relieving factors
	Associated symptoms
Experience with pain medications	Current pain medication regimen, including adjuvant medications, doses, interval
	Side effects experiences, currently and in the past, from pain medications
	Patient's perception of efficacy of medication
Integrative (nonpharmacologic) strategies	Relaxation, acupuncture, hypnosis, distraction, parent's touch, etc.
Parent personal experience with pain medications	Open discussion of parental concerns of pain management plan
	Discuss parental bias toward certain medications
Social factors	Which route would be most convenient and culturally appropriate for child and family
Spiritual factors	Influence on medication choice or treatment plan

Table 2
Neonatal pain assessment scale

CRIES	Indicators	Scoring		
		0	1	2
Neonatal postoperative pain	Crying	No	High pitch but consolable	Inconsolable
Score < 4: initiate nonpharmacologic measures	Requires oxygen for Sat >95%	No	<30%	>30%
Score >4: initiate pharmacologic and nonpharmacologic measures	Increased vital signs	No	HR or BP increased <20%	HR or BP increases >20%
	Expression	None	Grimace	Grimace & Grunt
	Sleepless	No	Wakes frequently	Constantly awake

Abbreviations: BP, blood pressure; HR, heart rate.
Data from Krechel SW, Bildner J. CRIES: a new neonatal postoperative pain measurement score. Initial testing of validity and reliability. Pediatric Anesthesia 1995;5:53–61.

psychologic, or spiritual pain is rarely incorporated into standardized pain assessment tools. Practioners caring for these children must be aware of these dimensions of pain and their relationship to the child's physical pain.

The use of opioids

Opioids are the mainstay for pain management in children at the end of life. As discussed above, obstacles from the patient, child, and provider can cause inadequate doses to be used in children [3,11].

Opioids work at many different receptors, including the five opioid receptors: mu, kappa, sigma, delta, and epsilon. Opioids work at the supraspinal and spinal levels and outside the central nervous system. When opioids attach to receptors at the spinal level or in the peripheral nervous system, they modify the transmission of painful signals, diminishing pain perception [23–25]. Each opioid may act at several receptors. At the supraspinal level, opioid receptors send descending inhibitory signals that modify incoming pain signals at the synaptic spinal level. In addition to inhibiting painful signal transmission, opioids work in the limbic system, which alters emotional response to pain. Each opioid has different affinities for different receptors, so patients may have different responses to different opioids with great intraindividual variability (Tables 5–7) [26,27].

Commonly used opioids in palliative care patients

Morphine

Morphine is the most commonly used and well-studied opioid used to treat moderate and severe pain in pediatric palliative care patients. As the

Table 3
Pediatric pain assessment scale for children who have difficulty verbalizing pain

FLACC SCALE
0 = Relaxed/comfortable
1–3 = Mild discomfort
4–6 = Moderate pain
7–10 = Severe pain

	Scoring		
Categories	0	1	2
Face	No particular expression or smile	Occasional grimace or frown, withdrawn, disinterested	Frequent to constant quivering chin, clenched jaw
Legs	Normal position or relaxed	Uneasy, restless, tense	Kicking, or legs drawn up
Activity	Lying quietly, normal position moves easily	Squirming, shifting back and forth, tense	Arched, rigid or jerking
Cry	No cry, (awake or asleep)	Moans or whimpers; occasional complaint	Crying steadily, screams or sobs, frequent complaints
Consolability	Content, relaxed	Reassured by occasional touching, hugging, or being talked to, distractible	Difficulty to console or comfort

From Merkes SI, Voepel-Lewis T, Shayevitz JR, et al. FLACC: a behavioral scale for scoring postoperative pain in young children. Pediatr Nurse 1997;23(3):293–7; used with permission from S. Merkel, MS, RN, T. Voepel-Lewis, MS, RN, and S. Malviya, MD, at C.S. Mott Children's Hospital, University of Michigan Medical Center, Ann Arbor, MI. Copyright © 2002, The Regents of the University of Michigan.

most well studied of the opioids, much is known about its pharmacokinetics and side effects. Studies in pediatric patients have demonstrated both its safety and efficacy [17,28,29]. Morphine is an opioid receptor agonist that binds and activates the μ-opioid receptors in the central nervous system. The activation of these receptors leads to euphoria, sedation, analgesia,

Table 4
Additional pediatric pain assessment scales

Scale	Age	Indicators	Score
CHEOPS (Children's Hospital of Eastern Ontario Pain Scale)	1–7years	Cry, facial expression, verbalization, torso movement, if child touches affectedsite, position of legs	≥4 signifies pain
NIPS (Neonatal/Infants Pain Scale)	Infants <1 year	Facial expression, cry, breathing pattern, arms, legs, and state of arousal are observed for 1-min intervals before, during, and after a procedure	>3 indicates pain

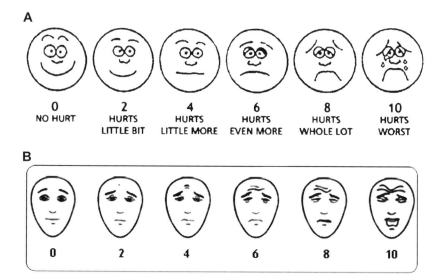

Fig. 2. Examples of visual analog scales to assess pain in pediatric patients 3 to 4 years and older. (*A*) Wong-Baker faces pain rating scale (*From* Hockenberry MJ, Wilson D, Winkelstein ML. Wong's essentials of pediatric nursing. 7th edition. St. Louis: Mosby; 2005. p. 125; used with permission. Copyright Mosby.) (*B*) The faces pain scale—revised (*From* Hicks CL, von Baeyer CL, Spafford P, et al. The Faces Pain scale—revised: Toward a common metric in pediatric pain measurement. Pain 2001;93:176; with permission.)

physical dependence, and respiratory depression. Almost all morphine is converted by hepatic metabolism to the 3- and 6-glucuronide metabolites (M3G and M6G). M6G has been shown to have a much stronger analgesic activity but crosses the blood-brain barrier poorly, while M3G has no significant analgesic activity [30,31]. Elevated concentrations of M3G as well as M3G/M6G ratios may play a role in hyperalgesia, allodynia, and myoclonus [32,33]. In patients who develop these side effects, it may be beneficial to switch to a structurally dissimilar opioid, such as methadone or fentanyl, to allow M3G to clear from the cerebral spinal fluid. Morphine can be given orally, sublingually, subcutaneously, intravenously, rectally, intrathecally, or via an epidural. The oral form comes in both an immediate release and sustained release preparation. It is important to remember that there is an increased half-life and diminished clearance in neonates that can produce a higher risk of respiratory depression. Thus the dose and dose intervals should be modified and titrated appropriately.

Hydromorphone

Hydromorphone has very similar properties to morphine. It is given in the same routes, although a long acting form is currently not available in the United States. Hydromorphone is more lipid soluble and more potent than morphine, but it is unclear what practical advantages exist. Adult

Table 5
Metabolism of common opioids

Opioid	Metabolism	Metabolites	Elimination route	Comments
Codeine	Cytochrome P-450 2D6[a]	Codeine-6-glucuronide Norcodeine Morphine (<10% -may account for analgesic properties of codeine)	Renal	Oral bioavailibilty 15%–80%; slow-metabolizers don't produce the active metabolite morphine
Morphine		Morphine-3-glucuronide (55%–75%); acts as a neuroexcitatory agent; contributes to adverse morphine effects such as myoclonus and confusion Morphine-6-glucuronide (5%–15%); exhibits opioid activity; up to 40 times more potent than morphine	Renal	Metabolites have a very extended half life in patients with renal failure
Hydromorphone	Cytochrome P-450 2D6[a]	Hydromorphone-3-glucuronide	Renal	Literature states no opioid active metabolite; however anecdotal evidence of increased neurotoxicity or renal failure with very high doses
Oxycodone	Cytochrome P-450 3A4 Cytochrome P-450 2D6[a]	Noroxycodone—major metabolite; weak mu agonist Oxymorphone (minor metabolite with marked opioid activity) Noroxymorphone	Renal, hepatic	Unlike codeine oxycodone is a potent analgesic itself
Fentanyl	Cytochrome P-450 3A4	Norfentanyl—inactive	Renal, hepatic	No active metabolites

[a] Metabolism affected by genetic polymorphisms in CYP 2D6 and drug interactions. It is estimated that 5% to 10% of Caucasians are CYP2D6 poor metabolizers.

Data from Refs. [26,27,24].

Table 6
Equianalgesic narcotic dosing

Medication	Parenteral dose (mg)	Oral or rectal dose (mg)
Codeine	120	200
Fentanyl	([a])	N/A
Hydrocodone	N/A	3
Morphine	10	30
Hydromorphone	1.5–2	6–8
Oxycodone	N/A	15–20
Methadone	10 mg	10 mg–20 mg

Converting patients from one opioid to methadone requires close observation for delayed sedation, which may occur 3 to 5 days following the initiation of the drug. Dose intervals need to be decreased after the initial 1 to 2 days of treatment to avoid late sedation.

[a] A child must be tolerant to 30 mg–60 mg per 24 hours oral morphine equivalent to be rotated to the smallest Fentanyl patch (12.5 mcg/hr). Conversion from oral morphine per drug supplier: 25 μg/h (oral morphine 30 mg/day–135 mg/day) 50 μg/h (135 mg/day–224 mg/day) 75 μg/h (225 mg/day–314 mg/day) 100 μg/h (315 mg/day–404 mg/day).

studies have not shown clear benefit over the use of morphine. It is metabolized in the liver by cytochrome P450 2D6 [34]. There have been some studies describing the drug's pharmacokinetics and metabolism in children [35,36]. It is advertised not to have any active opioid metabolites, which would improve its safety in patients with renal failure [37]. However, hydromorphone-3-glucoronide is a detectable metabolite and there is anecdotal evidence, including the authors' experience, that there is an increased neurotoxicity and incidence of jerking on high doses, especially in children with compromised renal function. Fentanyl or methadone are likely to be better choices in children with renal failure.

Fentanyl

Fentanyl is highly lipophilic and 80 to 100 times more potent than morphine in adults, less so in younger children (in neonates 13–20 times as potent). It is the only opioid available in a transdermal preparation in the United States, which makes it very useful in the palliative care patients who cannot take oral medications. Fentanyl has a shorter onset of action and shorter duration of action than morphine [38]. This has made the drug useful in conscious sedation for procedures in pediatric patients [39]. According to small studies, the pharmacokinetic parameters are similar in children as for adults [40,41]. The isoenzyme cytocrome P_{450} 3A4 (CYP 3A4) metabolises fentanyl in the liver and intestinal mucosa into the pharmacologic inactive metabolite norfentanyl, which is then eliminated by the kidney. Potent inhibitors of CYP 3A4, such as macrolide antibiotics (eg, erythromycin), certain protease inhibitors (eg, ritonavir), antimycotics (eg, ketoconacole), and grapefruit juice may decrease the systemic clearence of fentanyl, which may result in increased or prolonged opioid effects. When compared with other opioids, fentanyl is a relatively safe drug and adverse reactions are typical of the opioid group of drugs [42]. All patients receiving fentanyl must be monitored for respiratory depression, which may initially manifest as somnolence. Clinically significant respiratory depression can be antagonised with naloxone. Circulatory depression, hypotension, and shock seem to be caused less often by intravenous fentanyl than by other opioids. Thoracic rigidity may follow a rapid bolus of high dose intravenous fentanyl (greater than 5 mg/kg–15 mg/kg). This can be treated with naloxone, but may require a muscle relaxant.

It is also important to note that when using fentanyl as an infusion, tolerance may develop more quickly than with other opioids. Limitations of this medication include that the transdermal patch comes in set increments, which makes titration difficult. Routes of application include intranasal, intravenous, subcutaneous, sublingual, oral transmucosal, and transdermal.

Fentanyl patches must not be introduced as the first opioid in the treatment of pain and it cannot be used to manage the pain of opioid-naïve children. Because of a long onset time, inability to rapidly titrate drug delivery and long elimination half-life, transdermal fentanyl is contraindicated for acute pain management. It is better used for chronic, stable pain in the setting of an opioid rotation or finding an alternative route of administration.

Oxycodone

Oxycodone has similar properties to morphine. The pharmacokinetics of oral oxycodone differs from oral morphine in that it has a higher bioavailability, a slightly longer half-life, and is hepatically metabolized by cytochrome P450 to both active and inactive metabolites [25,43–45]. Noroxycodone is the major metabolite but has much weaker activity than oxycodone. The other significant metabolite, oxymorphone, is present in much smaller amounts but has potent opioid properties. Oxycodone is a mu and kappa opioid receptor agonist and its analgesia is characterized by a rapid onset of action without an analgesic ceiling. The relative potency of oral oxycodone is between 1.5 and two times that of oral morphine. Its doses can be escalated to effect even to very high doses. It has been shown that in children, clearance of the drug is up to 50% higher with a lower volume of distribution [46]. It comes in both an immediate release and sustained release formulation. There have been no significant safety studies in pediatrics using the extended release formulation. In addition, it is available both with and without acetaminophen.

Codeine

Codeine is often listed as a weak opioid. It is metabolized in the liver to morphine. However, it has been shown in recent literature that conversion

Table 7
Initial doses for common opioids

Drug	Routes	Oral dose	Parenteral dose	Infusion starting doses	Dosage forms
Codeine	PO	0.5 mg/kg–1 mg/kg codeine q 4–6 h (watch for acetaminophen doses to avoid toxicity)	N/A	N/A	Soln: 3 mg/mL Tabs: 15 mg, 30 mg
Fentanyl	IV Transdermal SQ Buccal Intranasal	N/A	0.5 mcg/kg–1 mcg/kg q 15–30 minutes	Init: 1 mcg/kg Basal: 0.5 mcg/kg/hour–1.5 mcg/kg/hr	Patches: 12.5 mcg/h, 25 mcg/h, 50 mcg/h, 75 mcg/h, 100 mcg/h
Hydromorphone	PO IV SQ SL	0.03 mg/kg/dose–0.06 mg/kg/dose q 3–4 hr (>50 kg: 1 mg–2 mg q 3–4 hr)	0.015 mg/kg/dose q 3–4 hr >50 kg: 1–1.5 mg/dose q3–4 hr	Init: 0.003 mg/kg/dose Basal:0.003 mg/kg/hr–0.005 mg/kg/hr	Inj: 2 mg/mL Tab: 2 mg, 4 mg, 8 mg
Morphine	PO SL PR SQ IV	Oral (Immediate release) >6mos: 0.15 mg/kg/dose–0.3 mg/kg/dose q 3–4 hr >50 kg: 10 mg–15 mg q 3–4 hr	0.05 mg/kg/dose–0.1 mg/kg/dose q3–4 hr >50 kg: 2.5 mg/dose–5 mg/dose q 2–4 hr	Init: 0.01 mg/kg/dose–0.02 mg/kg/dose Basal: 0.01 mg/kg/hr–0.03 mg/kg/hr	IV: 2 mg/mL, 15 mg/mL Tabs (IR): 15 mg Tabs (SR): 15 mg, 30 mg, 60 mg, 100 mg Soln: 10 mg/5 mL, 20 mg/mL

Oxycodone	PO SL	0.1 mg/kg–0.2 mg/kg q 4 h Adults: 5 mg –10 mg q 4 h	N/A	N/A	Soln: 1 mg/mL, 20 mg/mL: solution contains latex Tabs: 5 mg, 15 mg, 30 mg Capsule: immediate release: 5 mg Tablet, CR (OxyContin): 10 mg, 20 mg, 40 mg, 80 mg, 160 mg
Tramadol	PO	1–2 mg/dose q4 h; max. of 8 mg/kg/day (>50 kg max 400 mg/day)	N/A	N/A	Tabs: 50 mg, 100 mg (can be compounded to liquid)

Note that these merely represent starting doses, which need to be titrated to effect. Some children will require significantly larger doses to experience good pain control.

from codeine to the active analgesic form of morphine is suboptimal in the pediatric population and more than 10% of the white Caucasian population are slow metabolizers for the cytochrome P450 2D6, hence are unable to metabolize the prodrug codeine to morphine. This makes its use in the palliative care population, who often have moderate to severe pain, problematic [25,47]. Codein comes only with acetaminophen in the United States and is available in both liquid and pill forms. Its benefit is that it is widely available and most practioners and parents are familiar with the medication.

Methadone

Methadone is a unique long acting opioid that is a racemic mixture of two isomers. One acts primarily as a mu opioid and the other as an antagonist at the N-methyl-aspartate receptor in the brain, spinal cord, and peripheral nerves. It has a high oral bioavailability with slow metabolism in the liver [25,47–51]. Metabolites are inactive. It has a long and sometimes unpredictable half life ranging from 12 hours to almost 200 hours. To complicate things further, the duration of analgesia is much shorter than the half life, which requires dosing to be more frequent initially. This can cause delayed sedation and potentially life threatening respiratory depression. Because it comes in a liquid formulation, methadone can be used as an extended pain medication for children unable to swallow pills. However, it should be noted that little data is available regarding the pharmacokinetics in young children and infants [52,53]. In addition, conversion from standard opioids is highly dependent on the individual patient's metabolism and tolerance. The authors have found this medication extremely useful in the pediatric palliative care population when used cautiously. As mentioned below, it can be used in the management of neuropathic pain.

Managing opioid side effects

Opioids generally have a similar side effect profile. Side effects are common and, if left untreated, can greatly impact on the patient's quality of life [54–56]. It is important to be aware of the common opioid side effects and treat them aggressively [23,33,55,57]. Table 8 lists common side effects as well as management suggestions.

Adjuvant medications

Adjuvant pain medications are medications whose primary indication is not to treat pain, but that may have analgesic properties in specific circumstances. In the pediatric palliative care population, there have been few controlled trials showing significant efficacy. Most practitioners who use adjuvant regimens use anecdotal data or extrapolate from the adult studies. The most commonly used adjuvant medications include those used to treat

Table 8
Common opioid side effects

Side effect	Management	Notes
Constipation	• Prophylaxic stool softener (eg. lactulose) • Stimulant laxative • Low-dose naaloxone	• Almost universal • Should start prophylactically
Nausea/vomiting	• Opioid rotation • 5-HT3 receptor antagonist (Phenothiazine) • D2-Receptor Antagonists (eg. Metoclopramide, Haloperidol) • Antihistamins (Diphenhydramine, Cyclizine,	• Caused by activity at opioid receptors in the chemoreceptor trigger zone. Can decrease after 3–7 days
Pruritis	• Diphenhydramine • Hydroxizine • Opioid rotation	
Fatigue	• Opioid rotatation; if unsuccessful: psychostimulant trial	• Can decrease after 3–7 days
Confusion	• Opioid rotation • Or Consider trial of dose reduction	• Increased with renal or hepatic impairment
Myoclonus	• Opioid rotation • Benzodiazepine • Muscle relaxant	• Usually occurs in patients on high dose opioids because of the accumulation of neurotoxic metabolites.
Urinary retention	• Opioid rotation • External bladder pressure • bethanacol	• Anecdotally less common with fentanyl • Use of opioid mixed receptor agonist/antagonist such as nalbuphine may cause opioide withdrawal in children
Respiratory depression	• Opioid rotation, if poor pain control • Decrease dose interval of opioid, if good pain control • Oxygen • Repositioning • Use opioid receptor antagonists with caution	• Much less frequent than commonly thought • Can be more common in neonates due to longer opioid half life caused by immature enzyme systems

neuropathic pain and those used for specific disease related pain. Medications specifically for neuropathic pain are described in a later section. Disease related pain includes bone pain secondary to tumor metastasis, fracture, primary bone defects, bowel spasm from obstruction, or muscle pain from neurodegenerative disease, or other chronic diseases, such as cerebral palsy. Tables 9 and 10 [58] show examples of adjuvant pain regimens and dosing strategies for these conditions.

Management of neuropathic pain

The incidence and prevalence of neuropathic pain at the end-of-life of children is unclear, but in the authors' experience the majority of children or teenagers with cancer or neurodenegrative conditions suffer from this debilitating pain entity. Managing neuropathic pain in pediatric palliative care will likely require an interdisciplinary, holistic approach. This type of pain, not nociceptive in nature, and nonprotective, persists independent of ongoing tissue injury or inflammation. Verbal children may describe the quality of neuropathic pain as burning, shooting, or stabbing, but we are often entranced by the complexity of the child's own descriptors. It is of utmost importance to differentiate the different pain entities during pain assessment, as nociceptive, neuropathic, visceral, or spiritual pain may be scored by the child quite differently and needs to be treated individually as such. The authors suggest the following approach in managing neuropathic pain in children, which includes evaluation and the treatment of underlying causes through pharmacologic and nonphrmacologic approaches.

Evaluation

After a complete history has been taken, a child needs to be examined thoroughly, which includes a complete neurological examination. Clinical findings may include hyperalgesia, allodynia and cutaneous hypersthesia, motor dysfunction such as spasms, dystonia and fasciculations, and autonomic changes, such as cyanosis, hyperhidrosis, or swelling [59].

Treatment of underlying causes

Evaluate whether an underlying cause may be treatable in accordance with the treatment goals of the patient and his or her family. Underlying pathologies causing neuropathic pain may include neurodegenerative

Table 9
The use of adjuvant pain medications

Disease related pain	Adjuvant pain treatments
Bone pain	Bisphosphonate, calcitonin, steroids, radiotherapy
Bowel spasm	Octreotide, antichoinergic
Muscle pain	Benzodiazepine, Botulinum toxin A, baclofen

Table 10
Analgesia and adjuvant analgesia for managing neuropathic pain in children

Drug	Starting dose < 50 kg	Starting dose > 50 kg	Comments
Amitriptyline	0.2 mg/kg po once at night; titrated to a maximum of 1 mg/kg/day–2 mg/kg/day over 2–3 weeks	10 mg po once at night; titrated to a maximum of 50 mg/day–100 mg/day over 2–3 weeks	Majority of our patients remain at a dose < 0.5 mg/kg/day po
Gabapentin	2 mg/kg/dose–5 mg/kg/dose po qhs, then bid, then tid. increase over 2–4 weeks; maximum 10 mg/kg–20 mg/kg tid	100–300 mg po qhs, then bid, then tid. Increase over 2–4 weeks; maximum 600 mg–1200 mg po tid	Slow dose escalation may decrease onset of adverse effects
Ketamine (low-dose)	0.04 mg/kg/hr–0.15 mg/kg/hr IV/SC (titrated to effect: usually maximum 0.3 mg/kg/hr–0.6 mg/kg/hr)	2 mg/hr–5 mg/hr IV/SC; (titrated to effect in 2 mg/hr–4 mg/hr escalations every 24 hours)	Rectal, transmucosal, intranasal and transdermal application described [58]
	0.2 mg/kg/dose–0.4 mg/kg/dose po tid–quid and prn	10 mg–25 mg tid–quid and prn, increase dose in steps of 10 mg–25 mg up to 50 mg qid	
Tramadol	1 mg/kg–2 mg/kg q4–6 h (max. of 8 mg/kg/day)	50 mg–100 mg q4–6 h (max of 400 mg/day)	Opioid for mild to moderate pain with ceiling effect

conditions, raised intracranial pressure, postsurgical peripheral neuropathic pain, phantom limp pain, neuroirritabilty, and metabolic neuropathies. Children with malignancies may experience neuropathic pain caused by all aspects of tumor therapy (such as vinca-alkaloid induced neuropathy) and the tumor itself. Neuropathic pain caused by primary tumor or metastases involvement of the central or peripheral nervous system may respond to radiation, bisphosphonates for bone lesions, corticosteroids, palliative chemotherapy, or surgery. Anxiety, depression, and spiritual pain in the child and his caregivers need to be assessed and addressed.

Integrative, nonpharmacologic treatment modalities

State of the art pain management in the 21st century demands that pharmacologic management must be combined with supportive measures and integrative, nonpharmacologic treatment modalities. Physical methods include a cuddle or hug from the family, massage, transcutaneous electrical nerve stimulation, comfort positioning, heat, cold, and especially physical or occupational therapy, as well as rehabilitation. Cognitive behavioral techniques include guided imagery, hypnosis, abdominal breathing, distraction, story telling. Acupressure or acupuncture may be very helpful. An agreed upon plan of passive, and if possible, active coping skills, needs to be implemented considering the child's wishes and those of his or her family.

Pharmacologic approaches

There are no published randomized controlled trials (RCT) about the management of neuropathic pain in children, let alone in pediatric palliative care. A review of adult RCTs regarding drug approaches to neuropathic pain revealed that with a number-needed to treat (NNT) of 2.5, strong opioids (after carbamazepine – NNT 2.0) have the best evidence of efficacy. The NNT for tricyclic antidepressants was 3.1, lidocaine patch 4.4, gabapentin 4.7, and selective serotonine reuptake inhibitors 6.8 [60]. Traditional teaching that neuropathic pain is unresponsive to opioids cannot be upheld. In the authors' experience, the majority of children with life-limiting conditions experience a significant improvement of their neuropathic pain following the application of opioids.

Opioids

Opioids have become one of the mainstays of therapy in the pediatric management of neuropathic pain at end-of-life care. This is especially true if the pain is caused by tumor invasion of the spine, when doses of more than 1,000-mg intravenous morphine per hour may be required to achieve satisfactory pain control. Reported maximum morphine doses range between 73.9 mg/kg to 518 mg/kg per hour in pediatric palliative care [61–63]. If a dose escalation of morphine does not provide adequate pain control, or causes intolerable adverse effects, one should consider an opioid rotation (eg, to fentanyl, hydromorphone, or oxycodone on equianalgesic doses). Methadone is an opioid particularly useful in the management of neuropathic pain, with its combined activity as mu-receptor agonist and an N-methyl-D-aspertate (NMDA)-receptor antagonist.

Tramadol

The authors see a number of children with mitochondrial dysfunction and other degenerative conditions, who seem to experience prolonged episodes of inconsolability, which persist despite a thorough workup and initial management with simple analgesia, benzodiazepines, chloral hydrate, or anticonvulsants. In this subgroup we found the use of tramadol particularly helpful. This weak opioid (a synthetic 4-phenyl-piperidine analog of codeine) has a ceiling effect and a very good safety profile regarding respiratory depression. It is not only a weak mu-receptor antagonist, but also a serotonin and norepinephrine reuptake inhibitor and likely an alpha-2 agonist. This complementary action yields some theoretical benefit in the management of neuropathic and nociceptive pain. However, Finnerup and colleagues [60] rated tramadol in the above cited review merely with a NNT of 3.9.

N-methyl-D-aspertate-receptor antagonists

Strong pain stimuli activate NMDA receptors and produce hyper excit-ability of dorsal root neurons. This induces central sensitization, wind-up phenomenon, and pain memory. NMDA-receptor antagonist may be able to prevent the induction of central sensitizations caused by stimulation of peripheral nociception, as well as block the wind-up phenomenon.

Ketamine

Ketamine is an NMDA-receptor antagonist, but has other actions which may also contribute to its analgesic effect, including a mu-, delta-, and kappa-opioid like effect, interactions with calcium and sodium channels, cholinergic transmission, and noradrenergic and serotonergic reuptake inhi-bition (the latter ensuring intact descending inhibitory pathways necessary for analgesia). Evidence to guide its use at subanesthetic doses is limited and in part contradictory [64]. Pediatric experience has shown that ketamine is effective for the treatment of postoperative and nonsurgical acute nocicep-tive pain, as well as for neuropathic pain in low, subanesthetic doses, both alone or in combination with opioids [65–70]. Ketamine is unique among anesthetic agents in that it does not depress respiratory and cardiovascular systems. In subanesthetic (analgesic) doses, the typical anesthetic-dose side effects of ketamine, including nystagmus, lacrimation, salivation, tachycar-dia, and spontaneous movements are usually absent, and the patient can re-spond and interact coherently. Also, the vivid and oftentimes disturbing dreams and hallucinations are avoided. The clinical spectrum and variability with ketamine is much greater than with most other analgesics. Addition-ally, while some patients may tolerate enormous doses of the drug with an-algesic effect and no systemic side effects, others may have unacceptable side effects at a very low dose before experiencing any analgesic effect.

A large adult meta-analysis of 2,385 patients found that adverse effects were not increased with low-dose ketamine [51]. However, until there is bet-ter pediatric data, children should be watched for hypertension, tachycardia, euphoria or dysphoria, and hallucinations. Although one pediatric study could not appreciate an opioid sparing effect of ketamine, there is anecdotal evidence of significant opioid reductions in end-of-life pediatric cancer care with children on high doses of opioids after the initiation of ketamine [71].

The advantage of ketamine in comparison to other frequently used adju-vant analgesia, such as anticonvulsants or antidepressants, is its rather im-mediate onset of action [72].

Other N-methyl-D-aspertate-receptor antagonists

Methadone, as mentioned above, is an example of another NMDA-receptor antagonist (and mu-receptor agonist) frequently used in pediatric palliative care. Methadone's routes of application include intravenous, oral, subcutaneous, sublingual, and rectal. Other NMDA-receptor antagonists, such as dextromethorphan, amantadine, and mematine are not commonly used in pediatrics.

Tricyclic antidepressants

Tricyclic antidepressants have shown to be effective in the management of neuropathic pain in adults [73]. No pediatric RCTs were published yet. Tricyclic antidepressants exert their analgesic effects by blocking the presynaptic reuptake of serotonin and norepinephrine, thereby modulating the descending inhibiting pathways. They may also act as NMDA-receptor antagonists.

Common anticholinergic side effects include sedation (hence, to be give once at night), dry mouth, blurry vision, constipation, and urinary retention. Patients should receive an EKG before initiation of therapy to rule out QT-prolonging, Wolfe-Parkinsone-White-Syndrome, or other pre-existing rhythm disturbances, as tricyclic antidepressants may bear dysrhythmic qualities. Sudden discontinuation should be avoided.

Amitriptyline

Amitriptyline is among the oldest and most commonly used adjuvant analgesic for neuropathic pain in children, although the pediatric evidence is limited [74–77]. The authors use amitriptyline as the first-line tricyclic adjuvant analgesia for neuropathic pain. The sedating effect manifests immediately, which often proves helpful as sleeping through the night is a common problem among this pediatric patient group. The analgesic effect may commence to occur 3 to 7 days after initiation, occasionally even later. If distressing anticholinergic side effects occur, the authors usually reduce the dose by 50% and increase the dose slowly again over several days to weeks.

Other tricyclic antidepressants

Several major pediatric centers prefer nortriptyline (alternative: imipramine) with the notion that they may cause fewer anticholinergic side effects than amitriptyline. Desipramine, a secondary amine, may be considered an alternative, if small doses of the tertiary amines amitriptyline, nortriptyline, or imipramine cause over-sedation.

Anticonvulsants

Gabapentin

Gabapentin is commonly used in pediatric pain management. There are no RCTs and few case reports [78–85]. The exact mechanism of action is unclear, but it acts as a calcium-channel blocker, increases gamma-aminobutyric acid (GABA) synthesis and GABA release. Clinical pediatric experience seems to indicate, that gabapentin and amitriptyline are similar in efficacy. In our center, the authors use it second line to amitriptyline (or in combination). Reasons include its application three times per day, as compared with the tricyclic dose once per night, an (adult) NNT of 4.7, worse than those of tricyclic antidepressants (NNT of 3.1), and not infrequent incidence of side effects, such as nystagmus, thought disorder, hallucinations, headache, weight gain, and myalgia among the patient population.

To avoid pain or precipitating seizures, this anticonvulsant should be weaned off over one to two weeks.

Other anticonvulsants

Data to supporting the efficacy of other anticonvulsants in the management of pediatric neuropathic pain is less robust. Sodium channel modulators, such as carbamazepine, oxcarbazepine, phenobarbital, phenytoin, topimarate, lamotrigene, and valproic acid act as modulators of peripheral sensitization. Calcium-channel blockers, apart from gabapentin, include lamotrigene and oxcarbazepine, and inhibit central sensitization. There is no pediatric data on pregabaline.

Other pharmacological approaches

Lidocaine patch

The lidocaine 5% patch is effective in the management of adult neuropathic pain, including postherpetic neuralgia, painful diabetic neuropathy, painful idiopathic sensory polyneuropathy, and nonpostherpetic peripheral neuropathies (as well as osteoarthritis and lower back pain) [86–93]. There are no pediatric RCTs. The authors found the lidocaine patch useful in selected children.

Propofol

The authors have positive experiences in pediatric palliative care using the general anesthetic propofol in subanesthetic doses (starting dose 0.3 mg/kg–1 mg/kg per hour) for managing refractory (neuropathic) cancer pain in children [94].

Neurourgical interventions and nerve blocks

A small subgroup of children at the end-of-life may require invasive procedures, such as regional anesthesia (epidural or subarachnoid intrathecal infusions) with opioids, local anesthetics, or the alpha-2-agonist clonidine. Frequently, these agents are administered via an implantable catheter, alleviating the necessity of repeated punctures [95]. Rare interventions, such as implantable drug delivery systems, intraventricular morphine, or percutaneous cervical cordotomy may be considered, if pain is intractable using opioids, adjuvant analgesia, and integrative treatment modalities.

Nonpharmcologic pain management strategies

It is clear that pain in children is complex and modified based on the child's developmental level, temperament, previous experiences with pain,

Table 11
Nonpharmacological approaches to pediatric pain management

Age	Pain behaviors	Cognitive-behavioral approaches	Complementary therapies
Infants	• Avoiding eye contact • Grimacing • Difficulty sucking • High-pitched crying • Quivering chin • Difficulty calming • Wanting to be still • and ↑ hiccupping • and ↑or ↓ breathing	Use pacifier Swaddling Touch Distraction Music	Massage Sucrose solution Aromatherapy
Toddlers	• Difficulty in sleeping • Lose interest in play • and ↑ crying • and ↑ irritability • and ↑ restlessness • and ↓ eating or drinking	Story telling Blowing bubbles Toys Distraction Art & music therapy	Massage Warm/cool compress aromatherapy
Preschool	• Difficulty sleeping • Lose interest in play • Quiet or curled • Need to be held • Says something hurts • ↓ eating or drinking	Distraction (cartoons) Offer favorite toy/object to hold Art & music therapy	Massage Reiki Emotive imagery Warm/cool compress aromatherapy

School-age	• Difficulty sleeping • Moaning/crying • Hold or protect area of discomfort • Lose interest in play • Decrease activity level • ↓ eating or drinking	Create a safe environment Dim lights, decrease noise, approach using a calm manner Power of suggestion Counting Art & music therapy Breathing techniques Visualization/guided imagery	Massage Reiki Progressive muscle relaxation Warm/cool compress Hypnosis (> 10 y) Acupuncture (> 10 y) Aromatherapy Yoga/meditation/reflexology
Adolescent	• Increasingly quiet • Lose interest in friends and family • Decrease activity level • ↑ anger or irritability • Changes in eating habits	Create a safe environment Dim lights, decrease noise, approach using a calm manner Distraction TV, video game, read a book, music Art & music therapy Breathing techniques Visualization/guided imagery	Massage Reiki Warm/cool compress Hypnosis Acupuncture Aromatherapy Yoga/meditation/reflexology

anxiety, and other sources of distress, both physical, emotional, and spiritual. The use of nonpharacologic interventions in pain management strategies is crucial. Simple techniques, such as distraction and environmental changes, along with more complex cognitive behavioral therapies can be invaluable [96–99]. Table 11 lists examples of nonpharmacologic pain management strategies based on a child's age [98,100,101].

Summary

The management of pain in children with life-limiting illnesses is complex and, unfortunately, often not done effectively yet. Pain is a multidimensional symptom that can overshadow all other experiences of both the child and family. Frequent pain assessments and flexible treatment plans are essential. Further studies to better understand the safety, pharmacology, and effectiveness of medications used to treat pain in children is necessary. In addition, further exploration into the assessment and management of the emotional and spiritual components of pain needs to be done in this population. The authors believe that with an aggressive, consistent, and knowledgeable approach, pain suffered by children with life-limiting illnesses, regardless of etiology, can be treated effectively.

Acknowledgments

We would like to thank Gina Santucci, MSN, FNP, Faith Kim, and Somaly Srey for their assistance with the development of this article.

References

[1] Albano EA, Odom LF. Supportive care in pediatric oncology. Curr Opin Pediatr 1993;5: 131.
[2] Contro N, Larson J, Scofield S, et al. Family perspectives on the quality of pediatric palliative care. Arch Pediatr Adolesc Med 2002;156:14.
[3] Drake R, Frost J, Collins JJ. The symptoms of dying children. J Pain Symptom Manage 2003;26:594.
[4] Goldman A, Hewitt M, Collins GS, et al. Symptoms in children/young people with progressive malignant disease: United Kingdom Children's Cancer Study Group/Paediatric Oncology Nurses Forum survey. Pediatrics 2006;117:e1179.
[5] Jalmsell L, Kreicbergs U, Onelov E, et al. Symptoms affecting children with malignancies during the last month of life: a nationwide follow-up. Pediatrics 2006;117:1314.
[6] Wolfe J, Grier HE, Klar N, et al. Symptoms and suffering at the end of life in children with cancer. N Engl J Med 2000;342:326.
[7] Carter BS, Howenstein M, Gilmer MJ, et al. Circumstances surrounding the deaths of hospitalized children: opportunities for pediatric palliative care. Pediatrics 2004;114:e361.
[8] Schechter NL. The undertreatment of pain in children: an overview. Pediatr Clin North Am 1989;36:781.

[9] Brown RE Jr, Schmitz ML, Andelman PD. The treatment of pain in children. J Ark Med Soc 1993;90:112.

[10] Mack JW, Hilden JM, Watterson J, et al. Parent and physician perspectives on quality of care at the end of life in children with cancer. J Clin Oncol 2005;23:9155.

[11] Ellis JA, McCarthy P, Hershon L, et al. Pain practices: a cross-Canada survey of pediatric oncology centers. J Pediatr Oncol Nurs 2003;20:26.

[12] Hilden JM, Emanuel EJ, Fairclough DL, et al. Attitudes and practices among pediatric oncologists regarding end-of-life care: results of the 1998 American Society of Clinical Oncology survey. J Clin Oncol 2001;19:205.

[13] Fausett H. Anatomy and physiology of pain. In: Carol A, Warfield ZHB, editors. Principles and practice of pain medicine. 2nd edition. New York: McGraw Hill; 2004. p. 28.

[14] McGrath PA. Development of the World Health Organization Guidelines on cancer pain relief and palliative care in children. J Pain Symptom Manage 1996;12:87.

[15] Ventafridda V, Saita L, Ripamonti C, et al. WHO guidelines for the use of analgesics in cancer pain. Int J Tissue React 1985;7:93.

[16] Zech DF, Grond S, Lynch J, et al. Validation of World Health Organization guidelines for cancer pain relief: a 10-year prospective study. Pain 1995;63:65.

[17] Babul N, Darke AC. Evaluation and use of opioid analgesics in pediatric cancer pain. J Palliat Care 1993;9:19.

[18] Caraceni A, Cherny N, Fainsinger R, et al. Pain measurement tools and methods in clinical research in palliative care: recommendations of an Expert Working Group of the European Association of Palliative Care. J Pain Symptom Manage 2002;23:239.

[19] Clark JL, Kalan GE. Effective treatment of severe cancer pain of the head using low-dose ketamine in an opioid-tolerant patient. J Pain Symptom Manage 1995;10:310.

[20] Ducharme J. Acute pain and pain control: state of the art. Ann Emerg Med 2000;35:592.

[21] Franck LS, Greenberg CS, Stevens B. Pain assessment in infants and children. Pediatr Clin North Am 2000;47:487.

[22] Greco C, Berde C. Pain management for the hospitalized pediatric patient. Pediatr Clin North Am 2005;52:995.

[23] Choi YS, Billings JA. Opioid antagonists: a review of their role in palliative care, focusing on use in opioid-related constipation. J Pain Symptom Manage 2002;24:71.

[24] Inturrisi CE. Clinical pharmacology of opioids for pain. Clin J Pain 2002;18:S3.

[25] Zichterman A. Opioid pharmacology and considerations in pain management. In: Pharmacist U; 2007. Available at: https://www.uspharmacist.com/index.asp?page=ce/105473/default.htm. Accessed September 17, 2007.

[26] Armstrong SC, Cozza KL. Pharmacokinetic drug interactions of morphine, codeine, and their derivatives: theory and clinical reality, Part II. Psychosomatics 2003;44:515.

[27] Cohen S. Pathophysiology of pain. In: Warfield C, Bajwa Z, editors. Principles and practices of pain medicine. 2nd edition. New York: McGraw-Hill; 2004.

[28] Dampier CD, Setty BN, Logan J, et al. Intravenous morphine pharmacokinetics in pediatric patients with sickle cell disease. J Pediatr 1995;126:461.

[29] Koren G, Maurice L. Pediatric uses of opioids. Pediatr Clin North Am 1989;36:1141.

[30] Hunt A, Joel S, Dick G, et al. Population pharmacokinetics of oral morphine and its glucuronides in children receiving morphine as immediate-release liquid or sustained-release tablets for cancer pain. J Pediatr 1999;135:47.

[31] Hunt R, Fazekas B, Thorne D, et al. A comparison of subcutaneous morphine and fentanyl in hospice cancer patients. J Pain Symptom Manage 1999;18:111.

[32] Lugo RA, Kern SE. Clinical pharmacokinetics of morphine. J Pain Palliat Care Pharmacother 2002;16:5.

[33] Smith MT. Neuroexcitatory effects of morphine and hydromorphone: evidence implicating the 3-glucuronide metabolites. Clin Exp Pharmacol Physiol 2000;27:524.

[34] Chang SF, Moore L, Chien YW. Pharmacokinetics and bioavailability of hydromorphone: effect of various routes of administration. Pharm Res 1988;5:718.

[35] Babul N, Darke AC, Hagen N. Hydromorphone metabolite accumulation in renal failure. J Pain Symptom Manage 1995;10:184.

[36] Babul N, Darke AC, Hain R. Hydromorphone and metabolite pharmacokinetics in children. J Pain Symptom Manage 1995;10:335.

[37] Dean M. Opioids in renal failure and dialysis patients. J Pain Symptom Manage 2004;28: 497.

[38] Doyle L, Colletti JE. Pediatric procedural sedation and analgesia. Pediatr Clin North Am 2006;53:279.

[39] Noyes M, Irving H. The use of transdermal fentanyl in pediatric oncology palliative care. Am J Hosp Palliat Care 2001;18:411.

[40] Collins C, Koren G, Crean P, et al. Fentanyl pharmacokinetics and hemodynamic effects in preterm infants during ligation of patent ductus arteriosus. Anesth Analg 1985;64: 1078.

[41] Collins JJ, Dunkel IJ, Gupta SK, et al. Transdermal fentanyl in children with cancer pain: feasibility, tolerability, and pharmacokinetic correlates. J Pediatr 1999;134:319.

[42] Zernikow B, Michel E, Anderson B. Transdermal fentanyl in childhood and adolescence: a comprehensive literature review. J Pain 2007;8:187.

[43] Kokki H, Rasanen I, Reinikainen M, et al. Pharmacokinetics of oxycodone after intravenous, buccal, intramuscular and gastric administration in children. Clin Pharmacokinet 2004;43:613.

[44] Lugo RA, Kern SE. The pharmacokinetics of oxycodone. J Pain Palliat Care Pharmacother 2004;18:17.

[45] Sharar SR, Carrougher GJ, Selzer K, et al. A comparison of oral transmucosal fentanyl citrate and oral oxycodone for pediatric outpatient wound care. J Burn Care Rehabil 2002;23: 27.

[46] Taketomo C, Hodding J, Kraus D. Pediatric Dosage Handbook. 13th edition. Hudson (NH): 2006.

[47] Tobias JD. Weak analgesics and nonsteroidal anti-inflammatory agents in the management of children with acute pain. Pediatr Clin North Am 2000;47:527.

[48] Shir Y, Eimerl D, Magora F, et al. Plasma concentrations of methadone during postoperative patient-controlled extradural analgesia. Br J Anaesth 1990;65:204.

[49] Shir Y, Rosen G, Zeldin A, et al. Methadone is safe for treating hospitalized patients with severe pain. Can J Anaesth 2001;48:1109.

[50] Shir Y, Shenkman Z, Shavelson V, et al. Oral methadone for the treatment of severe pain in hospitalized children: a report of five cases. Clin J Pain 1998;14:350.

[51] Subramaniam K, Subramaniam B, Steinbrook RA. Ketamine as adjuvant analgesic to opioids: a quantitative and qualitative systematic review. Anesth Analg 2004;99:482.

[52] Berde CB, Beyer JE, Bournaki MC, et al. Comparison of morphine and methadone for prevention of postoperative pain in 3- to 7-year-old children. J Pediatr 1991;119:136.

[53] Brown R, Kraus C, Fleming M, et al. Methadone: applied pharmacology and use as adjunctive treatment in chronic pain. Postgrad Med J 2004;80:654.

[54] Drake R, Hain R. Pain-pharmacological management. New York: Oxford University Press; 2006.

[55] Drake R, Longworth J, Collins JJ. Opioid rotation in children with cancer. J Palliat Med 2004;7:419.

[56] Theunissen JM, Hoogerbrugge PM, van Achterberg T, et al. Symptoms in the palliative phase of children with cancer. Pediatr Blood Cancer 2007;49:160.

[57] Cherny N, Ripamonti C, Pereira J, et al. Strategies to manage the adverse effects of oral morphine: an evidence-based report. J Clin Oncol 2001;19:2542.

[58] Kronenberg RH. Ketamine as an analgesic: parenteral, oral, rectal, subcutaneous, transdermal and intranasal administration. J Pain Palliat Care Pharmacother 2002;16:27.

[59] Berde CB, Lebel A, Olsson G. Neuropathic pain in children. In: Schechter NL, Berde C, Yaster M, editors. Pain in infants, children, and adolescents. 2nd edition. Philadelphia: Lippincott Williams & Williams; 2003. p. 620.

[60] Faulkner KW, Thayer PB, Coulter DL, et al. Algorithm for neuropathic pain treatment: an evidence based proposal. Pain 2005;118:289.

[61] Collins JJ, Berde CB, Grier HE, et al. Massive opioid resistance in an infant with a localized metastasis to the midbrain periaqueductal gray. Pain 1995;63:271.

[62] Collins JJ, Grier HE, Kinney HC, et al. Control of severe pain in children with terminal malignancy. J Pediatr 1995;126:653.

[63] Siden H. Nalewajek. High dose opioids in pediatric palliative care. J Pain Symptom Manage 2003;25:397.

[64] Hocking G, Visser EJ, Schug SA, et al. Ketamine: does life begin at 40? In: Pain Clinical Updates International Association for the Study of Pain, vol. 15(3); 2007. p. 1.

[65] Aspinall RL, Mayor A. A prospective randomized controlled study of the efficacy of ketamine for postoperative pain relief in children after adenotonsillectomy. Paediatr Anaesth 2001;11:333.

[66] Finkel JC, Pestieau SR, Quezado ZM. Ketamine as an adjuvant for treatment of cancer pain in children and adolescents. J Pain 2007;8:515.

[67] Klepstad P, Borchgrevink P, Hval B, et al. Long-term treatment with ketamine in a 12-year-old girl with severe neuropathic pain caused by a cervical spinal tumor. J Pediatr Hematol Oncol 2001;23:616.

[68] Laufer M, Schippel P, Wild L, et al. [Treatment of extreme tumour pain with morphine and s-ketamine A case report of an 11-year old girl]. Schmerz 2005;19:220, [in German].

[69] Marcus RJ, Victoria BA, Rushman SC, et al. Comparison of ketamine and morphine for analgesia after tonsillectomy in children. Br J Anaesth 2000;84:739.

[70] Tsui BC, Davies D, Desai S, et al. Intravenous ketamine infusion as an adjuvant to morphine in a 2-year-old with severe cancer pain from metastatic neuroblastoma. J Pediatr Hematol Oncol 2004;26:678.

[71] Dix P, Martindale S, Stoddart PA. Double-blind randomized placebo-controlled trial of the effect of ketamine on postoperative morphine consumption in children following appendicectomy. Paediatr Anaesth 2003;13:422.

[72] Bell R, Eccleston C, Kalso E. Ketamine as an adjuvant to opioids for cancer pain. Cochrane Database Syst Rev 2003;1:CD003351.

[73] McQuay HJ, Tramer M, Nye BA, et al. A systematic review of antidepressants in neuropathic pain. Pain 1996;68:217.

[74] Chiu YK, Prendiville JS, Bennett SM, et al. Pain management of junctional epidermolysis bullosa in an 11-year-old boy. Pediatr Dermatol 1999;16:465.

[75] Collins JJ, Kerner J, Sentivany S, et al. Intravenous amitriptyline in pediatrics. J Pain Symptom Manage 1995;10:471.

[76] Guler N, Durmus E, Tuncer S. Long-term follow-up of patients with atypical facial pain treated with amitriptyline. N Y State Dent J 2005;71:38.

[77] Lauder GR, White MC. Neuropathic pain following multilevel surgery in children with cerebral palsy: a case series and review. Paediatr Anaesth 2005;15:412.

[78] Arvio M, Merikanto J. [A relief from neural pain–gabapentin helped against hip ache in a girl with cerebral palsy]. Duodecim 2001;117:1447, [in Finnish].

[79] Behm MO, Kearns GL. Treatment of pain with gabapentin in a neonate. Pediatrics 2001; 108:482.

[80] Butkovic D, Toljan S, Mihovilovic-Novak B. Experience with gabapentin for neuropathic pain in adolescents: report of five cases. Paediatr Anaesth 2006;16:325.

[81] Gay CT. An 8-year-old girl with unilateral facial and ear pain and isolated frontal headaches. Semin Pediatr Neurol 1999;6:182.

[82] Keskinbora K, Pekel AF, Aydinli I. The use of gabapentin in a 12-year-old boy with cancer pain. Acta Anaesthesiol Scand 2004;48:663.

[83] McGraw T, Kosek P. Erythromelalgia pain managed with gabapentin. Anesthesiology 1997;86:988.

[84] McGraw T, Stacey BR. Gabapentin for treatment of neuropathic pain in a 12-year-old girl. Clin J Pain 1998;14:354.

[85] Rusy LM, Troshynski TJ, Weisman SJ. Gabapentin in phantom limb pain management in children and young adults: report of seven cases. J Pain Symptom Manage 2001;21:78.

[86] Argoff CE, Galer BS, Jensen MP, et al. Effectiveness of the lidocaine patch 5% on pain qualities in three chronic pain states: assessment with the neuropathic pain scale. Curr Med Res Opin 2004;20(Suppl 2):S21.

[87] Davies PS, Galer BS. Review of lidocaine patch 5% studies in the treatment of postherpetic neuralgia. Drugs 2004;64:937.

[88] Galer BS, Jensen MP, Ma T, et al. The lidocaine patch 5% effectively treats all neuropathic pain qualities: results of a randomized, double-blind, vehicle-controlled, 3-week efficacy study with use of the neuropathic pain scale. Clin J Pain 2002;18:297.

[89] Gammaitoni AR, Galer BS, Onawola R, et al. Lidocaine patch 5% and its positive impact on pain qualities in osteoarthritis: results of a pilot 2-week, open-label study using the neuropathic pain scale. Curr Med Res Opin 2004;20(Suppl 2):S13.

[90] Herrmann DN, Barbano RL, Hart-Gouleau S, et al. An open-label study of the lidocaine patch 5% in painful idiopathic sensory polyneuropathy. Pain Med 2005;6:379.

[91] Meier T, Faust M, Huppe M, et al. [Reduction of chronic pain for non-postherpetic peripheral neuropathies after topical treatment with a lidocaine patch]. Schmerz 2004;18:172, [in German].

[92] Meier T, Wasner G, Faust M, et al. Efficacy of lidocaine patch 5% in the treatment of focal peripheral neuropathic pain syndromes: a randomized, double-blind, placebo-controlled study. Pain 2003;106:151.

[93] Rowbotham MC, Davies PS, Verkempinck C. Lidocaine patch: double-blind controlled study of a new treatment method for post-herpetic neuralgia. Pain 1996;65:39.

[94] Hooke MC, Grund E, Quammen H, et al. Propofol use in pediatric patients with severe cancer pain at the end of life. J Pediatr Oncol Nurs 2007;24:29.

[95] Faulkner KW, Thayer P, Coulter DL. Neurological and neuromuscular symptoms. In: Goldman A, Hain R, Liben S, editors. Oxford textbook of palliative care for children. New York: Oxford University Press; 2006. p. 409.

[96] Chen E, Joseph MH, Zeltzer LK. Behavioral and cognitive interventions in the treatment of pain in children. Pediatr Clin North Am 2000;47:513.

[97] Poltorak DY, Benore E. Cognitive-behavioral interventions for physical symptom management in pediatric palliative medicine. Child Adolesc Psychiatr Clin N Am 2006; 15:683.

[98] Rusy LM, Weisman SJ. Complementary therapies for acute pediatric pain management. Pediatr Clin North Am 2000;47:589.

[99] Zeltzer LK, Tsao JC, Stelling C, et al. A phase I study on the feasibility and acceptability of an acupuncture/hypnosis intervention for chronic pediatric pain. J Pain Symptom Manage 2002;24:437.

[100] Beider S, Moyer CA. Randomized controlled trials of pediatric massage: a review. Evid Based Complement Alternat Med 2007;4:23.

[101] Tsao JC, Meldrum M, Bursch B, et al. Treatment expectations for CAM interventions in pediatric chronic pain patients and their parents. Evid Based Complement Alternat Med 2005;2:521.

ELSEVIER
SAUNDERS

PEDIATRIC CLINICS
OF NORTH AMERICA

Pediatr Clin N Am 54 (2007) 673–689

Common Gastrointestinal Symptoms in Pediatric Palliative Care: Nausea, Vomiting, Constipation, Anorexia, Cachexia

Gina Santucci, MSN, APNP-BC[a],
Jennifer W. Mack, MD, MPH[b,c],*

[a]Pediatric Advanced Care Team, The Children's Hospital of Philadelphia,
3400 Civic Center Boulevard, 4th floor Wood Building, Philadelphia, PA 19104, USA
[b]Dana Farber Cancer Institute and Children's Hospital Boston,
Department of Pediatric Oncology, 44 Binney Street, Boston, MA 02115, USA
[c]Harvard Medical School, 25 Shattuck Street, Boston, MA 02115, USA

Many pediatric patients at the end of life experience significant suffering as a result of gastrointestinal symptoms [1,2]. Among children who have cancer, anorexia and cachexia (71%–100%), nausea and vomiting (50%–57%), constipation (incidence 39%–50%), and diarrhea (21%–40%) are reported most commonly [1–3]. The incidence of such symptoms in children who die of noncancer-related illnesses is unknown, but many children experience the underlying physiologic causes of gastrointestinal symptoms during the end-of-life period, regardless of diagnosis. Such symptoms may not be recognized fully by physicians [2–4], and even when attempts are made to alleviate such symptoms, treatment often is ineffective [2]. Attention to and management of such symptoms is fundamental to high quality care of children at the end of life.

Nausea and vomiting

In addition to the suffering associated with nausea and vomiting at the end of life, the presence of such symptoms has the potential to affect other

Dr. Mack was supported by the Glaser Pediatric Research Network.

* Corresponding author. Dana Farber Cancer Institute and Children's Hospital Boston, Department of Pediatric Oncology, 44 Binney Street, Boston, MA 02115.

E-mail address: jennifer_mack@dfci.harvard.edu (J.W. Mack).

important decisions about care. Patients who otherwise might prefer home-based care, for example, may choose inpatient care if nausea and vomiting are intractable or managed inadequately in the outpatient setting. As with other end-of-life symptoms, significant physical suffering from nausea and vomiting also may have an impact on the degree to which children can enjoy their life remaining and attend to spiritual and existential needs. Prompt attention to symptoms, therefore, should be a priority. See Fig. 1 for an algorithm in the treatment of nausea and vomiting in pediatric palliative care patients.

The brain's vomiting center, located in the medulla, produces the vomiting reflex in response to input from any of three possible sources: the chemoreceptor trigger zone in the area postrema, the cortex, and the gastrointestinal tract. The chemoreceptor trigger zone responds to toxins, such as metabolic products and drugs, in the blood and cerebrospinal fluid. Toxins commonly associated with nausea and vomiting in the end-of-life setting include medications (chemotherapeutic agents, antibiotics, and opioids) and metabolic byproducts of uremia or hepatic failure.

In contrast, the cortex stimulates the vomiting center in response to elevated intracranial pressure and emotional and sensory stimuli. Increased intracranial pressure is a particularly important cause of nausea and vomiting in patients who have central nervous system (CNS) tumors, and CNS metastases should be considered in patients who have vomiting and progressive cancer when the underlying disease has propensity for CNS spread. Anxiety and other psychologic symptoms can be important contributing factors to nausea and vomiting, also mediated by cortical mechanisms.

Gastrointestinal stimulation of the vomiting center occurs in response to local receptor stimulation in the gut by factors, such as obstruction, stasis, and toxins or drugs. Pharyngeal stimulation by mucous or mucosal breakdown also can stimulate the vomiting center.

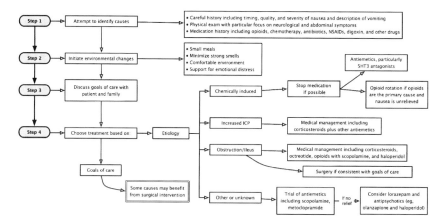

Fig. 1. Treatment of nausea and vomiting in pediatric palliative care patients.

Management of nausea and vomiting in pediatric patients can be challenging. It is important to consider possible causes before developing a management strategy (Table 1). This begins with a detailed evaluation of patients' history, including the timing, quality, and severity of nausea and a description of the vomiting. Small amounts of emesis after meals and associations with feelings of bloating, for example, should be differentiated from large volume bilious emesis that prevents any oral intake. Providers should ask about oral intake, hydration, and satiety. Any history of abdominal pain should be elicited, although young children may have difficulty differentiating between nausea and pain. Even older children may experience reflux as nausea, and symptoms of heartburn should be assessed. Other important elements of the history include headaches and other neurologic symptoms, constipation and diarrhea, and exacerbating psychologic factors, such as anxiety and depression. Children's medication lists also should be reviewed carefully for potentially causative agents.

Physical examination should include particular focus on the neurologic and abdominal examinations, with assessment for associated neurologic findings, including papilledema, and for abdominal findings, such as absent or hyperactive bowel sounds, abdominal tenderness, distention, and palpable stool or other masses.

Neurotransmitters in the vomiting center, including acetylcholine and histamine, and in the chemoreceptor trigger zone, including dopamine and serotonin, are targets of antiemetic therapy (Table 2 lists common antiemetics used in pediatric patients). Therapy often can be tailored based on the underlying cause of the nausea and vomiting. Whenever possible, the cause should be eliminated, but often even when the cause cannot be removed, the most effective palliation strategy is determined by the cause. For example, increased intracranial pressure caused by CNS tumors may be responsive to dexamethasone.

Table 1
Causes of nausea and vomiting in the end-of-life period

Central nervous system
Cortex
Increased intracranial pressure
Chemoreceptor trigger zone
Medications (chemotherapeutic agents, antibiotics, opioids)
Metabolic abnormalities (uremia, liver failure, hypercalcemia)
Vestibular
Vestibular nerve stimulation, sometimes increased by opioids
Gastrointestinal tract
Obstruction (gastric outlet or bowel)
Gastric ulcers or mucositis
Stasis/reduced motility
Constipation
Pharyngeal stimulation (mucous, mucosal irritation)

Table 2
Medications used in treatment of nausea and vomiting

Medication	Dose
Prokinetic/dopamine antagonist	
Metoclopramide	Prokinetic dose: 0.1 mg/kg/dose IV or orally every 6 hours
	Dopamine antagonist (antiemetic) dose: 0.5–1 mg/kg/dose IV or orally every 6 hours; use with diphenhydramine to prevent extrapyramidal symptoms
Serotonin receptor antagonists	
Ondansetron	0.45 mg/kg/d IV or orally; may be dosed once daily or divided every 8 hours
Anticholinergics	
Scopolamine	For children >40 kg: 1.5-mg patch behind ear every 72 hours
Antivertigo agents (piperazine)	
Meclizine	For children >12 years of age: 25–75 mg/d orally in up to 3 divided doses
Corticosteroids	
Dexamethasone	When used as antiemetic, 10 mg/m^2 IV or orally daily; maximum dose 20 mg daily. For increased intracranial pressure, increase dosing frequency to 2–4 times daily, with a maximum dose of 40 mg/d.
Somatostatin analogs	
Octreotide	5–10 μg/kg/d, either as continuous 24-hour IV infusion or divided twice daily and administered subcutaneously
Atypical antipsychotic	
Olanzapine	2.5–5 mg/d orally, may be increased to maximum 20 mg/d. Dosing in children not established but has been used in some adolescents.
Cannabinoid	
Dronabinol	For children ages 6 years and older; not recommended for children who have clinical depression; 2.5–5 mg/m^2/dose every 4–6 hours
Benzodiazepine	
Lorazepam	.025 mg/kg/dose IV or orally every 6 hours

Opioids are a common cause of nausea and vomiting in the end-of-life period. In addition to a direct effect of opioids on the chemoreceptor trigger zone, opioids can cause nausea and vomiting by decreasing gut motility with resultant gastroparesis and constipation. Patients are particularly susceptible to nausea and vomiting after initiation or dose escalation of opioids. Opioid-induced nausea and vomiting usually are responsive to antiemetic therapy, and after 3 to 4 days at a stable dose, nausea and vomiting typically resolve [5]. A minority of patients continue to experience chronic opioid-induced nausea. Nausea that persists for more than a week after initiation or escalation of opioids should be evaluated carefully for other causes. In a minority of patients who experience chronic opioid-related nausea, however, opioid rotation and ongoing antiemetic therapy can be effective. In addition, gastric motility agents, such as metoclopramide, in doses used for motility rather than the higher doses used for antiemesis, may be helpful.

Another important cause of refractory nausea and vomiting is intestinal obstruction [6], such as from an abdominal tumor. Surgery for bypass of the obstruction or placement of a venting gastrostomy should be a consideration, but in patients who cannot tolerate or do not wish for an invasive procedure, medical management is appropriate [7]. Corticosteroids may be effective in relieving intestinal obstruction [8]. In addition, octreotide can be effective in decreasing gastrointestinal secretions, such that nausea and vomiting diminish markedly [9]. Octreotide can be administered intravenously (IV) or subcutaneously, thus can be provided in the outpatient setting if needed. Other pharmacologic combinations, such as morphine with scopolamine and haloperidol, can relieve nausea and vomiting and the cramping associated with intestinal obstruction.

When a cause of nausea cannot be identified, empiric antiemetic therapy may be effective. Although many such agents are described in cancer patients receiving chemotherapy, such agents can be useful even if no antineoplastic agents are used. Metoclopramide and scopolamine are used successfully in this setting. Five-hydroxytryptamine antagonists, such as ondansetron, also can be effective [10,11], especially for opioid-induced nausea and vomiting. When symptoms are particularly difficult to control, lorazepam and antipsychotics, such as olanzapine [12] or haloperidol, also should be considered. Although dexamethasone often is used, its efficacy in an end-of-life setting may be limited [13], except when used for specific scenarios, such as increased intracranial pressure or edema associated with bowel obstruction. Diphenhydramine should be administered with phenothiazines to reduce the risk for extrapyramidal side effects. If nausea is exacerbated by motion, antivertigo agents, such as scopolamine or meclizine, can be useful. Some patients also benefit from dronabinol, which can stimulate the appetite in addition to minimizing nausea.

Nonpharmacologic therapy for nausea and vomiting also should be considered [5]. Smells, sights, and emotional state can be powerful inducers of nausea. Small meals at regular intervals may be tolerated best. Patients should be allowed to eat in a comfortable environment with other strong smells minimized, even smells associated with a patient's own body or care or a parent's meal. Some patients also may benefit from acupuncture or hypnosis. Because nausea also may be a symptom of psychologic distress, providers also should assess a child's emotional state carefully and provide any needed support or treatment.

Constipation

Constipation is a frequent cause of pain and distress in patients at end of life. In addition to associated discomfort, constipation and its assessment and treatment may contribute to feelings of loss of dignity, especially among older children and adolescents. Prevention should be a primary goal.

Constipation is prevalent particularly at end of life because of opioid use for pain. Opioids cause constipation by reducing bowel motility and secretions and by increasing colon transit time, resulting in increased fluid absorption in the colon. Constipation is common regardless of the strength or route of the opioid and, unlike many other opioid side effects, does not tend to diminish with ongoing use.

Patients who are experiencing significant pain may not consider regular bowel movements to be a priority, thus may go several days without a bowel movement before bringing it to medical attention, at which point aggressive measures may be required. Medical providers, therefore, should educate all patients (or parents of children) taking opioids about this side effect and take measures to prevent constipation at the time of initiation.

Other common causes of constipation in the end-of-life setting include effects of poor fluid and dietary intake. In addition, immobility contributes to constipation; colon peristalsis is stimulated in part by activity, and without activity, peristalsis slows. Similarly, children who have other neurologic impairments may have chronic constipation related to longstanding poor colonic tone and immobility. In cancer patients, intra-abdominal tumor causing direct compression of the gut or spinal cord compression also can cause constipation (Table 3).

A careful history should include frequency of evacuation, consistency of stools, and rectal pain associated with evacuation. Other constipation-related

Table 3
Causes of constipation in the end-of-life period

Inadequate fluid and fiber intake
Reduced activity
Neurologic impairment
Neuropathy (autonomic neuropathy or medication related, such as vinca alkaloid related)
Spinal cord compression (tumor or other spinal cord/cauda equina lesion)
Metabolic derangement
Hypercalcemia
Hypokalemia
Hypothyroidism
Uremia
Medication related
Opioids
Anticholinergics
Antiemetics
Anticonvulsants
Antidepressants
Antacids
Antihypertensive agents
Intestinal obstruction
Exacerbating conditions
Hemorrhoids
Anal fissure
Limited access to toilet

symptoms, including abdominal pain, nausea, vomiting, and anorexia, should be assessed. Neurologic symptoms, including urinary symptoms and numbness, weakness, or paresthesias of the lower extremities, also may be present and should be assessed carefully as signs of neurologic compromise as the primary cause of constipation. Patients may present with diarrhea resulting from obstipation with overflow. A history of diarrhea in patients who have a history of constipation or are at high risk for constipation, therefore, should prompt consideration of obstipation among possible causes. In patients who have limited ability to communicate, parents may describe an increase in general discomfort after several days of opioids, with an associated history of small loose stools or constipation. Some patients have a longstanding history of constipation, and such a history should be elicited along with a description of effective management used in the past.

A physical examination should include abdominal palpation and a neurologic examination. Hard stool may be palpable on abdominal examination. Abdominal palpation may cause some discomfort or cause grimacing in children who have limited ability to communicate verbally. Rectal examination can be used to establish rectal tone and the presence of rectal stool, although constipation often can be assessed and managed without a digital examination. Such an examination also places cancer patients who have neutropenia at risk for infection so should be avoided in that circumstance whenever possible. External examination for hemorrhoids and fissures may be useful when the history includes pain on passage of stool. An abdominal radiograph may be helpful in assessing for the possibility of intestinal obstruction and in identifying stool when the diagnosis is in question.

Medications used in treatment of constipation include stool softeners (docusate), osmotic agents (lactulose or magnesium sulfate), and stimulants (senna or bisacodyl) [5,14,15]. Stool softeners, such as docusate, have limited efficacy as single agents for patients who have significant constipation, although they can be useful in combination with stimulants, particularly when passage of hard stool causes pain. Osmotic agents can be helpful in the end-of-life setting and tend to be well tolerated, with little cramping. Agents, such as lactulose, magnesium sulfate, and polyethylene glycol, draw water into the bowel lumen through osmotic effects. Polyethylene glycol requires a patient to take 4 to 8 ounces of liquid and, therefore, should be prescribed only for patients who can take the requisite fluid. Lactulose can be escalated readily to relieve obstipation and is in a liquid form that can be used by young children and via gastrostomy tubes.

Stimulants, such as senna and bisacodyl, act by stimulating the myenteric plexus. Such agents often are necessary for relief of constipation and can be well tolerated, particularly when used in once-daily dosing for prophylaxis of constipation. Some patients experience cramping, particularly when these agents are used for evacuation. Senna is available in liquid or pill form and as a tea, which may be a preferred form for some patients. Bisacodyl is available as a pill, but the pill is small enough to be taken by some children who cannot swallow larger pills. A rectal form also is available.

Bulk forming agents can be effective by normalizing the consistency of the stool; however, such agents require significant liquid intake, so should be prescribed only when patients can take the necessary liquid. If fluid intake is inadequate, bulk-forming agents can increase constipation, so their usefulness in the end-of-life setting typically is limited.

Oral agents in adequate doses often are sufficient to relieve constipation, but rectal agents sometimes are needed in cases of impaction or severe constipation. Rectal agents include suppositories and enemas and, like the oral agents, work by softening stools or stimulating evacuation. In cancer patients who have neutropenia, use of rectal agents places such patients at risk for infection, an issue that should be considered carefully before administration. In select circumstances, manual disimpaction may be necessary, but in that case, comfort during the procedure should be a priority (Table 4 lists

Table 4
Medications used in treatment and prophylaxis of constipation

Prophylaxis	Dose
Docusate	10 times age in years orally daily, divided up to 4 times per day. Maximum dose 500 mg per day.
Lactulose	Ages 2–10: 2.5–7.5 mL orally daily
	Age >10 years: 15-30 mL orally daily
Polyethylene glycol	Ages 2–10 years: 8.5 g in 4 ounces liquid orally daily
	Age >10 years: 17 g in 8 ounces of liquid orally daily
Senna	Age <6 years: 2.5–5 mL, or 1 tablet orally daily
1.76 mg sennoside/mL	Age 6–12 years: 2 tablets orally daily
or 8.6 mg sennoside/tablet	Age >12 years: 3 tablets orally daily
Treatment	Consider combination of lactulose and senna
Lactulose	Age <2 years: 2.5 mL orally twice a day
	Ages 2–10 years: 2.5–7.5 mL orally twice a day
	Age >10 years: 15–30 mL orally twice a day
Polyethylene glycol	Ages 2–10 years: 8.5 g in 4 ounces liquid orally twice a day
	Age >10 years: 17 g in 8 ounces of liquid orally twice a day
Senna	Age <6 years: 2.5–5 mL or 1 tablet orally twice a day
	Age 6–12 years: 2 tablets orally twice a day
	Age > 12 years: 3 tablets orally twice a day
Evacuation	
Lactulose	Age <2 years: 3 mL orally 3 times a day
	Ages 2–10 years: 15–30 mL orally 3 times a day
	Age >10 years: 30 mL orally every 2 hours until patient has bowel movement
Senna	Age <6 years: 30 mL (6 tablets) orally × 1 dose
	Age 6–12 years: 45 mL (9 tablets) orally × 1 dose
	Age >12 years: up to 90 mL (18 tablets) orally × 1 dose
Magnesium citrate	Age <6 years: 2 mL/kg × 1 dose
1.745 g/30 mL solution	Age 6–12 years: 100 mL orally × 1 dose
	Age >12 years: 300 mL orally × 1 dose

medications used in treatment and prophylaxis of constipation in pediatric patients).

Once evacuation is accomplished, the risk for ongoing constipation should be considered and prophylaxis initiated if needed. In general, osmotic agents, such as lactulose or polyethylene glycol, may be adequate, but combination therapy with osmotic agents and stimulants may be necessary. A daily regimen that promotes daily bowel movements without excessive cramping or abdominal pain should be the goal. Oral medications usually are sufficient; in cases of significant neurologic impairment, such as a spinal cord lesion, maintenance therapy with rectal agents may be necessary.

Measures to prevent constipation in patients on opioids are important particularly from the time of initiation of opioids. Although many opioid-related side effects diminish over the first several days of use, constipation tends to remain a problem throughout the period of use [5]. Prophylaxis should be initiated at the time opioids are prescribed, and patients should be instructed to continue prophylactic agents daily to maintain soft bowel movements at least every other day and up to twice a day. Effective combinations include a softening or osmotic agent (such as polyethylene glycol or lactulose) in combination with a stimulant (such as senna). Instructions for increased measures to be taken when a patient has no bowel movement for one day also should be provided at the time of opioid initiation. For example, a change from once- to twice-daily dosing for the softener and stimulant may be effective. If such measures are ineffective, evacuation measures should be considered. Lactulose every 2 hours with senna up to 4 times daily until evacuation is achieved can be effective.

Some studies suggest that low oral doses of opioid antagonists, such as naloxone, can be effective in relieving opioid-induced constipation [16,17]. Existing studies are small and nonrandomized, and dosing has not been established definitively. Because most naloxone is metabolized hepatically, first-pass metabolism after gut absorption theoretically should prevent most systemic effects. Even small amounts of naloxone, however, available systemically can precipitate opioid withdrawal, particularly in patients who have physiologic dependence [18]. The authors, therefore, do not recommend use of oral naloxone in most circumstances. (See Fig. 2 for an approach to the treatment of constipation in this patient population).

Anorexia and cachexia

Weight loss and malnutrition often are unavoidable symptoms experienced by patients at the end of life and frequently are associated with poor clinical outcome and increased morbidity and mortality [19]. Eating and food can hold important meaning for patients and families; loss of appetite (anorexia) and involuntary weight loss (cachexia) can have a negative impact on quality of life beyond the symptoms that advancing poor

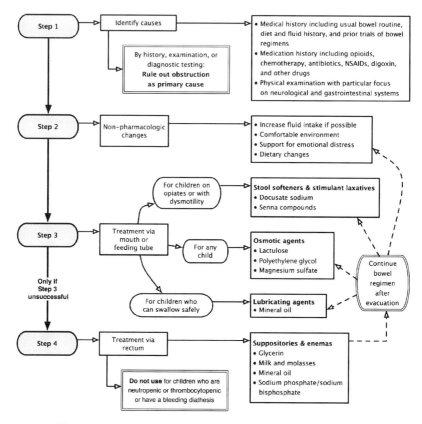

Fig. 2. Treatment of constipation in pediatric palliative care patients.

nutrition may cause. Mealtime frequently holds cultural, emotional, and religious significance and the inability to enjoy food can affect the entire family. Families may believe that providing nutrition may stave off or reverse wasting; however, given that children generally have higher energy and nutritional needs, those diagnosed with certain malignant tumors are particularly vulnerable to weight loss and malnutrition [20–24].

"Cachexia" is derived from the Greek word, "kakhexia," which means "bad or poor condition" [25]. It also is referred to as a "wasting syndrome [26] or "state of depletion" because patients often appear withered and debilitated [21–24]. Clinically, anorexia and cachexia may present as one entity; however, factors underlying each are multifactorial. Anorexia often is seen in patients who suffer from cachexia, although the reverse not always is true; additionally, the degree of cachexia correlates directly with prognosis and quality of life. Anorexia is a familiar symptom in children who have cancer and can occur anytime during the disease process [23]; most often it is a side effect of treatment (radiation or chemotherapy) or consequence of stomatitis, dysphagia, severe constipation, xerostoma, pain, or depression.

Cachexia and anorexia occur primarily in patients who have incurable neo-plasms (>80%) [27,28], but they also can be seen in end-stage acquired im-munodeficiency syndrome, chronic pulmonary disease, congestive heart failure, and other complex chronic and debilitating conditions [29,30]. Anorexia alone cannot wholly account for the overwhelming weight and muscle loss that occurs with progression of chronic disease [25].

There is no universal definition of cachexia, although it generally is accepted that a cluster of symptoms triggers a complex process that in turn affects metabolic, neurohormonal, and emotional states (Table 5). Cachexia is considered a metabolic disorder mediated by anabolic and cat-abolic changes, causing muscle wasting and protein and lipid loss that is not reversed by food intake [29–31]. Alterations in homeostasis, tumor cell ex-pression, lipolysis, appetite disruption, and hormonal dysregulation have been investigated as potential mediators in cachexia [21,30–33]. Proinflam-matory cytokines, including interleukin (IL)-6, interferon-γ, and tumor ne-crosis factor (TNF)-α, are known to play a major role in causing cachexia in debilitated patients [32]. For children diagnosed with malignant neoplasms, cachexia often is the end result of progressive disease (and the degree of mal-nutrition varies from 5% to more than 60% dependent on location and dis-ease stage) [19,22].

Primary versus secondary cachexia

Primary cachexia largely is a consequence of cancer, especially solid tumors, where proinflammatory cytokines lead to malnutrition, asthenia, sarcopenia, and, ultimately, decreased survival [28,34]. Cachexia that is caused by potentially treatable conditions and not necessarily chronic

Table 5
Factors involved in cachexia

Metabolic	Inflammatory cytokines	Carbohydrate alterations	Lipid alterations
	• TNF-α	• Insulin resistance	• Variable lipolysis
	• IL-1β, IL-6, IL-8	• Gluconeogenesis	• $\Downarrow$ Lipogenesis
	• Interferon-γ	• Increase lactate	• $\Downarrow$ HDL
	• Leukemia inhibiting factor		• $\Uparrow$ VLDL
	• Ciliary neurotrophic factor		
Hormonal	• Leptin		
	• Insulin		
	• Glucagon		
	• Toxohormone-L		
Neurotransmitters	• Neuropeptide Y		
	• Serotonin		
Psychologic	• Changes in body image		
	• Depression		
	• Low energy		

Abbreviations: HDL, high-density lipoprotein; VLDL, very low-density lipoprotein.

inflammation or infection is considered secondary cachexia (Table 6). Both can exist simultaneously, although primary cachexia typically is seen with advancing malignancy or disease. In chronic disease, cachexia usually is the end result not only of poor nutrition but also of a cluster of symptoms, including exhaustion, nausea, and decreased appetite, in which weight loss is related directly to the degree of debilitation [35]. Regardless of the cause, the result is massive skeletal muscle and lipid store loss [28] and increased resting energy expenditure in the face of declining caloric intake.

Identifying the cause of anorexia and cachexia is beneficial when planning a treatment approach (see Fig. 3 for an approach to the management of these symptoms in pediatric patients.) It is important to evaluate if symptoms of weight loss and wasting are the result of a potentially reversible process (ie, bowel obstruction, severe constipation, or pain) or a result of "normal" end-of-life progression, including progression of primary disease. There is no one test or laboratory finding that is solely diagnostic of a poor nutritional status consequent of cachexia. Instead, a combination of clinical assessment, dietary history, anthropometric measurements, and bioelectric impedance (when appropriate) can help in making a diagnosis. Serum albumin and prealbumin (transthyretin) are less reliable markers for protein loss in the face of chronic inflammation. Assessment tools can help clinicians monitor minute changes in nutritional status. The Patient-Generated Subjective Global Assessment is a simple tool that has become the standard for assessing nutritional needs in patients who have cancer [36,37].

Once treatable causes are ruled out, nonpharmacologic and pharmacologic therapies can be beneficial. When developing a treatment approach for cachexia, it is equally important to evaluate and treat the chronic nausea and psychologic distress that frequently is present. Therapeutic options currently available range from nutritional supplementation to appetite

Table 6
Primary versus secondary cachexia

Primary cachexia	Secondary cachexia
Host linked	Treatment linked (chemotherapy, radiation, surgery)
• Inflammatory cytokine production	• ⇓ Caloric intake
• Alterations in metabolism	• Xerostomia
Tumor linked	• Dysphagia
• Lipid and protein mobilizing factors	• Severe constipation or bowel obstruction
	• Severe pain
	• Malabsorption
	• Chronic inflammation
	• Ongoing deconditioning
	Psychologic linked
	• Depression
	• Food aversion
	• Odynophagia

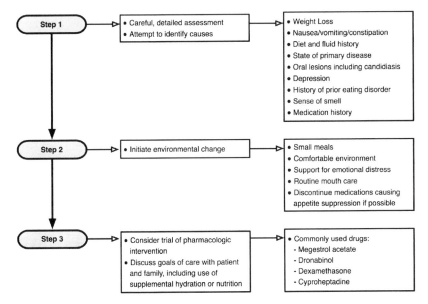

Fig. 3. Treatment of anorexia in pediatric palliative care.

stimulants and steroids. It often is difficult for a family to watch their child waste away from poor nutrition. Developing a treatment plan should include assessment of current disease stage, the child's and family's goals, and maximizing quality of life [38]. Unfortunately, the best treatment for cachexia is to cure the cancer or end-stage disease process. Several randomized clinical trials show that offering total parenteral nutrition to patients who have cachexia-anorexia has little to no beneficial effect and may increase morbidity [39,40]. Supplemental hypercaloric nutrition via a feeding tube or IV has little effect on increasing skeletal muscle mass and most weight gain can be attributed to an increase in adipose tissue. Some clinicians may agree to provide a time limited trial of supplemental nutrition (ie, parenteral therapy) in cases where there is an obstruction of the gastrointestinal tract. In these instances, enlisting a multidisciplinary approach may help address the broader issues—the psychologic and spiritual distress that frequently occurs with advanced progressive and incurable diseases. Given the risks and logistics of providing parenteral nutrition, in the absence of an obstruction, tube feedings may provide comfort for children and the families.

Several drugs show some benefit in palliating cachexia associated with advancing cancer and disease (see Table 6; Tables 7 and 8). Appetite stimulants (ie, progestational drugs, corticosteroids, and cannabinoids) can offer some improvement in weight gain albeit primarily in adipose not skeletal muscle tissue. Megestrol acetate and medroxyprogesterone, synthetic progestins, tend to increase a sense of well-being in addition to stimulating

Table 7
Pharmacologic treatments for cachexia

Appetite stimulants		
Corticosteriods		
Dexamethasone (preferred long half-life; minimal mineral effect)	Dosage by weight (kg) twice a day <10 kg 0.15 mg/mg/kg/dose 10–20 kg 2 mg 21–40 kg 4 mg >41 kg 8 mg	• Improves appetite and well-being. No lasting improvement in nutritional status Corticosteroid-type toxicity increased with Dexamethasone
Prednisone	0.05–2 mg/kg/d divided 1–4 times/d	• ↓ Proinflammatory cytokine • Inhibit prostaprime metabolism
Progestational		
Megestrol acetate	7.5–10 mg/kg/d in 1–4 divided doses; maximum 800 mg/d or 15 mg/kg/d.	• Titrate dose to response, weight gain seen in 2–4 weeks, limited data reported in children
Cannabinoids		
Dronabinol	Children ages 6 years and older; 2.5–5 mg/m²/dose every 4–6 hours.	• Not recommended for children who have clinical depression or hypersensitivity to sesame oil
Atypical antipsychotic		
Olanzapine (Zyrexa)	2.5–5 mg/d orally, may be increased to maximum 20 mg/d. Dosing in children not established, but is used in some adolescents	• Not recommended for children under 18 years. Appetite may increase 3%–6%.
Anti-inflammatory		
Immunomodulators		
Thalidomide	Not recommended for children under 12 years	• TNF blocking agent. Increased risk for deep vein thrombosis and pulmonary embolism when used in combination with dexamethasone
Prostaglandin inhibitors		
Indomethacin Ibuprofen	Unknown response in pediatric patients	• Reported to decrease C-reactive protein, increase weight in adult cancer patients
Hormone		
Melatonin	0.5–10 mg/d at night	• Antioxidant. May reduce weight loss in cancer patients [43]
Complementary		
Amino-acid derivative		
L-carnitine		
Essential fatty acids		
Omega 3		• Polyunsaturated fatty acids may inhibit IL-1 and TNF

Note that the majority of these treatments have not been studied in randomized clinical trials.

Dronabinol

2.5–5 mg/m²/dose every

Table 8
Nonpharmacologic treatments used in anorexia and cachexia

Relaxation and imagery
Provide favorite foods in desired amount
Reduce portion size
Eliminate foods with unpleasant odor
Explore emotional and spiritual issues related to weight loss

appetite. Randomized clinical trials in adults show high-dose progestestional drugs more effective than corticosteroids and cannabinoids as orexigenic agents [40,41]. In children, megestrol acetate may impair adrenal function and cause adrenal insufficiency; therefore, stress-dose glucocorticoids often are required [42]. Patients on progestational agents also need to be monitored for thromboembolic events, hypertension, and hyperglycemia. Corticosteriods usually are well tolerated for a short time and can help with nausea, pain, asthenia, and mood but show little to no benefit in increasing lean body mass [34,40]. Dronabinol is approved for use in weight loss associated with cancer; however, its effect is lesser than megestrol acetate and corticosteroids. Families can find a range of medications, including antipsychotics, anabolic steroids, and anti-inflammatory and complementary therapies, that are believed to increase weight in cachectic patients. The majority of these have not been studied in randomized clinical trials but are listed for reference in Table 7.

Given the multifactorial aspects of cachexia and anorexia, any treatment approach should consider its affect on children's physical, emotional, and psychosocial domains [28]. How treatments may have an impact on quality of life for children and families should be considered. Lastly, any plan of care should take into account cultural and religious preferences when appropriate.

Acknowledgment

We would like to thank Christopher Feudtner, MD, PhD, MPH, and Jordan Silberman, MAPP, for their assistance in developing the treatment algorithms.

References

[1] Jalmsell L, Kreicbergs U, Onelov E, et al. Symptoms affecting children with malignancies during the last month of life: a nationwide follow-up. Pediatrics 2006;117(4):1314–20.

[2] Wolfe J, Grier HE, Klar N, et al. Symptoms and suffering at the end of life in children with cancer. N Engl J Med 2000;342(5):326–33.

[3] Hongo T, Watanabe C, Okada S, et al. Analysis of the circumstances at the end of life in children with cancer: symptoms, suffering and acceptance. Pediatr Int 2003;45(1):60–4.

[4] Carter BS, Howenstein M, Gilmer MJ, et al. Circumstances surrounding the deaths of hospitalized children: opportunities for pediatric palliative care. Pediatrics 2004;114(3):e361–6.

[5] Abrahm J. A physician's guide to pain and symptom management in cancer patients. Baltimore (MD): Johns Hopkins University Press; 2000.

[6] Baines MJ. ABC of palliative care. Nausea, vomiting, and intestinal obstruction. BMJ 1997; 315(7116):1148–50.

[7] Ripamonti C, Bruera E. Palliative management of malignant bowel obstruction. Int J Gynecol Cancer 2002;12(2):135–43.

[8] Laval G, Girardier J, Lassauniere JM, et al. The use of steroids in the management of inoperable intestinal obstruction in terminal cancer patients: do they remove the obstruction? Palliat Med 2000;14(1):3–10.

[9] Ripamonti C, Mercadante S, Groff L, et al. Role of octreotide, scopolamine butylbromide, and hydration in symptom control of patients with inoperable bowel obstruction and nasogastric tubes: a prospective randomized trial. J Pain Symptom Manage 2000;19(1):23–34.

[10] Mystakidou K, Befon S, Liossi C, et al. Comparison of the efficacy and safety of tropisetron, metoclopramide, and chlorpromazine in the treatment of emesis associated with far advanced cancer. Cancer 1998;83(6):1214–23.

[11] Currow DC, Coughlan M, Fardell B, et al. Use of ondansetron in palliative medicine. J Pain Symptom Manage 1997;13(5):302–7.

[12] Srivastava M, Brito-Dellan N, Davis MP, et al. Olanzapine as an antiemetic in refractory nausea and vomiting in advanced cancer. J Pain Symptom Manage 2003;25(6):578–82.

[13] Bruera E, Moyano JR, Sala R, et al. Dexamethasone in addition to metoclopramide for chronic nausea in patients with advanced cancer: a randomized controlled trial. J Pain Symptom Manage 2004;28(4):381–8.

[14] Fallon M, O'Neill B. ABC of palliative care. Constipation and diarrhoea. BMJ 1997; 315(7118):1293–6.

[15] Mancini I, Bruera E. Constipation in advanced cancer patients. Support Care Cancer 1998; 6(4):356–64.

[16] Liu M, Wittbrodt E. Low-dose oral naloxone reverses opioid-induced constipation and analgesia. J Pain Symptom Manage 2002;23(1):48–53.

[17] Sykes NP. An investigation of the ability of oral naloxone to correct opioid-related constipation in patients with advanced cancer. Palliat Med 1996;10(2):135–44.

[18] Choi YS, Billings JA. Opioid antagonists: a review of their role in palliative care, focusing on use in opioid-related constipation. J Pain Symptom Manage 2002;24(1):71–90.

[19] Nelson KA, Walsh D. The cancer anorexia-cachexia syndrome: a survey of the prognostic inflammatory and nutritional index (PINI) in advanced disease. J Pain Symptom Manage 2002;24(4):424–8.

[20] den Broeder E, Lippens RJ, van 't Hof MA, et al. Nasogastric tube feeding in children with cancer: the effect of two different formulas on weight, body composition, and serum protein concentrations. JPEN J Parenter Enteral Nutr 2000;24(6):351–60.

[21] Ladas EJ, Post-White J, Hawks R, et al. Evidence for symptom management in the child with cancer. J Pediatr Hematol Oncol 2006;28(9):601–15.

[22] Ladas EJ, Sacks N, Meacham L, et al. A multidisciplinary review of nutrition considerations in the pediatric oncology population: a perspective from children's oncology group. Nutr Clin Pract 2005;20(4):377–93.

[23] Lai JS, Cella D, Peterman A, et al. Anorexia/cachexia-related quality of life for children with cancer. Cancer 2005;104(7):1531–9.

[24] Picton SV. Aspects of altered metabolism in children with cancer. Int J Cancer Suppl 1998; 11:62–4.

[25] Delano MJ, Moldawer LL. The origins of cachexia in acute and chronic inflammatory diseases. Nutr Clin Pract 2006;21(1):68–81.

[26] Camps C, Iranzo V, Bremnes RM, et al. Anorexia-cachexia syndrome in cancer: implications of the ubiquitin-proteasome pathway. Support Care Cancer 2006;14(12):1173–83.

[27] Jatoi A. Pharmacologic therapy for the cancer anorexia/weight loss syndrome: a data-driven, practical approach. J Support Oncol 2006;4(10):499–502.

[28] Strasser F, Bruera ED. Update on anorexia and cachexia. Hematol Oncol Clin North Am 2002;16(3):589–617.

[29] Dahlin C, Lynch M, Szmuilowicz G, et al. Management of symptoms other than pain. Anesthesiol Clin 2006;24(1):39–60.

[30] Del Fabbro E, Dalal S, Bruera E. Symptom control in palliative care–part II: cachexia/anorexia and fatigue. J Palliat Med 2006;9(2):409–21.

[31] Laviano A, Russo M, Freda F, et al. Neurochemical mechanisms for cancer anorexia. Nutrition 2002;18(1):100–5.

[32] Morley JE, Thomas DR, Wilson MM. Cachexia: pathophysiology and clinical relevance. Am J Clin Nutr 2006;83(4):735–43.

[33] Tisdale MJ. Clinical anticachexia treatments. Nutr Clin Pract 2006;21(2):168–74.

[34] Martignoni ME, Kunze P, Friess H. Cancer cachexia. Mol Cancer 2003;2:36–8.

[35] Witte KK, Clark AL. Nutritional abnormalities contributing to cachexia in chronic illness. Int J Cardiol 2002;85(1):23–31.

[36] Bauer J, Capra S, Ferguson M. Use of the scored patient-generated subjective global assessment (PG-SGA) as a nutrition assessment tool in patients with cancer. Eur J Clin Nutr 2002; 56(8):779–85.

[37] Isenring E, Bauer J, Capra S. The scored patient-generated subjective global assessment (PG-SGA) and its association with quality of life in ambulatory patients receiving radiotherapy. Eur J Clin Nutr 2003;57(2):305–9.

[38] McKinlay A. Nutritional support in patients with advanced cancer: permission to fall out? Proc Nutr Soc 2004;63:431–5.

[39] Bruera E. ABC of palliative care: anorexia, cachexia, and nutrition. BMJ 1997;315:1219–22.

[40] Inui A. Cancer anorexia-cachexia syndrome: current issues in research and management. CA Cancer J Clin 2002;52(2):72–91.

[41] maltoni M, Nanni O, Scarpi E, et al. High-dose progestins for the treatment of cancer anorexia-cachexia syndrome: a systematic review of randomised clinical trials. Ann Oncol 2001;12:289–300.

[42] Meacham L, Mazewski C, Krawiecki N. Mechanisms of transiet adrenal insufficeincy with megestrol acetate treatment of cachexia in children with cancer. J Pediatr Hematol Oncol 2003;25(5):414–7.

[43] Lissoni P, Paolorossi F, Tancini G, et al. Is there a role for melatonin in the treatment of neoplastic cachexia? Eur J Cancer 1996;32A(8):1340–3.

ELSEVIER
SAUNDERS

PEDIATRIC CLINICS

OF NORTH AMERICA

Pediatr Clin N Am 54 (2007) 691–708

Depression and Anxiety in Children at the End of Life

Leslie S. Kersun, MD, MSCE[a,b,*],
Eyal Shemesh, MD[c,d]

[a]Division of Oncology, The Children's Hospital of Philadelphia,
4th Floor Wood Building, 34th and Civic Center Boulevard,
Philadelphia, PA 19104, USA
[b]Department of Pediatrics, The University of Pennsylvania School of Medicine, 4th Floor
Wood Building, 34th and Civic Center Boulevard, Philadelphia, PA 19104, USA
[c]Behavioral Health Integrated Program, Behavioral Health Center,
The Children's Hospital of Philadelphia, 3440 Market Street, Suite 410,
Philadelphia, PA 19104, USA
[d]Department of Child and Adolescent Psychiatry, The Children's Hospital of Philadelphia,
3440 Market Street, Suite 410, Philadelphia, PA 19104, USA

This article discusses the manifestations and treatment of symptoms of anxiety and depression in children at the end of life. It demonstrates that these symptoms are common, treatable, and associated with distress and significant morbidity, and yet are underrecognized and, thus, undertreated. Therefore, it is important that clinicians who are faced with the challenges of caring for these children become familiar with the symptoms (in particular, with the way that they present in a chronically ill child) and understand the different ways that these symptoms can be addressed in this unique population [1,2].

Symptoms versus disorders

Two different, albeit overlapping, constructs are important to distinguish. A child may be anxious or sad, but may not reach the threshold of a psychiatric disorder (ie, is not suffering from a major depressive disorder or a generalized anxiety disorder). Sadness and grief may be normal and expected,

This work was partially supported by National Institutes of Health award MH063755-05 (Eyal Shemesh, MD).

* Corresponding author. Division of Oncology, The Children's Hospital of Philadelphia, 4th Floor Wood Building, 34th and Civic Center Boulevard, Philadelphia, PA 19104.

E-mail address: segall@email.chop.edu (L.S. Kersun).

whereas a major depressive disorder is a psychiatric disorder that needs to be treated. Symptoms of depression and grief may be similar (ie, crying, decreased appetite, difficulty sleeping, and decreased concentration and attention). The normal grief reaction is self-limited, responds to reassurance, and is not associated with self-blame or worthlessness, as in depression. Similarly, some level of anxiety or distress may be expected, or even healthy, in response to a stressor, but at some point, anxiety is of sufficient magnitude and duration that it warrants the designation of a psychiatric disorder (ie, generalized anxiety disorder). For the relevant *Diagnostic and Statistical Manual of Mental Disorders, Fourth Edition* (DSM-IV) diagnostic criteria, see Table 1. The reader should recognize the difference between symptoms that do not constitute a disorder, and a full-blown disorder. It is sometimes extremely difficult to determine, in a given child, whether the symptoms are indeed at a point where they need to be addressed by psychopharmacotherapy or psychotherapy. In the opinion of the authors of this article, undertreatment (ie, erroneously not treating a disorder) and overtreatment (ie, erroneously treating symptoms that are healthy, expected, and do not constitute a disorder) are often encountered in settings in which medically ill children are treated. Although the dilemma of whether to diagnose a disorder or not, given a specific constellation of symptoms, is hardly going to be resolved in these several pages, the authors describe some recent research and clinical findings that may help make this determination easier for practitioners. For the sake of clarity, when the authors discuss treatment options in this article, they always refer to the treatment of a true psychiatric disorder rather than a constellation of symptoms.

The importance of open communication and consideration of the child's understanding of death

The first step in determining whether a child is suffering from excessive symptoms of distress or depression is the ability to engage the child and parent in a discussion of these symptoms. Thus, it is important to establish clear and open communication with children at the end of life. The kind of discussion one would have with a child depends on his/her developmental age and understanding of death, parental wishes in the cases of younger children, and level of interest for older children [3]. For example, preschool children feel that death is not permanent and they may be most concerned with parental separation or physical pain; those in school understand that death is permanent and are most upset about being different than their peers; and adolescents have a more adult view of the irreversibility of death and are concerned about loss of control and independence [4]. The authors briefly summarize what is known about children's understanding of death, and demonstrate that lack of adequate communication increases the distress experienced by dying children.

Table 1
Diagnostic criteria for depression and anxiety disorders

Major depressive disorder	Characterized by the presence of depressed mood or anhedonia for 2 or more weeks, associated with symptoms such as weight change, sleep disturbance, psychomotor agitation or retardation, fatigue, feelings of worthlessness or guilt, decreased concentration, or recurrent thoughts of death or suicidal ideation.
Dysthymia	A less acute disorder than MDD. Chronically depressed or irritable mood that lasts for at least 1 year with at least two of the following: change in appetite, sleep disturbance, fatigue, low self-esteem, poor concentration, and feelings of hopelessness.
Generalized anxiety disorder	Excessive worry for a period of at least 6 months. The worry is not specific to a circumstance or one event or type or event (hence "generalized"). In children, this anxiety is accompanied by neurovegetative symptoms such as restlessness, fatigue, difficulty concentrating, irritability, muscle tension, and disturbed sleep.
Anxiety disorder due to a general medical condition	A disorder where the anxiety is due to the direct physiologic effects of a general medical condition or its treatment. Symptoms can include generalized anxiety symptoms, panic attacks, or obsessions/compulsions, and it must be evident from the history, physical, or laboratory findings that the disturbance is the direct physiologic consequence of a general medical condition.
Adjustment disorder with anxiety or depressed mood	A response to an identifiable stressor that results in the development of clinically significant emotional or behavioral symptoms after the onset of the stressor. Distress is marked and is in excess of what would be expected. A reaction to a stressor that might be considered normal or expected can still qualify for a diagnosis of adjustment disorder if the reaction is sufficiently severe to cause significant impairment.
Posttraumatic stress disorder	Re-experiencing symptoms ("flashbacks"), avoidance of reminders of the stressor, and heightened anxiety after being exposed to an emotionally traumatic event. These symptoms should be present for at least 1 month before the diagnosis can be entertained. ("Acute stress disorder" is the designation for a similar constellation of symptoms in the immediate aftermath of traumatic exposure).

Adapted from American Psychiatric Association. Diagnostic and statistical manual of mental disorders: text revision. 4th edition. Washington, DC: American Psychiatric Association; 2000.

It was thought originally that children with life-limiting illness do not understand death and should be shielded from prognosis, disease progression, and decisions at the end of life because this information would be harmful to them. However, early studies demonstrated that healthy children consider death and have organized thought about this process, progressing through stages of understanding [5]. Current information suggests that a complete understanding of the concept of death is achievable by 8 years of age. The irreversibility, universality, and finality of death are understood between ages 5 and 7 [6]. Withholding information about death is not in the child's best interest, and lack of communication about death increases children's fears and anxiety [7,8]. Furthermore, children who are not being given information about their illness nevertheless systematically learn about their disease in predictable stages that begin with the understanding that their illness is serious, and over time they comprehend that relapses can result in death. These stages are determined by their experiences, not by age or cognitive ability, so a 4-year-old child may understand more about a disease and prognosis than a 10 year-old [9]. Later studies demonstrated that dying children know more about their disease than expected, when one is considering the type of information given to them [10–12]. In addition, children were found to be aware of the significance of their illness, to be more distressed than controls, and to sense isolation from family.

Failure to establish effective communication between patients/families and caregivers influences the development of symptoms of distress in the patient [13]. An ideal time to establish communication is at diagnosis, so patients are able to trust their providers throughout the illness [14,15]. The "day 1 talk" and the "final stage conference" are examples of including the patient and the family in open communication at the beginning of the illness, and when the child is unresponsive to further therapy. Other, more general, methods of communication have been described and include engaging the child at a time of struggle, exploring the child's current knowledge and level of information desired, empathizing with the child's reaction, and allowing the child to understand that the physician role includes listening to his/her concerns and serving as a support [13].

Prevalence of symptoms of distress in children at the end of life

No large epidemiologic studies specifically evaluate the prevalence of depressive symptoms or anxiety disorders in children at the end of life [1,16,17]. However, data exist regarding the presence of physical and general psychologic symptoms of distress of dying children [18,19]. Theunissen and colleagues [18] administered a questionnaire to 32 parents of children in palliative care. Thirteen of forty-five items questioned symptoms of distress. The mean number of symptoms was 3.2 per child. The most common symptoms were sadness, difficulty talking about feelings, fear of being alone, loss of perspective, and loss of independence. Drake and colleagues [19] evaluated the symptoms of 30 children in the last week of life using the Memorial Symptom Assessment Scale (MSAS). One half the subjects rated their degree of distress as "quite a bit/very much" and 14% and 10% of subjects reported nervousness or worry, respectively. It may be difficult to generalize this information because the samples were small and the data from one study were derived from parental recall of psychologic symptoms of their dying children (as opposed to direct evaluation of these symptoms). Even so, the data suggest that a subset of children who experience distress exists and that it would be important for their physicians to recognize and treat these symptoms.

Diagnostic considerations

It is hard to tell the difference between medically ill children who are sad, anxious, depressed, or panicked. In fact, the diagnosis of mental health symptoms, especially "internalizing" ones (ie, depression and anxiety) has been shown to be suboptimal in medically ill patients [2]. The difficulty with recognition may stem from patient and physician factors. Physical symptoms associated with a psychiatric disorder may be attributed to the illness or the treatment. Physicians may think that feelings of depression and anxiety are a normative response in the setting of palliative care and therefore overlook them [20]. Perhaps owing to the lack of clarity about what constitutes a normal reaction versus a psychiatric disorder, a survey of pediatric oncologists found that this group is less comfortable with the management of mental health symptoms than they are with the management of physical symptoms [21]. Furthermore, a recent study evaluating pediatric oncology staff assessment of depression and anxiety in adolescent cancer patients found that this group underestimates psychosocial symptoms [22]. Parent and clinician underestimation of patient depression has also been found in other pediatric populations with chronic illness [23].

What can clinicians do to distinguish between normal sadness and true depression? First and foremost, experience is important. Familiarity with the general course of an illness can inform a decision about whether a given child's symptoms are expected or excessive (given the norm) [24]. Also, specific training workshops for the purpose of developing interviewing and communication skills have succeeded in increasing physician awareness and in teaching medical providers to identify adult patients with psychologic difficulty [25–27]. Pediatricians might benefit from a similar intervention.

With regard to specific symptom recognition, symptoms of anhedonia (lack of interest in pleasurable activities) are considered to be more specific to the diagnosis of depression in medically ill patients and are less influenced by medical status [28]. The use of standardized screening measures is also an option. It was originally thought that self-report screening measures, which are sometimes used in the general pediatric population, were invalid in chronically ill patients [29–31]. However, the Children's Depression

Inventory (CDI) and other similar measures have been evaluated in medically ill children and were found to be reasonably accurate in predicting depression and distress [23,32–34].

Another option for assessment is the MSAS, which has been used in pediatric cancer patients as young as 7 [35,36]. This scale and the CDI are best viewed as measures of distress, rather than specific measures of depression in this population. If items regarding sadness or worries suggest that the patient is symptomatic, this may prompt the physician to consider a more specific evaluation. Clinician-rated assessment scales or measures can be reserved for patients who display prominent symptoms or who are identified by a screening self-report instrument. These measures include structured interview tools (ie, Children's Depression Rating Scale) and semistructured interviews (Schedule for Affective Disorders and Schizophrenia for School-Age Children, Present and Lifetime version) [37,38].

No tools specifically assess anxiety in the pediatric palliative care setting. However, the CDI and the MSAS have a few items that relate to general worry. These items would not be sufficient to make the diagnosis of an anxiety disorder, but may direct the provider to consider more focused diagnostic testing. The only self-report instrument targeting symptoms of a specific anxiety disorder for which validity data are available in medically ill children is the UCLA Posttraumatic Stress Disorder Reaction Index, which assesses symptoms of posttraumatic stress [39]. However, its performance was far from ideal in this group [40]. Other self-report measures include the Spence Children's Anxiety Scales, the Screen for Child Anxiety Related Emotional Disorders and the Multidimensional Anxiety Scale for Children, although none have been validated in chronically ill children [41–43]. Validated diagnostic interviews include the Anxiety Disorders Interview Schedule for Children and the Schedule for Affective Disorders and Schizophrenia for School-Age Children [38,44]. For children younger than 8, the interviews are primarily for the caregivers; however, developmentally appropriate assessments in younger children have been reported [45].

Several general principles are worthy of consideration when evaluating children in palliative care for psychiatric morbidity [46]. First, it is critical to establish open communication among the physician, patient, and family because the general reactions of family and others around the child significantly impact that child's mental state [3]. Second, it is important to consider various comorbid psychiatric disorders that can co-occur with, or present in a similar way as, anxiety or depressive disorders in youth [45]. Finally, understanding the child's developmental level and comprehension of his/her illness may inform a better understanding of the context and severity of the symptoms.

The previous section discussed the psychiatric symptoms of distress, including depression and anxiety, together. In the following section, the authors emphasize issues that may be unique or more characteristic of depression or anxiety alone.

Depression

Definition

Several depressive disorders may be encountered in children at the end of life. All result in impaired social and academic functioning. The most common include major depressive disorder, dysthymia, and adjustment disorder with depressed mood. Symptom duration for a major depressive disorder is at least 2 weeks. Dysthymia is less severe (but can be as debilitating) and is defined by a chronically depressed or irritable mood over a longer period of time. An adjustment disorder with depressed mood is characterized by a response to an identifiable stressor that is associated with clinically significant change in emotion or mood in excess of what would be expected normally. Relevant definitions paraphrased from the DSM-IV are shown in Table 1 [47]. Prominent symptoms differ by age group. Because younger children may not be able to describe their symptoms clearly, diagnosis of a depressive disorder in these patients relies more heavily on observable behavior such as temper tantrums. On the other hand, older children might be able to report, like adults, lower self-esteem, guilt, hopelessness, and suicidal ideation.

Management

No studies specifically evaluate treatment for depression in children at the end of life. The authors briefly review the principles of psychotherapeutic and psychopharmacologic therapy for depression in youth, describe the available data on the management of depression in chronically ill children, and suggest a general treatment approach for these patients.

Psychotherapy

Although no data exist regarding the impact of psychotherapy on end-of-life pediatric patients who have anxiety and depression, it is possible that some of the benefits of psychotherapy to medically healthy children might be applicable to this population. A recent meta-analysis of 35 studies reviewed the effects of psychotherapy (cognitive or noncognitive, such as family therapy, group therapy, interpersonal psychotherapy, relaxation training, role playing) for depression in healthy children and adolescents [48]. The mean effect size for the overall effect of psychotherapy on youth depression was 0.34, or a small-medium treatment effect. The use of cognitive-behavioral therapy in the management of physical symptoms has been studied in medically ill patients and has been shown to decrease nausea, fatigue, insomnia, and pain [46,49]. It is quite possible that improved physical symptom control decreases depression and anxiety.

Anecdotal evidence suggests that psychotherapy can be helpful for some patients in addressing anticipatory grief, loss of identity, loss of control, anger, jealousy of siblings, and patient-family conflicts at the end of life [4,50].

Psychopharmacotherapy

The use of medication for depression in adults with cancer has had some success. However, published experience is limited regarding the use of anti-depressants, including selective serotonin reuptake inhibitors (SSRIs), in the pediatric oncology population [51–53]. Only one study examined the safety of an SSRI in a small number of medically ill children; it demonstrated that it was safe and well tolerated, but stopped short of concluding that it was also effective [53]. In healthy children, concern about the safety of SSRIs, especially related to suicidal risk, led to a "black box" warning by the Food and Drug Administration (FDA) (www.fda.gov). Furthermore, most SSRIs have not demonstrated efficacy in randomized clinical trials, with the exception of fluoxetine, which has shown efficacy in three studies [54]. Until more data are available, most SSRIs should be regarded as experimental and unproven treatments for depression in youth, and especially in medically ill children. Dying children have complex medical issues and may be vulnerable to medication side effects and drug–drug interactions. Therefore, the use of additional, potentially nonhelpful medications should be considered with caution.

Stimulants such as methylphenidate and dextroamphetamine have been used to counteract sedation secondary to opiates and for the treatment of depression in medically ill adults, but have not been studied for these indications in children [55,56]. The rapid onset and short half-life may be helpful in the palliative care setting, but potential disadvantages include exacerbation of anxiety, anorexia, and cardiovascular side effects. Tricyclic antidepressants are often used for neuropathic pain in adult and pediatric cancer patients [57,58]. Given the narrow therapeutic window, potential for cardiac toxicity, lowering of the seizure threshold, and interaction with other medications (ie, fluconazole), the authors would not recommend their routine use for depression in children [59].

General approach to the palliative care patient who has depression

If the medical team diagnoses symptoms of depression in a palliative care patient, it is prudent to consult the psychosocial team if they are not already evaluating the patient. In the opinion of the authors, if a psychiatric disorder is present, safety (ie, lack of suicidal ideation) should be assessed and addressed first. Second, an assessment of psychosocial risks might identify areas in which the team may be able to focus specific treatment efforts (ie, lack of contact with a primary caretaker who can be brought into the picture). The next line of treatment, if available and applicable to the specific case, should be a trial of either cognitive behavioral therapy (CBT) or supportive psychotherapy. Some psychotherapeutic approaches (such as those aimed at procedural pain and distress) have a fair amount of empiric support, but many others have not been examined extensively in medically ill children [60]. However, even the psychotherapeutic interventions that were not extensively studied are probably the safest among the other potential options, and therefore should be tried first. If psychotherapy appears to be ineffective, an SSRI can be considered because this is the safest class of antidepressant medication, and some safety data in medically ill children are emerging [53]. However, their use has a number of caveats.

First, SSRIs take several weeks to work and are better suited for ongoing, not emergent, therapy. Second, the patient and family must be presented with the risks and benefits of SSRI therapy. They should be informed that the use of these medications has only been examined in a small number of patients in this setting, they may lead to an increased risk of suicidality, and they are not more effective than placebo, with the exception of fluoxetine. If a medication is going to be used off-label, the rationale for this approach should be reviewed with the family. Third, patients should be adequately screened for a family history of bipolar disorder because antidepressants are thought to play a role in precipitating manic episodes in this patient group [61]. Fourth, the close monitoring recommended by the FDA includes evaluating patients for possible worsening of depression or suicidality at the beginning of therapy and at times of dose adjustment to determine if drug discontinuation or dose modification is required. To that, in medically ill patients, should be added close monitoring of biologic indices such as liver function testing, and drug level monitoring for other medications that are administered concomitantly with the SSRI. Some palliative care patients are seen less often in the clinic (they may be treated primarily at home), so a provider needs to be in close contact with the family or performing home visits to evaluate the patient. Health care providers should be attentive and instruct families to be alert for symptoms including anxiety, agitation, panic attacks, insomnia, irritability, hostility, impulsivity, akathisia, hypomania, and mania because these may be a precursor for worsening of depression or suicidal impulses. Fifth, clinicians who are prescribing SSRIs must be aware of a serious complication: the "serotonin syndrome," which can manifest with nausea, fever, tachycardia, tachypnea, sweating, and agitation, in addition to more severe symptoms including confusion, coma, seizures, hallucinations, hyperthermia, and hypertension [62]. Clinical management necessitates stopping the medication and providing life-support. The 5H2 antagonists (cyproheptadine, chlorpromazine, and ketanserin) may also be useful [63].

Suicidality and requests for euthanasia

Suicidal wishes and suicidal ideation may occur in dying patients, whether or not they are prescribed an SSRI [64]. Brief thoughts about hastening death are common in adults; however, persistent requests in the palliative care setting are unusual and should prompt a psychiatric evaluation [65]. Patients most likely to request or attempt suicide are adolescents, and they may have other risk factors, including a history of attempted suicide, a clear plan of suicide, family history of depression or suicidality, comorbid psychiatric illness, intractable pain, insomnia, lack of social support, inadequate coping skills, recent improvement in depressive symptoms, and impulsivity [66]. Only one retrospective study specifically evaluates suicidality in cancer patients on therapy [67]. Over a 17-year period, clinicians at a large institution identified 10 patients with suicidal events, of which 4 were on therapy. Most patients had advanced illness and inadequate pain management. Psychosocial risk factors such as depression and hopelessness, stressful family events such as divorce, illness, or financial pressures were present in most. Although this study has limitations, it does imply that attempted suicide does not occur often, and suicide does not appear to be a common coping strategy during the dying process.

As described in the American Academy of Pediatrics Consensus Statement on Palliative Care for Children, a request for euthanasia from a child or adolescent must be handled in an empathic manner with the goal of reviewing the sources of distress, which could include a concern about abandonment, depression, loneliness, physical symptoms, and difficulty with communication [68]. Furthermore, the choice of the patient or family to discontinue life-sustaining medical treatment under these circumstances is not equivalent to euthanasia or suicide and must be distinguished as such. These requests are often short-lived if they are followed by compassionate and competent palliative care focusing on improving symptom management and communication efforts.

Anxiety

Definition

Anxiety disorders that may be seen at the end of life include

1. Generalized anxiety disorder, which denotes a heightened level of anxiety in general
2. Specific phobia, which denotes anxiety related to a specific circumstance
3. Anxiety disorder due to a general medical condition, which denotes anxiety symptoms that are caused by a biologic effect of the medical condition or its treatment
4. Posttraumatic stress disorder, which is a specific response to a stressor that may be related to the illness or its treatment
5. Adjustment disorder with prominent symptoms of anxiety, which is also a disorder that is related to the presence of an identifiable stressor

Relevant definitions paraphrased from the DSM-IV are shown in Table 1 [47]. It can be difficult to distinguish a full-blown anxiety disorder from fear or worry secondary to life circumstances. Knowledge of the developmental differences in presentation can be helpful. Younger children often have specific worries relating to separation, strangers, loud noises, and injury, whereas the concerns of adolescents are more abstract [45]. Subclinical symptoms can include overconcern about competence, increased need for reassurance, fear of the dark, concern about harm to self or parent, and somatic complaints [66].

Anxiety in the palliative care setting

Early work by Spinetta and colleagues demonstrated that children with life-limiting illness had symptoms of anxiety [10–12]. In the early 1970s, this group found that children with leukemia related significantly more stories preoccupied with bodily threat and integrity, when compared with normal children [11]. They also demonstrated that, compared with controls, children at the end of life expressed greater general anxiety and decreased adaptability, resulting in escalating anxiety over subsequent outpatient visits [12]. However, these studies were conducted before the acceptance of the new nomenclature for psychiatric illnesses (*Diagnostic and Statistical Manual of Mental Disorders, Third Edition* [DSM-III, 1983]). Therefore, their results cannot be interpreted easily in the context of the newly defined psychiatric disorders referred to in this article. A number of issues can contribute to the development of anxiety, and include uncontrolled or worrisome physical symptoms, being away from home, potential separation from caregivers, parental reaction, fear of death, and lack of adequate communication of relevant information [66].

Management

Psychotherapy

Variations of cognitive-behavioral approaches have been used in the treatment of anxiety disorders in children, including systematic and prolonged exposure to situations causing anxiety for the alleviation of post-traumatic stress symptoms [69]; cognitive restructuring; and improvement of coping mechanisms by teaching relaxation, problem solving, assertiveness, and stress management [45]. Trauma-focused psychotherapy to alleviate distress in medically ill patients has recently been described in adults [70] and children [71], but its efficacy has not been established. Different approaches may be helpful for each developmental level [72].

Psychopharmacotherapy

Psychotropic medications have not been studied for the treatment of anxiety disorders in children in the palliative care setting. However, the safety of benzodiazepine (BDZ) medications has, in fact, been established in children because these agents are being used for the induction of conscious sedation [73,74] and in the treatment of seizure disorders [75]. A retrospective study reported an increase in morphine and BDZ use in the last 3 days of life in children with cancer [76]. The investigators conclude that the increased use of these medications is related to neuropathic pain; however, it is much more likely that the increase in BDZ use is related to agitation and anxiety [77]. The authors briefly summarize studies evaluating BDZs, SSRIs and tricyclic antidepressants in the treatment of anxiety disorders.

Although safety has been established, studies that evaluated the efficacy of BDZ for pediatric anxiety disorders have reported mixed results [78–80]. Because of the paucity of data and the fact that dependence can result from long-term use, they are usually not chosen as a long-term treatment [81].

In treating palliative care patients clinically, BDZs such as lorazepam or diazepam ameliorate symptoms of anxiety in the short-term because they have a rapid onset of action and are fairly safe. They are most helpful for conscious sedation in painful procedures, for insomnia, and sometimes for general anxiety [82]. Disadvantages include sedation, delirium in patients who have central nervous system involvement, and withdrawal if not tapered upon discontinuation. The authors caution against the use of BDZ for long-term treatment.

SSRIs have been studied in a number of anxiety disorders in children [78,83]. These agents are particularly helpful in obsessive-compulsive disorders [84]. SSRIs have been suggested as helpful in the treatment of panic disorder, but no randomized clinical trials have been conducted in this setting [78,83]. Both sertraline and paroxetine have been found to be effective in the treatment of posttraumatic stress disorder in adults [85], but SSRIs have not been rigorously evaluated for this indication in children.

Tricyclic antidepressants are not used commonly for the initial treatment of pediatric anxiety disorders, except in obsessive-compulsive disorders where clomipramine is effective and approved by the FDA. Because of its purported ability to block the formation of traumatic memories, propranolol has been evaluated for the prevention of posttraumatic stress disorder symptoms in a small group of adults [86] and in one small study in children [87]. Until more data are available, the authors do not recommend the use of tricyclic antidepressants or propranolol in the palliative care setting because of concerns about serious side effects.

In the authors' opinion, the short-term use of medications for the treatment of various anxiety disorders in children is justified and can constitute a valid alternative to psychotherapy. SSRIs and BDZs may be used cautiously, given the potential for side effects and dependency (BDZ only) (Table 2).

Psychotherapy, pharmacotherapy, or both?

Because excellent psychotherapeutic treatment options for anxiety disorders exist (see earlier discussion), the authors recommend psychotherapy (CBT) as a first line of treatment in dying patients whenever a qualified therapist is available and patients are motivated. If CBT is not possible (ie, a therapist is not available), or is not likely to be helpful (ie, a child with cognitive deficits), a medication may be considered. For short-term, acute treatment, or for short-term prevention of symptoms (ie, right before

Table 2
Medications commonly used for the treatment of pediatric anxiety disorders

Medication	FDA-approval (for any indication) from age	Dose (oral route)
BDZs		
Lorazepam	12 years	0.5–6.0 mg/day
Diazepam	6 months	1.0–2.5 mg/dose, 3–4 times a day, for older children
Oxazepam	12 years	10–30 mg three times a day (adolescents)
SSRIs		
Fluoxetine	18 years	10–80 mg/day
Fluvoxamine	8 years[a]	25–200 mg/day
Paroxetine	18 years	20–50 mg/day
Sertraline	6 years[a]	25–200 mg/day
Citalopram	18 years	20–40 mg/day

[a] Pediatric use is approved only for the treatment of obsessive-compulsive disorder.

a painful procedure), a short-acting BDZ is preferred. For more generalized anxiety and longer treatment duration, an SSRI may be considered.

Few studies have looked at the sequential use of psychologic and pharmacologic therapy for anxiety in children, but some data regarding combination therapy exist [88,89]. For patients who have obsessive-compulsive disorders, combination treatment with sertraline and CBT were superior in the short-term, compared with sertraline or CBT alone [90]. Additionally, CBT, with or without imipramine, was evaluated in a randomized, controlled trial of adolescents with school refusal, depression, and anxiety, and the combination was shown to improve depressive symptoms more than CBT alone [91]. Although combination treatment therefore seems to be a promising avenue, more information is needed before this approach can be recommended routinely in the palliative care setting.

General approach for the treatment of anxiety disorders in the palliative care setting

Anxiety disorders are a heterogeneous group of disorders with several potential causes and remedies. In medically ill children, it is likely that the anxiety is caused, or at least exacerbated, by a stressor. Hence, an important task in management is to try to identify the stressor and, if possible, minimize it. Thus, alleviating pain and discomfort, anticipating the anxiety that follows a painful procedure and trying to prepare the patient for it, and ensuring that the parent's own anxiety is addressed may all be very effective approaches to reducing anxiety symptoms in the child. The use of relaxation techniques (a part of many standard CBT treatments), when applicable, may be helpful in specific circumstances. The judicious use of medications to alleviate pain, induce sedation when appropriate, or reduce anxiety in stressful situations may also be helpful. Finally, for the few patients who are found to be suffering from a full-blown anxiety disorder, prompt referral is advisable. Medical care providers should realize that most anxiety disorders are treatable; it is therefore important to screen for them, identify them, and refer or treat promptly.

Summary

   The principles of an integrated and ideal model of pediatric chronic illness and palliative care include the consideration, assessment, prevention, and management of symptoms of distress, depression, and anxiety in the entire family [2,68,92,93]. As described, several options exist for the treatment of anxiety and depression in children. At the end of life, appreciation of the child's understanding of death, clear and open communication with the child and family, and the alleviation of distress can significantly improve the patient's, and the family's, quality of life. Treatment should be at least attempted; it is as unacceptable to allow patients to suffer from psychiatric symptoms at the end of life as it is to refrain from treating their pain. A clear understanding of the issues involved in screening and diagnosis, and the benefits and risks associated with each treatment modality, can lead to a rational approach to the diagnosis and management of depression and anxiety in this setting.

References

 [1] Wolfe J, Grier HE, Klar N, et al. Symptoms and suffering at the end of life in children with cancer. N Engl J Med 2000;342(5):326–33.
 [2] Gothelf D, Cohen IJ. Pediatric palliative care. N Engl J Med 2004;351(3):301–2 [author reply 301–2].
 [3] Lewis M. Dying and death in childhood and adolescence. In: Lewis M, editor. Child and adolescent psychiatry. 2nd edition. Baltimore (MD): Williams & Wilkins; 1996. p. 1066–73.
 [4] Sourkes B. Psychotherapy with the dying child. In: Chochinov H, Breitbart W, editors. Handbook of psychiatry in palliative medicine. New York: Oxford University Press; 2000. p. 265–72.
 [5] Nagy M. The child's theories concerning death. J Genet Psychol 1948;73:3–27.
 [6] Stevens MM, et al. Psychological adaptation of the dying child. In: Doyle D, Hanks G, Cherny N, editors. Oxford textbook of palliative medicine. 3rd edition. Oxford (UK): Oxford University Press; 2004. p. 798–806.
 [7] Waechter E. Children's awareness of fatal illness. Am J Nurs 1971;71:1168–72.
 [8] Waechter E. Children's reactions to fatal illness. In: Krulik T, Holaday B, Martinson I, editors. The child and family facing life-threatening illness. Philadelphia: J.B. Lippincott Company; 1972. p. 108–19.
 [9] Bluebond-Langer M. The private worlds of dying children. Princeton (NJ): Princeton University Press; 1978.
[10] Spinetta JJ. The dying child's awareness of death: a review. Psychol Bull 1974;81(4):256–60.
[11] Spinetta JJ, Rigler D, Karon M. Anxiety in the dying child. Pediatrics 1973;52(6):841–5.
[12] Spinetta J, Maloney L. Death anxiety in the outpatient leukemic child. Pediatrics 1975;56(6): 1034–7.
[13] Beale EA, Baile WF, Aaron J. Silence is not golden: communicating with children dying from cancer. J Clin Oncol 2005;23(15):3629–31.

[14] Mack JW, Grier HE. The day one talk. J Clin Oncol 2004;22(3):563–6.

[15] Nitschke R, Meyer WH, Sexauer CL, et al. Care of terminally ill children with cancer. Med Pediatr Oncol 2000;34(4):268–70.

[16] Postovsky S, Ben Arush MW. Care of a child dying of cancer: the role of the palliative care team in pediatric oncology. Pediatr Hematol Oncol 2004;21(1):67–76.

[17] Hinds PS, Schum L, Baker JN, et al. Key factors affecting dying children and their families. J Palliat Med 2005;8(Suppl 1):S70–8.

[18] Theunissen JM, Hoogerbrugge PM, van Achterberg T, et al. Symptoms in the palliative phase of children with cancer. Pediatr Blood Cancer 2007;49(2):160–5.

[19] Drake R, Frost J, Collins JJ. The symptoms of dying children. J Pain Symptom Manage 2003;26(1):594–603.

[20] Block SD. Assessing and managing depression in the terminally ill patient. ACP-ASIM End-of-Life Care Consensus Panel. American College of Physicians—American Society of Internal Medicine. Ann Intern Med 2000;132(3):209–18.

[21] Hilden JM, Emanuel EJ, Fairclough DL, et al. Attitudes and practices among pediatric oncologists regarding end-of-life care: results of the 1998 American Society of Clinical Oncology survey. J Clin Oncol 2001;19(1):205–12.

[22] Hedstrom M, Kreuger A, Ljungman G, et al. Accuracy of assessment of distress, anxiety, and depression by physicians and nurses in adolescents recently diagnosed with cancer. Pediatr Blood Cancer 2006;46(7):773–9.

[23] Shemesh E, Annunziato RA, Shneider BL, et al. Parents and clinicians underestimate distress and depression in children who had a transplant. Pediatr Transplant 2005;9(5):673–9.

[24] Shemesh E, Yehuda R, Rockmore L, et al. Assessment of depression in medically ill children presenting to pediatric specialty clinics. J Am Acad Child Adolesc Psychiatry 2005;44(12):1249–57.

[25] Passik SD, Donaghy KB, Theobald DE, et al. Oncology staff recognition of depressive symptoms on videotaped interviews of depressed cancer patients: implications for designing a training program. J Pain Symptom Manage 2000;19(5):329–38.

[26] Maguire P, Booth K, Elliott C, et al. Helping health professionals involved in cancer care acquire key interviewing skills—the impact of workshops. Eur J Cancer 1996;32A(9):1486–9.

[27] Fallowfield L, Jenkins V, Farewell V, et al. Efficacy of a cancer research UK communication skills training model for oncologists: a randomised controlled trial. Lancet 2002;359(9307):650–6.

[28] Shemesh E, Bartell A, Newcorn JH. Assessment and treatment of depression in medically ill children. Curr Psychiatry Rep 2002;4(2):88–92.

[29] Canning EH, Kelleher K. Performance of screening tools for mental health problems in chronically ill children. Arch Pediatr Adolesc Med 1994;148(3):272–8.

[30] Phipps S, Srivastava DK. Approaches to the measurement of depressive symptomatology in children with cancer: attempting to circumvent the effects of defensiveness. J Dev Behav Pediatr 1999;20(3):150–6.

[31] Harris ES, Canning RD, Kelleher KJ. A comparison of measures of adjustment, symptoms, and impairment among children with chronic medical conditions. J Am Acad Child Adolesc Psychiatry 1996;35(8):1025–32.

[32] Yang YM, Cepeda M, Price C, et al. Depression in children and adolescents with sickle-cell disease. Arch Pediatr Adolesc Med 1994;148(5):457–60.

[33] Kuttner M, Delamater A, Santiago J. Learned helplessness in diabetic youths. J Pediatr Psychol 1990;15:581–94.

[34] Kovacs M. Children's Depression Inventory (CDI). New York: Multi-Health Systems, Inc.; 1992.

[35] Collins JJ, Byrnes ME, Dunkel IJ, et al. The measurement of symptoms in children with cancer. J Pain Symptom Manage 2000;19(5):363–77.

[36] Collins JJ, Devine TD, Dick GS, et al. The measurement of symptoms in young children with cancer: the validation of the Memorial Symptom Assessment Scale in children aged 7–12. J Pain Symptom Manage 2002;23(1):10–6.

[37] Poznansky E, Mokros H. Children's Depression Rating Scale–Revised (CDRS-R). Los Angeles: Western Psychological Services; 1995.

[38] Kaufman J, Birmaher B, Brent D, et al. Schedule for affective disorders and schizophrenia for school-age children–present and lifetime version (K-SADS-PL): initial reliability and validity data. J Am Acad Child Adolesc Psychiatry 1997;36(7):980–8.

[39] Rodriguez N, Steinberg A, Pynoos R. UCLA Post traumatic stress disorder reaction index for DSM-IV, child, adolescent and parent versions. Los Angeles (CA): University of California; 1998.

[40] Shemesh E, Annunziato RA, Newcorn JH, et al. Assessment of posttraumatic stress symptoms in children who are medically ill and children presenting to a child trauma program. Ann N Y Acad Sci 2006;1071:472–7.

[41] Spence SH. A measure of anxiety symptoms among children. Behav Res Ther 1998;36(5):545–66.

[42] Birmaher B, Khetarpal S, Brent D, et al. The Screen for Child Anxiety Related Emotional Disorders (SCARED): scale construction and psychometric characteristics. J Am Acad Child Adolesc Psychiatry 1997;36(4):545–53.

[43] March J. Multidimensional Anxiety Scale for Children (MASC). North Tonawanda (NY): Multi-Health Systems Inc.; 1997.

[44] Silverman WK, Nelles WB. The anxiety disorders interview schedule for children. J Am Acad Child Adolesc Psychiatry 1988;27(6):772–8.

[45] Lyneham HJ, Rapee RM. Evaluation and treatment of anxiety disorders in the general pediatric population: a clinician's guide. Child Adolesc Psychiatr Clin N Am 2005;14(4):845–61, x.

[46] Steif BL, Heiligenstein EL. Psychiatric symptoms of pediatric cancer pain. J Pain Symptom Manage 1989;4(4):191–6.

[47] Diagnostic and statistical manual of mental disorders: text revision. 4th edition. Washington, DC: American Psychiatric Association; 2000.

[48] Weisz JR, McCarty CA, Valeri SM. Effects of psychotherapy for depression in children and adolescents: a meta-analysis. Psychol Bull 2006;132(1):132–49.

[49] Poltorak DY, Benore E. Cognitive-behavioral interventions for physical symptom management in pediatric palliative medicine. Child Adolesc Psychiatr Clin N Am 2006;15(3):683–91.

[50] Sourkes B. Psychotherapy. In: Holland J, editor. Psycho-oncology. New York: Oxford University Press; 1998. p. 946–53.

[51] Kersun LS, Kazak AE. Prescribing practices of selective serotonin reuptake inhibitors (SSRIs) among pediatric oncologists: a single institution experience. Pediatr Blood Cancer 2006;47(3):339–42.

[52] Porrteus A, Ahmad N, Tobey D, et al. The prevalence and use of antidepressant medications in pediatric cancer patients. J Child Adol Psychopharm 2006;16(4):467–73.

[53] Gothelf D, Rubinstein M, Shemesh E, et al. Pilot study: fluvoxamine treatment for depression and anxiety disorders in children and adolescents with cancer. J Am Acad Child Adolesc Psychiatry 2005;44(12):1258–62.

[54] Whittington CJ, Kendall T, Fonagy P, et al. Selective serotonin reuptake inhibitors in childhood depression: systematic review of published versus unpublished data. Lancet 2004;363(9418):1341–5.

[55] Wilwerding MB, Loprinzi CL, Mailliard JA, et al. A randomized, crossover evaluation of methylphenidate in cancer patients receiving strong narcotics. Support Care Cancer 1995;3(2):135–8.

[56] Pereira J, Bruera E. Depression with psychomotor retardation: diagnostic challenges and the use of psychostimulants. J Palliat Med 2001;4(1):15–21.

[57] Collins JJ, Kerner J, Sentivany S, et al. Intravenous amitriptyline in pediatrics. J Pain Symptom Manage 1995;10(6):471–5.

[58] Berger A, Dukes E, Mercadante S, et al. Use of antiepileptics and tricyclic antidepressants in cancer patients with neuropathic pain. Eur J Cancer Care (Engl) 2006;15(2):138–45.

[59] Robinson RF, Nahata MC, Olshefski RS. Syncope associated with concurrent amitriptyline and fluconazole therapy. Ann Pharmacother 2000;34(12):1406–9.

[60] Kazak AE. Evidence-based interventions for survivors of childhood cancer and their families. J Pediatr Psychol 2005;30(1):29–39.

[61] Cheung AH, Emslie GJ, Mayes TL. The use of antidepressants to treat depression in children and adolescents. CMAJ 2006;174(2):193–200.

[62] Mills KC. Serotonin syndrome. A clinical update. Crit Care Clin 1997;13(4):763–83.

[63] Isbister GK, Buckley NA. The pathophysiology of serotonin toxicity in animals and humans: implications for diagnosis and treatment. Clin Neuropharmacol 2005;28(5): 205–14.

[64] Wolf S. Assisted suicide and euthanasia in children and adolescents. In: Emanual L, editor. Regulating how we die: the ethical, medical and legal issues surrounding assisted suicide. Cambridge (UK): Harvard University Press; 1998. p. 92–119.

[65] Block SD, Billings JA. Patient requests for euthanasia and assisted suicide in terminal illness. The role of the psychiatrist. Psychosomatics 1995;36(5):445–57.

[66] Stuber M, Bursch B. Psychiatric care of the terminally ill child. In: Chochinov H, Breitbart W, editors. Handbook of psychiatry in palliative medicine. New York: Oxford University Press; 2000. p. 255–64.

[67] Kunin H, Patenaude A, Grier HE. Suicide risk in pediatric cancer patients: an exploratory study. Psychooncology 1995;4(2):149–55.

[68] American Academy of Pediatrics. Committee on Bioethics and Committee on Hospital Care. Palliative care for children. Pediatrics 2000;106(2 Pt 1):351–7.

[69] Cohen J. Practice parameters for the assessment and treatment of children and adolescents with posttraumatic stress disorder. J Am Acad Child Adolesc Psychiatry 1998;37(10 Suppl): 4S–26S.

[70] Shemesh E, Koren-Michowitz M, Yehuda R, et al. Symptoms of posttraumatic stress disorder in patients who have had a myocardial infarction. Psychosomatics 2006;47(3): 231–9.

[71] Shemesh E, Lurie S, Stuber ML, et al. A pilot study of posttraumatic stress and nonadherence in pediatric liver transplant recipients. Pediatrics 2000;105(2):E29.

[72] Compton SN, March JS, Brent D, et al. Cognitive-behavioral psychotherapy for anxiety and depressive disorders in children and adolescents: an evidence-based medicine review. J Am Acad Child Adolesc Psychiatry 2004;43(8):930–59.

[73] Averley PA, Lane I, Sykes J, et al. An RCT pilot study to test the effects of intravenous midazolam as a conscious sedation technique for anxious children requiring dental treatment— an alternative to general anaesthesia. Br Dent J 2004;197(9):553–8 [discussion: 549].

[74] Hosey MT. UK national clinical guidelines in paediatric dentistry. Managing anxious children: the use of conscious sedation in paediatric dentistry. Int J Paediatr Dent 2002;12(5): 359–72.

[75] McIntyre J, Robertson S, Norris E, et al. Safety and efficacy of buccal midazolam versus rectal diazepam for emergency treatment of seizures in children: a randomised controlled trial. Lancet 2005;366(9481):205–10.

[76] Dougherty M, DeBaun MR. Rapid increase of morphine and benzodiazepine usage in the last three days of life in children with cancer is related to neuropathic pain. J Pediatr 2003; 142(4):373–6.

[77] Berde C, Wolfe J. Pain, anxiety, distress, and suffering: interrelated, but not interchangeable. J Pediatr 2003;142(4):361–3.

[78] Waslick B. Psychopharmacology interventions for pediatric anxiety disorders: a research update. Child Adolesc Psychiatr Clin N Am 2006;15(1):51–71.

[79] Simeon JG, Ferguson HB, Knott V, et al. Clinical, cognitive, and neurophysiological effects of alprazolam in children and adolescents with overanxious and avoidant disorders. J Am Acad Child Adolesc Psychiatry 1992;31(1):29–33.

[80] Graae F, Milner J, Rizzotto L, et al. Clonazepam in childhood anxiety disorders. J Am Acad Child Adolesc Psychiatry 1994;33(3):372–6.

[81] Witek MW, Rojas V, Alonso C, et al. Review of benzodiazepine use in children and adolescents. Psychiatr Q 2005;76(3):283–96.

[82] Spiegel L. Pediatric psychopharmacology. In: Holland J, editor. Psycho-oncology. New York: Oxford University Press; 1998. p. 954–61.

[83] Reinblatt SP, Walkup JT. Psychopharmacologic treatment of pediatric anxiety disorders. Child Adolesc Psychiatr Clin N Am 2005;14(4):877–908, x.

[84] Flament MF, Geller D, Irak M, et al. Specificities of treatment in pediatric obsessive-compulsive disorder. CNS Spectr 2007;12(2 Suppl 3):43–58.

[85] Opler LA, Grennan MS, Opler MG. Pharmacotherapy of post-traumatic stress disorder. Drugs Today (Barc) 2006;42(12):803–9.

[86] Pitman RK, Sanders KM, Zusman RM, et al. Pilot study of secondary prevention of post-traumatic stress disorder with propranolol. Biol Psychiatry 2002;51(2):189–92.

[87] Famularo R, Kinscherff R, Fenton T. Propranolol treatment for childhood posttraumatic stress disorder, acute type. A pilot study. Am J Dis Child 1988;142(11):1244–7.

[88] Klein RG, Koplewicz HS, Kanner A. Imipramine treatment of children with separation anxiety disorder. J Am Acad Child Adolesc Psychiatry 1992;31(1):21–8.

[89] Fluvoxamine for the treatment of anxiety disorders in children and adolescents. The Research Unit on Pediatric Psychopharmacology Anxiety Study Group. N Engl J Med 2001; 344(17):1279–85.

[90] Cognitive-behavior therapy, sertraline, and their combination for children and adolescents with obsessive-compulsive disorder: the Pediatric OCD Treatment Study (POTS) randomized controlled trial. JAMA 2004;292(16):1969–76.

[91] Bernstein GA, Borchardt CM, Perwien AR, et al. Imipramine plus cognitive-behavioral therapy in the treatment of school refusal. J Am Acad Child Adolesc Psychiatry 2000; 39(3):276–83.

[92] Himelstein BP, Hilden JM, Boldt AM, et al. Pediatric palliative care. N Engl J Med 2004; 350(17):1752–62.

[93] Kazak AE. Pediatric Psychosocial Preventative Health Model (PPPHM): research, practice and collaboration in pediatric family systems medicine. Fam Syst Health 2006;24(4):381–95.

Management of Common Neurologic Symptoms in Pediatric Palliative Care: Seizures, Agitation, and Spasticity

Courtney J. Wusthoff, MD, Renée A. Shellhaas, MD, Daniel J. Licht, MD*

Division of Child Neurology, The Children's Hospital of Philadelphia, 6th Floor Wood Building, 34th and Civic Center Boulevard, Philadelphia, PA 19104, USA

Palliative care increasingly is recommended throughout treatment for a variety of illnesses, including those for which cure remains possible or even likely [1,2]. This is emphasized in guidelines issued by the Royal College of Paediatrics and Child Health, which identify four groups of conditions as particularly appropriate for palliation. The first group is life-threatening diseases for which curative treatment is possible but might fail, such as cancer. The second group is conditions with long periods of treatment devoted to prolonging life, with premature death still possible. An example is muscular dystrophy. The third is progressive conditions without curative treatments, such as mucopolysaccharidosis. The last group, and perhaps the one relevant to the greatest number of children, is conditions with severe neurologic disability. Although not progressive in themselves, these conditions put children at risk for unpredictable critical illness and death. Examples are brain or spinal cord injuries and severe cerebral palsy [3]. Primary neurologic disease affects many children in each of these categories. Considering cerebral palsy alone, of the approximately 2 in 1000 children known to have cerebral palsy at 12 months of age, 15% die before age 7 [4]. Secondary neurologic illnesses affect even more children. These include a variety of conditions, such as seizures in the setting of infection or motor agitation in the last days of life. When taken as a whole, the need for pediatric palliative care

---

Dr. Licht is supported by grant 1K23NS052380 from the National Institute of Neurological Disorders and Stroke.

* Corresponding author.
E-mail address: licht@email.chop.edu (D.J. Licht).

for neurologic symptoms is significant. As illustrated in the following cases, among the most common of these symptoms are seizures, agitation, and spasticity.

Seizures

> JF is a 16-year-old boy who has had relapsed nasopharyngeal carcinoma. He came to the emergency department via ambulance after his brother found him unresponsive, lying on the floor, with clonic jerking of the face, arms, and legs. The episode lasted 8 minutes, after which it took JF several hours to return to his baseline mental status. Serum electrolytes and cerebrospinal fluid studies did not reveal a cause for his seizure. A brain MRI demonstrated, however, extension of the tumor to the extradural space surrounding his left temporal lobe.

Many children who require end-of-life care experience seizures, as part of a primary neurologic illness, as part of an overwhelming systemic illness (chronic or acute), as a metabolic derangement (eg, hypo/hypernatremia or hypoglycemia), or as a reflection of disease progression (eg, cerebral metastases). Seizures are an indication of central nervous system disease and typically cause significant stress on patients and families. Parents who have witnessed a child convulsing commonly state they believed their child was dying and that they never want to see their child have another seizure [5,6]. Patients are more likely to express the fear of future mental handicap, embarrassment about losing control of consciousness during a seizure, and especially bladder or bowel function in front of friends and family [7].

When considering how to treat this distressing symptom, the following systematic approach may be helpful:

1. Confirm that the events of concern are epileptic seizures. Conditions in children that mimic seizures include syncope (eg, breath holding spells, vasovagal syncope, and cardiac arrhythmias), gastroesophageal reflux, transient ischemic attacks or strokes, complicated migraines, tics or other dyskinesias, behavioral events (eg, tantrums or daydreaming), conversion disorders, and parasomnias. Usually, history alone is sufficient, but on occasion a video-electroencephalogram (EEG) may be helpful to confirm the diagnosis.
2. Determine if the seizures are provoked. Common provoking factors include fever, electrolyte abnormalities (eg, hypoglycemia, hyponatremia, hypernatremia, hypocalcemia, or hypomagnesemia), central nervous system infection, and acute head trauma.
3. Describe the clinical features of the episode from the beginning (aura) to the end (postictal state). Look for signs of focal onset, including any type of aura, focal twitching, posturing, or sensory phenomena, such as dysesthesias or visual or auditory symptoms. Determine the degree

of responsiveness during the episode. Note the duration of the seizure. Describe clinical manifestations of the postictal state, such as transient focal weakness.

4. If the episode is nonconvulsive (ie, staring, behavioral arrest, or unresponsiveness), try to distinguish between focal seizures with altered awareness (complex partial seizures) and generalized nonconvulsive seizures (absence seizures). Focal seizures with altered awareness often have a postictal state, whereas generalized nonconvulsive seizures usually do not. Also, complex partial seizures typically are longer and occur less frequently than absence seizures. Most palliative care patients have focal-onset seizures. Some may have pre-existing primary generalized epilepsy, however, which is treated with a different set of medications than focal seizures.

5. Assess for any clear precipitating factors, such as sleep deprivation or medication changes (additions or withdrawals). Note anything predictable about the timing of the seizures: Do they always occur during sleep or within a few minutes of awakening? Because the unpredictability of seizures is anxiety provoking, identification of a reliable trigger can be helpful to patients and families.

6. Determine the frequency of seizures and their impact on physical health (injuries and hospitalizations) and psychosocial well-being (embarrassment of seizures in public places, anxiety over the next seizure, and stress on the family).

Although advanced seizure classification is beyond the scope of this article, as alluded to previously, it is important to clarify whether or not a patient has generalized or partial-onset seizures. If there is doubt, a routine EEG may be helpful. Patients who have generalized epilepsy typically have generalized epileptiform patterns on EEG. Patients who have partial-onset seizures may show focal epileptiform discharges on EEG, or the EEG may be normal.

Once a diagnosis of seizure is made, the physician and family must decide whether or not and how to treat this symptom. If a clear provoking factor can be identified, treatment may be straightforward (eg, correction of hypoglycemia by adding glucose to feeds or fluids). If not, and the seizures are interfering with a patient's quality of life, daily antiepileptic drugs (AEDs) likely are indicated.

AEDs can be classified into three categories: narrow spectrum, broad spectrum, and syndrome specific (Table 1) [8–11]. Broad-spectrum AEDs usually are required for generalized or mixed epilepsy syndromes. In general, partial epilepsies may be treated with narrow- or broad-spectrum AEDs. Note that partial seizures with secondary generalization are treated in the same manner as partial seizures without generalization. Syndrome-specific AEDs, such as ethosuximide for absence seizures, typically are required for patients who need palliative care.

Table 1
Antiepileptic drug spectrum of action, site of clearance, effect on hepatic enzymes, dosing formulations, and pediatric dosing ranges

Antiepileptic drug	Spectrum of action[a]	Site of clearance hepatic induction or inhibition	Pediatric friendly formulation	Initial dose (mg/kg/d)	Range of maintenance dose[b] (mg/kg/d)	Reference range for serum level (mg/L)
Carbamazepine (Tegretol, Tegretol XR, Carbatrol)	Narrow	• >95% hepatic • Inducer	Chewable tablets (100 mg) Suspension (100 mg/5 mL) Extended-release sprinkle capsule (100, 200, or 300 mg)	• 5–10	• 15–40	• 4–12[c]
Clobazam (Frisium)	Broad	• Hepatic		• <2 y: 0.5–1 • 2–16 y: 5 mg/d	• Maximum 40 mg/d	• Not available
Clonazepam (Klonopin)	Broad	• Hepatic	Orally disintegrating wafers (0.125, 0.25, 0.5, 1, or 2 mg)	• 0.01	• 0.1–0.2	• Not available
Gabapentin (Neurontin)	Narrow	• 100% renal • None		• 30–40 1 months–3 y • 10–20 3–12 y	• 30–100	• 2–12
Lamotrigine (Lamictal)	Broad	• 90% hepatic • None	Chewable tablet (2 mg, 5 mg, or 25 mg)	• Monotherapy: 0.5 for 2 weeks, then increase by 1 every 1–2 weeks • Added to VPA: 0.15 for 2 weeks, then 0.3 for 2 weeks, then increase by 0.3 every 1–2 weeks • Added to enzyme-inducing AED: with inducer: 0.6 for 2 weeks, then 1.2 for 2 weeks, then increase by 1.2 every 1–2 weeks	• With VPA: 1–5 • Monotherapy or with inducer: 5–20	• 4–20
Levetiracetam (Keppra)	Broad	• 66% renal • None	Suspension (500 mg/5 mL)	• 10–20	• 30–90	• 5–40
Oxcarbazepine (Trileptal)	Narrow	• 45% renal • 45% hepatic	Suspension (300 mg/5 mL)	• 8–10	• 30–50	• 12–30

Drug	Spectrum[a]	Clearance	Formulations	Starting dose	Maintenance dose[b]	Level
Phenobarbital	Broad	• 75% hepatic • 25% renal • Inducer	Suspension (20 mg/5 mL)	• 2–5 neonates • 3–7 children	• 2–5 neonates • 3–7 children	• 15–40[c]
Phenytoin (Dilantin)	Narrow	• >90% hepatic • Inducer	Chewable tablets (50 mg) Suspension (125 mg/5 mL)	• 4–5	• 4–8	• 10–20[c] • Free level 0.5–3
Pregabalin (Lyrica)	Narrow	• 100% renal • None		• Adult (150 mg/d)	• Adult maximum (600 mg/d)	• Not available
Topiramate (Topamax)	Broad	• 30%–50% hepatic • 50%–70% renal	Sprinkle capsule (15 mg, 25 mg)	• 1–3	• 2–15 (higher for infantile spasms)	• 4–10
Valproate (Depakote, Depakene)	Broad	• >95% hepatic • Inhibitor	Sprinkle capsule (125 mg) Suspension (250 mg/5 mL)	• 15	• 15–60	• 50–130[c]
Zonisamide (Zonegran)	Broad	• Hepatic and renal clearance	Capsule only, powder is freely soluble in water or apple juice	• 2–4	• 8–12 (higher for infantile spasms)	• 15–40

Note—extended-release and sprinkle formulations are not intended for use with enteral feeding tubes; choose liquid or dispersible formulations instead.

Abbreviations: VPA, valproic acid, Depakote.

[a] Narrow-spectrum AEDs are used for partial-onset seizures only and may exacerbate generalized epilepsies. Broad-spectrum AEDs can be used for partial and generalized-onset seizures.

[b] For some patients, the usual maintenance dose may not be sufficient. AED dosing should be titrated individually for each patient according to efficacy and tolerability.

[c] Indicates AED levels that typically are available with rapid turnaround. The others may not be available or may take days to receive results.

Data from Refs. [8–11].

In addition to the spectrum of action, certain AEDs have clear advantages and disadvantages, depending on a patient's situation (Table 2) [8,12]. Special consideration of children's other medical conditions and symptoms, such as pain, anxiety, mood disorder, and level of alertness, clearly is important.

Selection of an AED also depends on a medicine's formulation—Is a child able to swallow liquid, sprinkles, or pills, or does he need medication to be administered via gastrostomy tube, rectally, or intravenously (IV) (see Table 1)? Immediate-release tablets can be crushed, dissolved in water, and given via feeding tubes. Extended-release preparations, however, should not be crushed, and sprinkle formulations clog feeding tubes and stick to bottles or cups. In general, liquid AEDs can be given rectally, if necessary. In addition, IV formulations of certain medications are available and may be used interchangeably with enteral formulations in children who have IV access who cannot tolerate or absorb enterally administered medications (eg, levetiracetam, 200 mg orally, is equal to levetiracetam, 200 mg IV). Dosing guidelines are listed in Table 1.

For children who have recurrent seizures, physicians and caregivers must plan for the possibility of status epilepticus. Enabling caregivers to initiate treatment of prolonged or repetitive seizures can improve outcome or decrease anxiety and may prevent visits to an emergency department [13]. Several abortive therapies are available. The one used most widely is rectal diazepam gel (Diastat), although intranasal and buccal midazolam increasingly are prescribed. A study comparing rectal diazepam and buccal midazolam shows that midazolam may be more effective in treating status epilepticus than rectal diazepam [14]. Both medications, however, remain good options in the appropriate clinical settings. Although there are theoretic risks to administering rectal diazepam or intranasal/buccal midazolam outside a hospital setting, these medications seem safe when used according to prescribing guidelines (Table 3) [15,16]. The risk for respiratory compromise is smaller with rectal diazepam than with IV administered formulations of the same medication, because absorption is slower and peak concentrations remain lower [16].

In addition to the safety and efficacy of abortive AEDs used in a home setting, there is an additional benefit of empowerment of the caregiver. A study of childhood epilepsy patients demonstrated that education about seizures and about the administration of the rescue medication for status epilepticus may reduce standardized measures of parental stress significantly [13].

In some cases, patients continue to have breakthrough seizures despite an appropriate AED selection. In this situation, an assessment of the seizures' impact on patient and family is essential. For some children, occasional simple partial seizures may be tolerated better than the sedative effects of multiple AEDs. For others, this is not the case. Addition of a second agent may be warranted, in consultation with a neurologist. In addition, just as rescue medication should be available for children in case of prolonged of

Table 2
Advantage and disadvantages of specific antiepileptic drugs

Drug	Advantages	Disadvantages
Carbamazepine (Tegretol, Tegretol XR, Carbatrol)	• Possible mood stabilization • Sustained-release formulation • Readily available blood levels	• Bone marrow suppression • Idiosyncratic leukopenia and aplastic anemia • May be sedating initially • Hepatic enzyme inducer • May aggravate generalized epilepsies • No IV formulation • Rash and hypersensitivity reactions
Clobazam (Frisium)	• Fewer cognitive side effects than other benzodiazepines	• Not approved for use in the United States
Clonazepam (Klonopin)	• Available as orally disintegrating wafer • Effective treatment for anxiety	• Sedation and cognitive effects • Increased drooling
Gabapentin (Neurontin)	• Well tolerated • Rapid escalation if needed • Effective treatment for neuropathic pain	• 3 times per day dosing • Weight gain • No IV formulation
Lamotrigine (Lamictal)	• Favorable central nervous system profile (not sedating) • Twice-daily dosing • Possible mood stabilization	• Slow titration (8 weeks or more) • Interaction with VPA (VPA increases LTG levels) • Rash and hypersensitivity reactions • May exacerbate myoclonic epilepsy • No IV formulation
Levetiracetam (Keppra)	• Well tolerated, usually not sedating • Twice-daily dosing • Rapid titration if needed • No drug interactions • IV formulation • Liquid may be given rectally	• May exacerbate behavioral problems • Renal dosing required
Oxcarbazepine (Trileptal)	• Twice-daily dosing • Possible mood stabilization • Well tolerated • Effective treatment for neuropathic pain	• Can cause hyponatremia • Rash and hypersensitivity reactions • May exacerbate generalized epilepsy • No IV formulation • Possible bone marrow suppression
Phenobarbital	• IV formulation • Can quickly load and bolus • Long half-life • Readily available blood levels	• Sedation • Hyperactivity in younger children • Cognitive concerns • Hepatic enzyme inducer • Rash and hypersensitivity reactions

(*continued on next page*)

Table 2 (*continued*)

Drug	Advantages	Disadvantages
Phenytoin (Dilantin)	• IV formulation • Can quickly load and bolus • Long half-life • Readily available blood levels	• Hepatic enzyme inducer • Unpredictable pharmacokinetics at higher dosages • Difficult to maintain therapeutic levels using oral dosing in infants • Rash and hypersensitivity reactions, especially in combination with radiation therapy
Pregabalin (Lyrica)	• Twice-daily dosing • Effective against neuropathic pain • Possibly effective against bone pain	• No pediatric-friendly formulation • Not FDA approved for children
Topiramate (Topamax)	• Twice-daily dosing • Effective for migraine prevention • Mild diuretic • May reduce intracranial pressure	• Adverse cognitive effects, especially word-finding difficulties • Weight loss • Metabolic acidosis • Renal stones, hypohydrosis • Rare acute angle closure glaucoma • No IV formulation
Valproate (Depakote, Depakene)	• IV formulation • Can quickly load and bolus • Possible mood stabilization • Effective for migraine prevention • Once-daily dosing with extended-release formulation • Readily available blood levels	• Idiosyncratic reactions (pancreatitis, hepatic failure especially in children under 2 years old who have polypharmacy) • Dose-related thrombocytopenia • Weight gain • Tremor, hair loss • Links to polycystic ovarian syndrome • High protein binding • Hepatic enzyme inhibitor
Zonisamide (Zonegran)	• Freely soluble in water Once or twice daily dosing	• Similar to Topiramate, though milder and only at higher doses.

Abbreviations: LTG, Lamotrigine, Lamictal; VPA, valproic acid, Depakote.

Data from Sullivan J, Dlugos D. Antiepileptic drug monotherapy: pediatric concerns. Semin Pediatri Neurol 2005;12:88–96 and Sander J. The use of antiepileptic drug—principles and practice. Epilepsia 2004;45(Suppl 6):28–34.

Table 3
Doses of antiepileptic drugs used for control of acute repetitive or prolonged seizures (status epilepticus)

Patient's age	Rectal diazepam[a]	Intranasal or buccal midazolam[b]
2 to 5 years	0.5 mg/kg/dose	0.5 mg/kg/dose
6 to 11 years	0.3 mg/kg/dose	0.5 mg/kg/dose
12 years and older	0.2 mg/kg/dose	0.5 mg/kg/dose
Maximum dose	20 mg	10 mg

[a] Because of the available dosing formats for Diastat (10-mg or 20-mg syringe, programmed to specified dose by the pharmacist), rectal diazepam doses should be rounded to the nearest 2.5 mg.

[b] Liquid midazolam is available as 5 mg/mL, supplied in 1-mL or 2-mL vials. Caregiver must draw required dose into syringe and administer in the buccal mucosa or attach an atomizer for intranasal administration.

repetitive seizures, intermittent dosing of additional AEDs may be appropriate for patients who have a "flare" in their seizure frequency. For example, a short course of chlorazepate, given twice per day for 3 to 5 days, during an acute reversible illness may prevent a flurry of seizures in a vulnerable patient. As always, consideration must be given to a patient's level of arousal, ability to take enteral medications, and so forth.

Agitation

RH is a 3-year-old boy who has had severe cerebral palsy and chronic lung disease. After recurrent pneumonias complicated by prolonged sepsis, he now has significant respiratory decompensation. RH's parents recognize he is not likely to recover and wish to focus on his quality of life. Recently they have been frightened by behavioral spells. He cannot communicate with words but has been having sporadic bouts of crying, thrashing, and increased arching for no clear reason. They wonder if he is in pain or having more trouble breathing.

"Agitation" is used to describe collectively several signs and symptoms. In essence, agitation is an unpleasant state of increased arousal. It may present as loud or angry speech, crying, increased muscle tension, increased autonomic arousal (such as diaphoresis and tachycardia), or irritable affect [17,18]. In the early stages, agitation may start as frequent, nonpurposeful motor activity, disturbance in sleep-rest patterns, or an inability to concentrate or relax [19]. Although symptoms of agitation overlap with manifestations of anxiety, agitation is considered to include a greater element of motor, rather than psychologic, symptoms. The term, "terminal restlessness," is used to describe the constellation of agitation with or without delirium, occurring in 25% to 88% of adults at the end of life [19,20]. Frequency of this pattern of symptoms in children is unknown.

Treatment of agitation begins with identification of symptoms, and consideration of possible causes. The following steps are helpful groundwork in managing agitation:

Address possible causes of discomfort, such as pain, dyspnea, muscle tension/spasm, bladder fullness, constipation, and improper positioning. Evaluate for anxiety and situational/environmental stressors.

Evaluate for treatable medical components. For example, symptoms resulting from neuromotor excitation, such as myoclonus or increased nonpurposeful movements, may reflect raised intracranial pressure, renal or hepatic failure, hypercalcemia, cerebral irritation, hypoxia, or hypercapnia. Consider triggers of clinical signs, such as infection, changes in cardiac or respiratory status, and medication effect.

Assess for the presence of delirium. Although pediatric delirium may include an element of agitation, it is characterized further by sleep problems, impaired attention, mood lability, and confusion [21].

Consider mimics, such as movement disorders. Tremor, for example, may not truly reflect agitation but may appear otherwise to some observers. Akathisia is an unpleasant state of motor restlessness or compulsion to move that may appear primarily as "agitation." Exposure to antidopaminergic medications and some opiates and anticonvulsants increases the odds of developing akathisia up to 18 times in adults receiving palliative care [22].

Review medications. Identify agents that might cause akathisia, such as antidopaminergics. Consider possible paradoxic reactions to sedatives or unusual responses to corticosteroids. Autonomic signs may result from adrenergic medications, such as albuterol. Certain opiates, such as hydromoprhone, cause myoclonus or symptoms of agitation in up to a third of hospice patients [23]. Finally, withdrawal from alcohol, anticonvulsants, clonidine, corticosteroids, opioids, nicotine, and sedative-hypnotics all also can cause agitation.

Nonpharmaceutical treatment of agitation

Initial management of agitation almost always is nonpharmaceutical. Intuitively and appropriately, caregivers attempt to soothe children through gentle touch or with a calming voice. Familiar objects from home may provide comfort. Frequent reminders of orientation, such as a bulletin board or calendar, may help older children who are experiencing confusion or delirium. Unfortunately, agitation may continue despite these measures. In cases in which a child is in danger of self-harm, such as when agitated movements might dislodge a central line or a tracheal airway, physical restraints may be indicated. These have the advantage of immediately protecting the child without sedation. The minimal amount of restraint needed should be used, such as solely covering one arm with a soft "no-no" to prevent removal of a line. Judicious use of selective measures can be preferable to additional medication, although the appropriateness of these measures must be evaluated carefully in discussion with families.

Pharmaceutical treatment of agitation

Nonpharmaceutical treatments have minimal side effects and interactions but may be insufficient treatment for agitation. For many, the addition of a medication is required for symptom management. Largely because of the multifactorial nature of agitation, there is disagreement as to the drug of choice. Furthermore, most recommendations are based on experience in treating adults who have severe or life-limiting illness or in managing behavior problems for children who have other medical problems. Unfortunately, there are no prospective, randomized trials to study the use of pharmacologic agents for the treatment of agitation in the end of life in adults or children. The medications used most commonly for these groups are benzodiazepines and antipsychotics, although other sedatives sometimes are used. These are described later and summarized in Tables 4–6 [24–33].

Benzodiazepines

Benzodiazepines are central nervous system depressants, acting via modulation of γ-aminobutyric acid (GABA) signaling. Because of their effects on arousal and anxiety, many prefer benzodiazepines for treating agitation in pediatric palliative care [34]. Although not as well studied for agitation in terminally ill children, benzodiazepines are recommended for agitation and "terminal restlessness" in adult palliative care [35,36]. Furthermore, these medications are recommended for anxiolysis, amnesia, and sedation in various settings for children [37–39]. Benzodiazepines have the advantage of prior experience in the very ill and in children, with well-described dosing, risks, and side effects (see Table 4). Benzodiazepines generally are fast-acting and effective sedatives; most also have anterograde amnesic properties.

Drawbacks of benzodiazepines result primarily from their sedative effects. These medicines can decrease alertness and induce sleep in many children, which may be unacceptable for some families. Dose-related respiratory depression, especially in combination with opioids, can limit use. In severe cases, a benzodiazepine may be cautiously reversed with flumazenil. Risks for chronic benzodiazepine use include habituation and physical dependence. Finally, in some children, paradoxic reactions of worsened agitation and hyperactivity, or even delirium, may occur with these medications. Treatment decisions must balance these possible benefits and drawbacks in terms of the goals of care for individual children.

When choosing an agent in this class and a dose, titrate to the minimally effective duration of sedation with an adequate dose to treat a patient's level

Table 4
Benzodiazepines in the treatment of agitation

Drug	Dose	Duration	Advantages	Cautions
Midazolam	By mouth: 0.2–0.75 mg/kg up to 20 mg IV: 0.025–0.1 mg/kg every 2–4 h up to 6 mg/d Infusions range 0.03–0.12 mg/kg/h titrated to effect SC, intranasal (IN), buccal, and rectal dosing is reported	Peak effect: 30–60 min IV; 10 min IN Duration: IM 2–6 h; IN 1 h	• Onset of action within 1–5 min IV, 10–20 min orally • Multiple routes of administration available • Metabolite half-life 3–12 h • 3–4 times as potent as diazepam • Used widely in pediatric palliative care [24] • Evidence for efficacy in pediatric and adult palliation [25–27]	• Higher risk for respiratory depression than other benzodiazepines • Side effects may include hypotension, respiratory depression, drowsiness, dizziness • Up to 8% of neonates have myoclonus as a side effect • Liquid has a low pH and can cause burning when given nasally; buccal administration seems better tolerated [28]
Lorazepam	By mouth/IV/intramuscularly: 0.025 mg/kg/dose up to 2 mg every 4–8 h up to 0.1 mg/kg/dose	8–24 h	• Onset of effect within 60 min orally, 30 min IV • Less hypotension than midazolam	• Side effects may include hypotension, respiratory depression, drowsiness, dizziness

Drug	Dose	Half-life	Comments	Side effects
				• Neurotoxicity and myoclonusis reported in neonates
Diazepam	By mouth: 0.12–0.8 mg/kg/d divided every 6–12 h up to 10 mg/dose Intramuscularly/IV: 0.05–0.2 mg/kg/dose every 6–12 h up to 0.6 mg/kg every 8 h Rectal preparation has been given at 0.5 mg/kg/dose for anticonvulsant uses	12–24 h	• More predictable clearance in renal/hepatic impairment than diazepam • No active metabolite • Used widely in pediatric palliative care [24] • Used commonly for a variety of pediatric indications • Onset of effect almost immediate when given IV • Used widely in pediatric palliative care [24]	• Reports of pain and high rates of thrombophlebitis at injection site when given IV [44] • Side effects may include hypotension, respiratory depression, drowsiness, dizziness • Active metabolites with half-life up to 100 h
Clonazepam	By mouth: 0.01 mg/kg/d divided up to 4 times a day, increase to effect, maximum of 0.2 mg/kg/d divided 3 times a day or 20 mg/d	6–8 h	• Onset of effect 20–60 min • Pediatric experience in safety as anticonvulsant	• Side effects may include hypotension, respiratory depression, drowsiness, dizziness • Metabolite half-life up to 50 h

Table 5
Neuroleptics in the treatment of agitation

Drug	Dose	Advantages	Cautions
Haloperidol	By mouth: 0.01–0.03 mg/kg every day up to maximum 6 mg/d divided 3 times a day Intramuscularly: 1–3 mg/dose every 4–8 h up to 0.1 mg/kg/d (Not labeled for IV or subcutaneous use, although haloperidol lactate has been given this route)	• Used widely for agitation in critically ill children • Safety and efficacy established as young as 3 y • Evidence for efficacy in seriously ill children [29]	• Significant incidence of extrapyramidal side effects in children
Thioridazine	By mouth: 0.5–3 mg/kg/d divided 2 to 3 times a day	• Fewer extrapyramidal effects than chlorpromazine • Used in children as young as 2 y	• Sedation and anticholinergic side effects common • Extreme caution due to associated side effect of prolonged QTc interval; some suggest checking EKG before starting and on treatment [17].
Chlorpromazine	By mouth: 0.5–1 mg/kg/dose every 4–6 h up to 200 mg/d Intramuscularly/IV: 0.5–1 mg/kg/dose every 6–8 h up to 40 mg/d if <5 y, 75 mg/d 5–12 y Rectal: 1 mg/kg/dose every 6–8 h	• Used widely in children as young as infancy [17] • Less sedating than thioridazine • Antiemetic properties • Evidence for efficacy in adults at end of life [30]	• Side effects may include hypotension, sedation, and tardive dyskinesia • More autonomic effects than newer agents • Extrapyramidal effects are more common in children than adults; although can be treated with antihistamines
Risperidone	By mouth: 0.25–1 mg every 6–12 h	• Fewer extrapyramidal effects at low doses	• Side effects may include hypotension at higher doses

of distress [40]. Short-acting benzodiazepines avoid problems of prolonged sedation or the accumulation of toxic metabolites in the liver. Some patients, however, need longer coverage or a combination of a longer-acting medicine with a shorter-acting agent for acute episodes. Selection of a particular benzodiazepine thus is based largely on pharmacodynamics, with some consideration of availability and agent familiarity [36,41].

Neuroleptics

Neuroleptics, or antipsychotics, are more controversial in treatment of agitation (see Table 5). Through an antidopaminergic mechanism, neuroleptics have treated delirium and psychosis effectively for several decades. Accordingly, many consider neuroleptics the drug of choice for agitation in adults at the end of life [19,35]. Neuroleptics are less sedating and may be useful particularly in patients who cannot take benzodiazepines because of tolerance or respiratory depression. They also may be more helpful when delirium is a prominent feature of agitation [34,42]. Widespread neruoleptic use, however, has been limited by concerns for side effects in children. These include extrapyramidal symptoms, such as dystonia, tardive dyskinesias, neuroleptic malignant syndrome, and lowered seizure threshold. Dystonic reactions occur in up to 10%, especially young men. These generally can be treated with diphenhydramine, given every 30 minutes until symptoms resolve, but are troubling nonetheless. Individual drugs confer different degrees of risk and some unique side effects. The neuroleptics are approximately comparable in efficacy, so these side-effect profiles often dictate the choice of agent [43]. Although neuroleptics are used widely in other pediatric settings, there is a paucity of evidence for their use specifically in children at the end of life. Neuroleptics might be helpful particularly for agitation with features of delirium in palliative care, but their potential benefits must be balanced against their known risks.

Adrenergic agonists and antagonists

β-Adrenergic antagonists (β-blockers) have been used successfully in various settings to treat agitation. Although somewhat sedating, these medicines have a benign side-effect profile, making them appealing for long-term use. They may be useful especially when there is a prominent autonomic component to chronic agitation (see Table 6). Unfortunately, β-blockers generally do not reach full effect for 2 to 6 weeks, making them less useful in an acute setting. The α_2-adrenergic agonist, clonidine, is believed to work through a similar mechanism although with faster results. There is less evidence available to support its use, however.

Other agents for treatment of agitation

When other treatments are insufficient, or contraindicated, several other medications are used for agitation (see Table 6). Barbiturates, such as phenobarbital or pentobarbital, are used for severe cases of agitation refractory to other treatments. They generally are, however, not a first choice as they cause heavy sedation. Chloral hydrate is a sedative-hypnotic with a long history of use in young children. Diphenhydramine and hydroxyzine frequently are used in the management of acute agitation of inpatients who have various medical problems because of their sedative properties and relatively benign side-effect profile [17,40]. Finally, in

Table 6
Other drugs in the treatment of agitation

Drug	Dose	Duration	Advantages	Cautions
Propranolol	By mouth: 0.5 mg/kg/d divided every 6–8 h titrated up to maximum of 5 mg/kg/d IV: 0.01 mg/kg/dose 2–3 times a day	6 h	• Less sedating than benzodiazepines • More benign side-effect profile than neuroleptics • Some effects of beta-blockade are seen within 1 h • Efficacious in akathisia [43] • Evidence for efficacy in cognitively disabled adults and children [17,31,32]	• Hypotension may occur • May take 2–6 weeks to reach full effect • Side effects may include cardiovascular depression, dizziness, sedation
Phenobarbital	By mouth: 2 mg/kg 3 times a day IV/intramuscularly/ subcutaneously: 3–5 mg/kg at bedtime	4–10 h	• Abundant experience with use in children as young as neonates • Onset of action within 5 min when given IV, 20–60 min by mouth • Can test blood levels to assess if in therapeutic/toxic range • Evidence for efficacy at the end of life [33]	• Can cause respiratory depression • Not reversible • More heavily sedating than benzodiazepines • Metabolites with prolonged half-life • Tolerance can develop • Hepatic enzyme inducer

Chloral hydrate	By mouth/rectally: 20–75 mg/kg/d divided 3 times a day	4–8 h	• Oldest sedative agent used in children • Peak effect within 1 h • Less efficacious in children >3 y [37] • Can cause paradoxic excitement
Diphenhydramine	By mouth/IV/intramuscularly: 1 mg/kg/dose every 4–6 h up to 75 mg every 4 h	4–7 h	• Maximum sedative effect 1 h after administration, with gradual onset • Used commonly in children • Anticholinergic side effects, such as dry mouth, dizziness, common
Hydroxyzine	By mouth: 0.6 mg/kg/dose every 6 h Intramuscularly: 0.55–1.1 mg/kg/dose every 4–6 h up to maximum 50 mg for <6 y, 100 mg for >6 y	4–6 h	• Onset of effect within 15–30 min • Side effects may include drowsiness, dizziness, dry mouth • Peripheral IV and subcutaneous routes are used but have a high risk for thrombosis and extravasation
Propofol	IV: low infusion rates of 0.5 mg/kg/h are used for anxiolysis without complete sedation	3–10 min (bolus dose)	• Onset of effect in less than a minute from bolus dose • Rapid emergence, especially when used less than 10 days • Evidence for efficacy at subanesthetic doses in children at the end of life [45] • Can be heavily sedating; may require intubation and mechanical ventilation • Metabolic acidosis with fatal cardiac failure has occurred in pediatric ICU patients • May worsen agitation at higher doses • Not for use <3 y of age

agitation refractory to all other agents, propofol is an option to ensure comfort at the end of life [44,45].

Spasticity

> LM is a 5-year-old girl who has had a progressive metabolic disease. Over the past 2 years, she has had developmental deterioration and worsening spasticity. Her parents hope to spend as much time as possible with her at home but have increasing difficulties in caring for her. Specifically, LM's mother asks about her child's increasing stiffness. This has made dressing her and proper positioning difficult, as her arms and legs no longer move easily. LM's mother worries this is painful and that her joints might become even more restricted with time.

Spasticity is a velocity-dependent increase in resistance to passive muscle stretch. Associated findings include increased tone, hyperactive reflexes, extensor plantar responses, muscle spasm, and lack of motor control and agility [46]. Although spasticity is common, particularly in neurologic disease, it can result from several conditions. Any disease process causing disinhibition of cerebral or spinal motor mechanisms can cause spasticity and rigidity. Thus, not only diseases affecting brain but also illness, such as cancer cell infiltration or mechanical compression of the spinal cord, can result in spasticity. In the most severe cases, spasticity causes rigidity and contractures of the limbs. This can be painful to patients and make the mechanics of caregiving, such as changing and positioning, difficult. Although these consequences make improvement of spasticity desirable, treatment must be adjusted to the needs of individual patients. For some children, removing the stiffness of spasticity may uncover profound underlying weakness. In these cases, a small degree of spasticity actually may be helpful in maintaining extension of lower extremities to allow for weightbearing and mobility [35]. In other cases, as in younger children or of advanced disease, mobility is less of a concern, and maximal reduction of muscle tone is desirable. Treatments must be selected and adjusted according to the goal most important for each child and family.

Nonpharmaceutical treatments of spasticity

Nonpharmaceutical treatments for spasticity should be optimized before adding medication. This includes physical therapy, positioning, and durable medical equipment [47]. Studies of stretching in children who have cerebral palsy show passive stretching increases range of movements and reduces spasticity [48]. These therapies can confer significant benefit without the side effects and interactions inherit in drug treatment.

Pharmaceutical treatments of spasticity

Until recently, central acting muscle relaxants were by far the treatment used most commonly for spasticity in most settings. Baclofen, tizanidine, and dantrolene are used commonly in adults. Although there are some differences in their side-effect profiles, their overall tolerabilites are comparable. Selection of a particular agent often is based on potential side effects and familiarity to the prescriber. As with drugs for anxiety and agitation, the guiding principle is to start at a low dose and titrate gradually to the desired effect. Specific agents are discussed further later and summarized in Table 7 [49,50].

Baclofen

Baclofen is a central acting muscle relaxant (GABA-B agonist), among the agents used most commonly in treating pediatric spasticity. Baclofen is shown efficacious in a variety of settings [51]. Although often sedating, oral dosing is fairly reliable and guidelines for titration are available. Long term, baclofen can be delivered via intrathecal pump to improve spasticity without systemic effects and sedation. This method, however, is used uncommonly in palliative care, as pump placement is a surgical procedure, and substantial benefits generally do not appear until months into slowly titrated therapy [46].

α_2-Adrenergic agonists

Tizanidine, a central α_2-adrenergic agonist, is effective in spasticity in adults [46,51,52]. Furthermore, it has mild antinocicoptive properties via substance P modulation, making it useful in chronic conditions, such as low back pain and tension headaches. There are no clear studies, however, of tizanidine in children who have spasticity [46]. Clonidine is an agent with a similar mechanism to tizanidine; it is used for hypertension, pain, and behavior modification in children. It does have sedating effects for some, although not usually as pronounced as with baclofen or benzodiazepines. Although often used in practice, little data are published regarding clonidine use in children to treat spasticity [53]. Commonly used doses are described, however, and are included in Table 7.

Benzodiazepines

Longer-acting benzodiazepines, such as diazepam and clonazepam, also are used for spasticity. These agents are considered by many as efficacious as other treatments and have the advantage of more extensive experience in children [46,51]. As with all drugs in this class, their use is limited mainly by sedation and the potential for tolerance and dependence. Thus, for children not able to tolerate, or not responsive to baclofen, diazepam and the other benzodiazepines are attractive alternatives.

Dantrolene

Dantrolene has a unique mechanism of action directly on the skeletal muscle rather than in the central nervous system. As such, it has fewer sedating side effects than other muscle relaxants Some experts recommend its use

Table 7
Drugs used in the treatment of spasticity

Drug	Dose	Advantages	Cautions
Baclofen	2–7 y by mouth: start 10 mg/d, increase by 5–15 mg/d every 3 days as needed up to maximum of 40 mg/d divided 3 times a day >8 y: as above to maximum 60 mg/d divided 3 times a day	• Considerable experience in children • Also may ameliorate muscle spasm and dystonia [49] • Excreted primarily by kidneys; useful in hepatic impairment	• Can cause significant sedation • Side effects may include drowsiness, psychiatric disturbance, urinary frequency, retention, constipation, vomiting • Reports of weakness emerging at higher doses [50]
Tizanidine	Dosage not established in children Adult by mouth: initial 2 mg every h, up to 8 mg 4 times a day	• Less likely to cause weakness than baclofen • Less sedating than diazepam • Mild antinociceptive properties	• Not well studied in children • Risk for hepatotoxicity • Side effects include dry mouth, dizziness, fatigue, possible hypotension
Clonidine	By mouth: 3–5 µg/kg/d divided 3–4 times a day. Start 0.05 mg every day, increase every 7 days, up to maximum 0.3 mg/d SR patch: start 0.1 mg/24-h patch, applied weekly, 0.2 mg and 0.3 mg also available	Similar mechanism of action to tizanidine, but more experience with use in children, particularly in attention-deficit/hyperactivity disorder and hypertension	• Not as well studied as tizanidine for spasticity • Can cause significant hypotension • Side effects include dry mouth, dizziness, fatigue
Diazepam	By mouth: 0.12–0.8 mg/kg/d divided every 6–12 h, maximum 10 mg/dose Intramuscularly/IV: 0.05–0.2 mg/kg/dose up to every 6–12 h, maximum 0.6 mg/kg in 8 h	Used widely in children for many years, in ages as young as infancy	• Risk for respiratory depression increased if used in combination with other sedatives • Side effects include drowsiness, dizziness • Tolerance may develop
Dantrolene	>5 y by mouth: start 0.5 mg/kg/d, then increase slowly by 0.5 mg/kg/d at 4–7 day intervals up to maximum 12 mg/kg/d or 400 mg/d divided 2–3 times a day until effective Also available in IV form	Less sedating due to direct action on skeletal muscle	• Not well tested in long-term use • Side effects include muscle weakness, drowsiness, dizziness, diarrhea, malaise, fatigue, hepatotoxicity • Contraindicated in hepatic impairment

Drug	Dosage	Notes	Side effects
Cyclobenzaprine	Dosage not established in children Adult by mouth: 5–10 mg 3 times a day, up to 60 mg/d	Labeled for use in as young as 15 y	• Side effects include drowsiness, dry mouth, dizziness • Agitation may occur at high doses.
Metaxolone	Dosage not established in children Adult by mouth: 400–800 mg 3–4 times a day	Labeled for use in muscle spasm as young as 12 y	• Side effects include drowsiness, dizziness, nausea • May be more useful for spasms than true spasticity [52]
Methocarbamol	Dosage not established in children Adult by mouth: 750–1500 mg 4 times a day up to 3 days, 4500 mg/d maximum maintenance dose Adult IV/intramuscularly: 1 g, may repeat every 8 h up to 3 days		• Not labeled for long-term use at high doses • Side effects include drowsiness, dizziness, gastrointestinal upset
Orphenadrine	Dosage not established in children Adult by mouth: 100 mg twice a day Adult IV/intramuscularly: 60 mg every 12 h	NMDA antagonist; unique mechanism of action may be useful in symptoms refractory to other agents	• Anticholinergic side effects, restlessness, agitation
Carisoprodol	Dosage not established in children Adult by mouth: 350 mg 3–4 times a day		• Side effects include drowsiness, dizziness, ataxia, tremor, gastrointestinal upset • Unreliable metabolism in hepatic impairment • Has potential for abuse

in combination with diazepam and suggest it might be more efficacious than baclofen in children [46].

Other central muscle relaxants

Several other central muscle relaxants used in adults, but not well-studied in children, are included in Table 7 [52]. Because of the paucity of data in the pediatric population, they are not advisable first-line treatments. They might be considered, however, in adolescent patients when other treatments fail.

Botulinum toxin

Intramuscular botulinum toxin is a temporary means of chemodenervation to control spasticity. It is used widely in children who have cerebral palsy. Initially proved efficacious for limited symptoms, botulinum toxin now is used safely and reliably in multiple muscle groups [54,55]. Onset of action is 12 to 72 hours after injection, with duration of effect up to 3 months [46]. Although this is an extremely useful treatment for chronic spasticity, it is not used often in palliative care because of children's preference to avoid intramuscular injection.

Muscle cramps

Although not a direct result of spasticity, painful muscle cramps are a common associated symptom. Treatments (described previously) that have some benefit for cramping are baclofen, tizanidine, dantrolene, diazepam, and botulinum toxin. Although quinine sulfate had been used widely for muscle cramps, in 2006 the Food and Drug Administration (FDA) issued a statement reaffirming the unapproved nature of this practice, stating the risks do not justify the use for this indication. Preliminary reports have suggested cannabinoids might be helpful for cramping secondary to neurologic disease in adults, but further study is needed before use for this indication in children.

Improving the palliation of neurologic symptoms

As described in this section, there are many alternatives for treating neurologic symptoms of children receiving palliative care. Although many options exist, further work is needed to help integrate experience from adult palliative care and general pediatrics into evidence on how to best provide palliation to children.

References

[1] Himelstein BP, Hilden JM, Boldt AM, et al. Pediatric palliative care. N Engl J Med 2004; 350(17):1752–62.

[2] Hain RD. Paediatric palliative medicine: a unique challenge. Pediatr Rehabil 2004;7(2): 79–84.

[3] Association for Children with Life-threatening or Terminal Conditions and their Families. A guide to the development of children's palliative care services. Bristol (London): Royal College of Paediatrics and Child Health; 1997.

[4] Paneth N, Hong T, Korzeniewski S. The descriptive epidemiology of cerebral palsy. Clin Perinatol 2006;33(2):251–67.

[5] van Stuijvenberg M, de Vos S, Tjiang GC, et al. Parents' fear regarding fever and febrile seizures. Acta Paediatr 1999;88(6):618–22.

[6] Baumer JH, David TJ, Valentine SJ, et al. Many parents think their child is dying when having a first febrile convulsion. Dev Med Child Neurol 1981;23(4):462–4.

[7] Arunkumar G, Wyllie E, Kotagal P, et al. Parent- and patient-validated content for pediatric epilepsy quality-of-life assessment. Epilepsia 2000;41(11):1474–84.

[8] Sullivan J, Dlugos D. Antiepileptic drug monotherapy: pediatric concerns. Seminars in Pediatric Neurology 2005;12:88–96.

[9] French J, Gidal B. Antiepileptic drug interactions. Epilepsia 2000;41(Suppl 8):S30–6.

[10] Perucca E, Dulac O, Shorvon S, et al. Harnessing the clinical potential of antiepileptic drug therapy: dosage optimisation. CNS Drugs 2001;15(8):609–21.

[11] Levy RH, Mattson RH, Meldrum BS, et al. Antiepileptic drugs. 5th edition. Philadelphia: Lippincott Williams & Wilkins; 2002.

[12] Sander J. The use of antiepileptic drugs—principles and practice. Epilepsia 2004;45(Suppl 6): 28–34.

[13] O'Dell C, Shinnar S, Ballaban-Gil KR, et al. Rectal diazepam gel in the home management of seizures in children. Pediatr Neurol 2005;33(3):166–72.

[14] McIntyre J, Robertson S, Norris E, et al. Safety and efficacy of buccal midazolam versus rectal diazepam for emergency treatment of seizures in children: a randomised controlled trial. Lancet 2005;366(9481):205–10.

[15] Pellock JM, Shinnar S. Respiratory adverse events associated with diazepam rectal gel. Neurology 2005;64(10):1768–70.

[16] Cloyd JC, Lalonde RL, Beniak TE, et al. A single-blind, crossover comparison of the pharmacokinetics and cognitive effects of a new diazepam rectal gel with intravenous diazepam. Epilepsia 1998;39(5):520–6.

[17] Cummings MR, Miller BD. Pharmacologic management of behavioral instability in medically ill pediatric patients. Curr Opin Pediatr 2004;16(5):516–22.

[18] Houlahan KE, Branowicki PA, Mack JW, et al. Can end of life care for the pediatric patient suffering with escalating and intractable symptoms be improved? J Pediatr Oncol Nurs 2006; 23(1):45–51.

[19] Kehl KA. Treatment of terminal restlessness: a review of the evidence. J Pain Palliat Care Pharmacother 2004;18(1):5–30.

[20] Travis SS, Conway J, Daly M, et al. Terminal restlessness in the nursing facility: assessment, palliation, and symptom management. Geriatr Nurs 2001;22(6):308–12.

[21] Turkel SB, Trzepacz PT, Tavare CJ. Comparing symptoms of delirium in adults and children. Psychosomatics 2006;47(4):320–4.

[22] Gattera JA, Charles BG, Williams GM, et al. A retrospective study of risk factors of akathisia in terminally ill patients. J Pain Symptom Manage 1994;9(7):454–61.

[23] Thwaites D, McCann S, Broderick P. Hydromorphone neuroexcitation. J Palliat Med 2004; 7(4):545–50.

[24] Drake R, Frost J, Collins JJ. The symptoms of dying children. J Pain Symptom Manage 2003;26(1):594–603.

[25] Bottomley DM, Hanks GW. Subcutaneous midazolam infusion in palliative care. J Pain Symptom Manage 1990;5(4):259–61.

[26] Henderson M, MacGregor E, Sykes N, et al. The use of benzodiazepines in palliative care. Palliat Med 2006;20(4):407–12.

[27] Burke AL, Diamond PL, Hulbert J, et al. Terminal restlessness—its management and the role of midazolam. Med J Aust 1991;155(7):485–7.

[28] Weisman SJ. Supportive care in children with cancer. In: Berger A, Portenoy RK, Weissman DE, editors. Principles and practice of supportive oncology. Philadelphia: Lippincott-Raven; 1998. p. 845–51.

[29] Harrison AM, Lugo RA, Lee WE, et al. The use of haloperidol in agitated critically ill children. Clin Pediatr (Phila) 2002;41(1):51–4.

[30] McIver B, Walsh D, Nelson K. The use of chlorpromazine for symptom control in dying cancer patients. J Pain Symptom Manage 1994;9(5):341–5.

[31] Fugate LP, Spacek LA, Kresty LA, et al. Measurement and treatment of agitation following traumatic brain injury: II. A survey of the Brain Injury Special Interest Group of the American Academy of Physical Medicine and Rehabilitation. Arch Phys Med Rehabil 1997;78(9): 924–8.

[32] Fleminger S, Greenwood RJ, Oliver DL. Pharmacological management for agitation and aggression in people with acquired brain injury. Cochrane Database Syst Rev 2006;4: CD003299.

[33] Stirling LC, Kurowska A, Tookman A. The use of phenobarbitone in the management of agitation and seizures at the end of life. J Pain Symptom Manage 1999;17(5):363–8.

[34] Collins JJ. Paediatric palliative medicine: symptom control in life-threatening illness. In: Doyle D, editor. Oxford textbook of palliative medicine. 3rd edition. Oxford (UK): Oxford University Press; 2004. p. 789–98.

[35] Hicks F, Pearse H. Palliative care for people with progressive neurological disorders. In: Faull C, Carter Y, Daniels L, editors. Handbook of palliative care. 2nd edition. Malden (MA): Blackwell Pub.; 2005. p. 256–72.

[36] Good PD, Cavenagh JD, Currow DC, et al. What are the essential medications in palliative care?—A survey of Australian palliative care doctors. Aust Fam Physician 2006;35(4):261–4.

[37] Krauss B. Management of acute pain and anxiety in children undergoing procedures in the emergency department. Pediatr Emerg Care 2001;17(2):115–22.

[38] Kang T, Hoehn KS, Licht DJ, et al. Pediatric palliative, end-of-life, and bereavement care. Pediatr Clin North Am 2005;52(4):1029–46, viii.

[39] Friebert S, Hilden JM. Palliative care. In: Altman AJ, Children's Oncology Group, editors. Supportive care of children with cancer: current therapy and guidelines from the children's oncology group. 3rd edition. Baltimore (MD): Johns Hopkins University Press; 2004. p. 379–96.

[40] Tremblay A, Breitbart W. Psychiatric dimensions of palliative care. Neurol Clin 2001;19(4): 949–67.

[41] Nauck F, Ostgathe C, Klaschik E, et al. Drugs in palliative care: results from a representative survey in Germany. Palliat Med 2004;18(2):100–7.

[42] Miser J, Miser A. Pain and symptom control. In: Armstrong-Dailey A, Goltzer SZ, editors. Hospice care for children. New York: Oxford University Press; 1993. p. 22–59.

[43] Mysiw WJ, Sandel ME. The agitated brain injured patient. Part 2: pathophysiology and treatment. Arch Phys Med Rehabil 1997;78(2):213–20.

[44] Shapiro BA, Warren J, Egol AB, et al. Practice parameters for intravenous analgesia and sedation for adult patients in the intensive care unit: an executive summary. Society of Critical Care Medicine. Crit Care Med 1995;23(9):1596–600.

[45] Hooke MC, Grund E, Quammen H, et al. Propofol use in pediatric patients with severe cancer pain at the end of life. J Pediatr Oncol Nurs 2007;24(1):29–34.

[46] Verrotti A, Greco R, Spalice A, et al. Pharmacotherapy of spasticity in children with cerebral palsy. Pediatr Neurol 2006;34(1):1–6.

[47] Himelstein BP. Palliative care for infants, children, adolescents, and their families. J Palliat Med 2006;9(1):163–81.

[48] Pin T, Dyke P, Chan M. The effectiveness of passive stretching in children with cerebral palsy. Dev Med Child Neurol 2006;48(10):855–62.

[49] Sibson K, Craig F, Goldman A. Palliative care for children. In: Faull C, Carter Y, Daniels L, editors. Handbook of palliative care. 2nd edition. Malden (MA): Blackwell Pub.; 2005. p. 295–316.

[50] Kurent JE. Neurological diseases. In: Taylor GJ, Kurent JE, editors. A clinician's guide to palliative care. Malden (MA): Blackwell Pub.; 2003. p. 104–27.

[51] Chou R, Peterson K, Helfand M. Comparative efficacy and safety of skeletal muscle relaxants for spasticity and musculoskeletal conditions: a systematic review. J Pain Symptom Manage 2004;28(2):140–75.

[52] Smith HS, Barton AE. Tizanidine in the management of spasticity and musculoskeletal complaints in the palliative care population. Am J Hosp Palliat Care 2000;17(1):50–8.

[53] Lubsch L, Habersang R, Haase M, et al. Oral baclofen and clonidine for treatment of spasticity in children. J Child Neurol 2006;21(12):1090–2.

[54] Berweck S, Heinen F. Use of botulinum toxin in pediatric spasticity (cerebral palsy). Mov Disord 2004;19(Suppl 8):S162–7.

[55] Heinen F, Molenaers G, Fairhurst C, et al. European consensus table 2006 on botulinum toxin for children with cerebral palsy. Eur J Paediatr Neurol 2006;10(5–6):215–25.

PEDIATRIC CLINICS

OF NORTH AMERICA

Pediatr Clin N Am 54 (2007) 735–756

Assessment and Management of Fatigue and Dyspnea in Pediatric Palliative Care

Christina K. Ullrich, MD[a,b], Oscar H. Mayer, MD[c,d]

[a]Harvard Medical School, 25 Shattuck Street, Boston, MA 02115, USA
[b]Department of Pediatric Oncology, Children's Hospital Boston,
Dana Farber Cancer Institute, 44 Binney Street, Boston, MA 02115, USA
[c]Division of Pulmonology, 5th Floor Wood Center, The Children's Hospital of Philadelphia,
34th Street and Civic Center Boulevard, Philadelphia, PA 19104, USA
[d]The Pediatric Advanced Care Team, 5th Floor Wood Center, The Children's Hospital
of Philadelphia, 34th Street and Civic Center Boulevard, Philadelphia, PA 19104, USA

Fatigue
Christina K. Ullrich, MD

Fatigue is one of the most prevalent symptoms in patients with life-threatening illness, occurring in more than 75% of adult cancer patients [1,2] and in 81% of adult palliative care patients [3]. Fatigue is the most common symptom in children who have advanced cancer and accounts for the greatest degree of suffering [4–6]. For example, Wolfe and colleagues [6] found fatigue to be the most common symptom in children with advanced cancer in the last month of life, with 96% of children experiencing fatigue and 57% of them suffering significantly from it. In another study, Jalmsell and colleagues [5] reported that of 449 parents of children who had died of cancer, 86% reported that fatigue significantly affected their child's well-being.

According to adult patients who have cancer, fatigue is the most distressing of all the symptoms they experience. Fatigue is a unique symptom in that it can create a combination of profound physical, psychologic, and financial burdens [7]. In the Fatigue II trial of 379 adults undergoing treatment for cancer, 60% ranked fatigue as the symptom impacting their life the most [7]. In pediatrics, a small descriptive study of eight adolescents who had cancer demonstrated that fatigue impacted their physical, social,

Corresponding authors:
Fatigue: Christina K. Ullrich, MD (christina_ullrich@dfci.harvard.edu).
Dyspnea: Oscar H. Mayer, MD (mayero@email.chop.edu).

0031-3955/07/$ - see front matter © 2007 Elsevier Inc. All rights reserved.
doi:10.1016/j.pcl.2007.07.006   *pediatric.theclinics.com*

and psychologic well-being [8]. In adults and children, fatigue may lead to decreased activity, loss of control in a situation that likely already feels out of control, and a sense of loneliness and isolation. Untreated fatigue can impair quality of life and prohibit addressing practical needs, psychosocial and spiritual distress, and opportunities for growth and closure at life's end. To this end addressing fatigue is a crucial component of the provision of effective palliative care.

Impact of fatigue on treatment in patients with life-threatening illness

Concerns regarding fatigue as a side effect of disease-directed or symptom-directed treatment may limit these interventions. As a common opioid dose-limiting side effect, concerns regarding fatigue can also inhibit adequate opioid administration, thereby preventing optimal pain relief [9,10]. In this situation patients and families must choose between well-controlled pain with attendant fatigue, somnolence, and mental clouding, and less sedation, with less impaired interactions with others but at the expense of increased pain. Fatigue is the most common side effect of chemotherapy and radiotherapy [11,12]. In adults, treatment-related fatigue can be severe enough to prevent maximal treatment and disease control [13,14].

Features of fatigue in patients with life-threatening illness

Fatigue is a complex and multifaceted symptom that patients may experience and describe in a wide variety of ways (Box 1). Regardless of the varied characteristics of the experience of fatigue, patients almost universally report that (1) it is not responsive to rest, (2) it is not proportional to activity, and (3) it pervades their life and can serve as a significant source of distress. Cancer-related fatigue is the best-studied type of disease-associated fatigue, particularly in pediatrics. Cancer-related fatigue has been defined by The National Comprehensive Cancer Network (NCCN) as a "distressing persistent, subjective sense of tiredness or exhaustion related to cancer or cancer treatment that is not proportional to recent activity and interferes with usual functioning" [13]. Based on these characteristics it is clear that this kind of fatigue is not the fatigue of everyday life. The toll that fatigue takes on physical, cognitive, and emotional stamina and the degree to which is can impair quality of life can diminish a patient's hope and desire to continue living [7]. Recent studies in adults who have completed treatment for cancer also reveal that fatigue can last for months to years after treatment.

Case study

B.H. is 19-year-old female college student who has osteosarcoma of the humerus. She was treated with intensive chemotherapy and surgery, with

---

Box 1. Manifestations of fatigue

Physical
Weakness
Physical tiring
Heaviness

Cognitive
Mental clouding
Poor concentration
Impaired memory

Emotional
Depression
Apathy
Irritability
Decreased motivation

Energy
Tiredness
Lethargy
Low energy
Decreased endurance

Sleep
Insomnia
Hypersomnia
Somnolence
Nonrestorative sleep

---

remission of her disease, and she resumed her studies at college. She was an excellent student and a star athlete, playing on the varsity soccer team. B.H. was also active in swimming, outdoor activities at school, and her sorority. A pulmonary relapse was detected at the end of the academic year, and she began additional chemotherapy. She was determined to pass her exams during treatment, but found it difficult to concentrate on her studies. She was discouraged by the potential setback of not being able to complete the school year and missed participating in the activities and connections that gave her life such meaning. With tears in her eyes she remarked, "I just can't concentrate and am so tired that I can't get my work done. I try to get extra sleep but it just doesn't help. It's all I can do to get out of bed. I just don't know what's wrong with me...I've never felt like this before...I don't even have energy to be with my friends and I really miss that."

On review of systems, B.H. reported no problems with chest pain in the region of the tumor recurrence that responded well to oxycodone taken as needed. She stated that she slept relatively well, with no difficulties falling asleep or with early morning awakening. On further exploration of her sleeping habits, she stated that the chest pain did awaken her from sleep most nights but she usually tried to "sleep through the pain." B.H. also had chemotherapy-induced nausea and vomiting, which was controlled with an intensive multiagent prophylaxis regimen consisting of ondansetron, lorazepam, metoclopramide, and diphenhydramine. Although she described sadness and frustration regarding her recent relapse, she expressed determination to overcome her illness and remained hopeful that she would return to school.

Physical examination revealed normal vital signs, no cardiac or thyroid abnormalities, and no pallor. She had previously been very muscular, and was notably less so than before. She was able to ambulate independently without difficulty and had a normal neurologic examination. She was alert and oriented, with a normal affect. Laboratory studies included a complete blood count with a hemoglobin of 12 g/dL, normal chemistries and liver function studies, and normal thyroid studies. Based on these findings, a plan was made with BH to address her fatigue.

A clinical approach to the patient with fatigue

Diagnosis and assessment of fatigue

In contradistinction to other symptoms, the impact of fatigue on patients is frequently underappreciated by clinicians. Although oncologists believe that pain adversely affects their patients to a greater degree than fatigue (61% versus 37%), cancer patients felt that fatigue adversely affected their daily lives more than pain (61% versus 19%) [2]. Fatigue also seems to be underrecognized by palliative care physicians. In one study of adults admitted to a palliative care unit, although 96% experienced significant fatigue, only 42% of palliative care physicians noted this symptom in the medical record [15]. This notation is in contrast to the report of pain, which was documented in at least 96% of cases.

Patients, too, rarely broach the topic of fatigue with their care team. Vozelgang [2] found that 50% of patients did not discuss treatment of fatigue with their physicians. In a large multicenter study of 1317 adults who had cancer, 52% of those who had fatigue reported it to their physician [16]. Barriers to discussion between clinicians and patients may include (1) lack of appreciation for its profound effects, in part because of the clinician's lack of experiential reference; (2) a belief that fatigue is "normal" or "to be expected;" (3) a paucity of descriptors for the various manifestations of fatigue; (5) lack of familiarity with options to ameliorate fatigue; (6) system-related problems, such as time pressures or reimbursement difficulties; and (7) a primary focus on disease-directed treatment.

The NCCN provides guidelines for fatigue management in adults and although not intended for fatigue management in children they provide an excellent framework [13]. These guidelines call for screening for fatigue at every visit using a 1 to 10 scale. Such a scale has recently been shown to have good discrimination when compared with a well-validated measure of fatigue, the FACIT-F. Scores between 3 and 5 provided optimal discrimination in diagnosing fatigue [17]. In the pediatric population in general, children 7 years and older can reliably use a 1 to 10 scale, although use for measuring fatigue has never been studied. Regular inquiry regarding a child's experience of fatigue, regardless of the specific screening tool use, may be a first step in increasing awareness of this symptom.

Because fatigue is highly subjective and unique to the individual, we rely on the child's or parent's report to measure and assess it. Several unidimensional and multidimensional scales for fatigue assessment in adults are available. Hockenberry and colleagues [18] have developed instruments for children who have cancer. Three separate instruments were developed to measure fatigue in pediatric oncology patients from the child, parent, and staff perspective. In addition, the PedsQL Multidimensional Fatigue Scale measures child and parent perceptions of fatigue in pediatric patients and has been studied in healthy children and children who have cancer [19].

Hinds and colleagues [20] have found that children tend to conceptualize fatigue as a physical sensation, whereas adolescents alternate or merge the physical concept with mental tiredness. Parents and staff conceptualize fatigue as a symptom that interferes with the child's ability to participate in various activities and may be manifested by physical, emotional, and mental changes. A useful approach to fatigue may be to explore various possible manifestations of fatigue that the child or adolescent and the adult caregiver may identify. Exacerbating and alleviating factors, pattern of fatigue, and the degree to which the symptom is impacting the child's life can then be explored. Investing the time to explore these characteristics may reveal important clues regarding the cause of the fatigue. This is particularly important because few diagnostic tests exist to determine the cause of fatigue.

Factors associated with fatigue

Just as the presentation of fatigue may be varied, so too are the underlying conditions that may contribute to fatigue. Fatigue may stem from multifactorial and interrelated causes, including physical factors, psychosocial factors, and disrupted sleep (Fig. 1). Inroads have been made in the understanding of how and to what degree such factors may play a role in the genesis of fatigue in adults. The likely inciting factors may be categorized into physical and psychosocial factors to simplify the diagnostic process, recognizing that many patients experience fatigue resulting from a combination of factors.

For example, Irvine and colleagues [21] found that in adults undergoing chemotherapy or radiotherapy, fatigue correlated with symptom distress

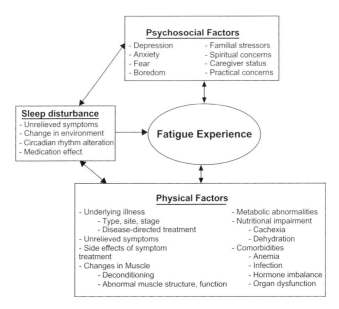

Fig. 1. A conceptual model of fatigue in life-threatening illness.

(based on 13 symptoms) and mood disturbance (defined as depression, anxiety, anger, or confusion). A controlled study of adult patients who had cancer found that fatigue was associated with severity of pain, dyspnea, and psychologic symptoms (anxiety and depression) [1]. One study that also evaluated several sociodemographic factors found that in addition to performance status and depression, the demographic factors of being employed or living alone were significantly associated with the symptom of fatigue in adults [22]. Within the palliative care population, overall symptom distress, depression, anxiety, and performance status are associated with fatigue [23]. There have been no published analyses of objective factors associated with fatigue in the pediatric oncology or palliative care realm.

Physical factors

Physical factors contributing to fatigue include direct effects of the underlying disease and side effects of treatment of the underlying illness. Unrelieved symptoms are also likely to contribute to a patient's fatigue, as are treatments for symptoms such as pain or dyspnea. A thorough examination of the patient's medication list should be undertaken because medications, such as opioids, benzodiazepines, antiemetics, antihistamines, and psychotropic medications, may cause fatigue. Other potential causes, such as infection, organ dysfunction, electrolyte imbalance, dehydration, and nutritional impairment, should also be considered.

Anemia

Anemia is frequently associated with fatigue and impaired quality of life. However, it does not by itself always account for the fatigue observed in patients. In one study, anemia did not fully account for perceived fatigue in adults who had cancer, with pain, dyspnea and sleep disturbance also contributing to fatigue [24]. In the palliative care population, anemia has not been shown to be significantly related to fatigue [25] suggesting that at least in some patients, such as those who have more extensive disease, factors beyond anemia may contribute to fatigue.

Muscle abnormalities

Cachexia (anorexia, weight loss, and muscle wasting) is associated with fatigue. Cytokines believed to mediate cachexia, such as tumor necrosis factor and interleukin-1, may also contribute to the sensation of fatigue [26]. Even in the absence of cachexia, abnormalities in muscle structure and function may lead to fatigue [27]. Finally, prolonged immobility may lead to deconditioning that reduces endurance and produces a sensation of fatigue.

Endocrine dysfunction

Hypothyroidism is associated with fatigue in various patient populations. Alterations in the hypothalamic–pituitary axis have also been proposed as contributors to fatigue [26]. Hypogonadism, which may cause negative mood and cachexia, has also been recently shown to be associated with fatigue [28,29]. The development of fatigue in men undergoing hormonal ablation for prostate cancer further strengthens the association between fatigue and hypogonadism [30].

Psychologic factors

Psychologic factors, such as depression and anxiety, may be contributors or consequences of fatigue. Fatigue (presenting, for example, as lack of motivation and difficulty concentrating) may be a manifestation of depression. Conversely, the limitations caused by fatigue that can result in isolation, loneliness, and decreased work capacity or enjoyment of life may serve as potential contributors to depression. By impairing the ability to accomplish even minor tasks, fatigue may diminish a patient's sense of efficacy and control, thereby contributing to anxiety. Furthermore, existential or spiritual suffering along with practical concerns, such as schoolwork, may contribute to fatigue.

Sleep impairment

Decreased quantity or quality of sleep may stem from physical, emotional, or spiritual distress along with environmental factors, such as sleep disruption for medical care and alteration of sleep architecture by medications. For these reasons and others, sleep disturbance is common in the palliative care population. Among adults admitted to palliative care units, 70%

reported insomnia. Of these patients, 60% cited physical problems as the cause, 37% attributed their insomnia to worry, and 38% felt that improved symptom control would improve their sleep (as opposed to an alternative intervention, such as a hypnotic) [31]. Sleep deprivation may worsen other factors, such as unrelieved physical or emotional distress, further exacerbating fatigue. Although sleep impairment and circadian rhythm disruption frequently are associated with fatigue, this is not universally true, such as in some instances of cancer-related fatigue [32].

Interventions for fatigue

Correction of the underlying factors believed to contribute to fatigue should be undertaken when possible and when consistent with the patient's goals. Less specific interventions, such as exercise and stimulants, seek to reduce fatigue, optimize function, and promote adaptation, even when the exact underlying causes may not be determined. Whatever the approach, educating the patient and their family about fatigue is important in helping them understand the ways in which it can impact their lives and that although common, it need not be simply endured. Discussing strategies that facilitate adaptation to fatigue, such as realistic goal setting, modifying activities, conserving energy, and prioritizing goals, may also be helpful.

Exercise

Decreasing activity is an anticipated reaction to fatigue and is in fact a frequent remedy prescribed by oncologists [2]. Randomized controlled trials have demonstrated that exercise actually alleviates fatigue in adults, however. For example, a 6-week walking program for women undergoing radiotherapy for breast cancer improved fatigue along with anxiety, depression, and sleep disturbance [33]. Exercise can also provide various physiologic benefits, including improved range of motion, strength, and overall function.

Psychosocial interventions

Strategies to address psychologic factors include pharmacologic and nonpharmacologic approaches. Psychotherapy and support group participation may reduce fatigue [34]. Pharmacologic agents to treat underlying depression and anxiety may also lessen fatigue.

Complementary and alternative therapy

To date, no complementary and alternative therapies have been conclusively shown to reduce fatigue. Some interventions may ameliorate other symptoms, such as pain or nausea, thereby reducing fatigue, but no studies documenting this have been published.

Sleep

The first step should be to address sleep hygiene and reduce factors disrupting sleep. Pharmacologic therapy, including benzodiazepines, benzodiazepine receptor agonists (eg, zolpidem), sedating antidepressants, and antihistamines, may also be considered, keeping in mind that benzodiazepines and antihistamines may have paradoxic effects in children, and that benzodiazepine receptor agonists have not been well studied in children.

Pharmacologic interventions

Correction of anemia

Some studies have demonstrated that correction of anemia in adults undergoing therapy for cancer with erythropoietin may reduce fatigue and enhance quality of life [35,36]. In children who have cancer, erythropoietin improved anemia but failed to improve health-related quality of life [37]. Although there are several possible explanations for this observation, it suggests that correcting anemia alone may not fully address fatigue. If untreated anemia is suspected to be a significant contributor to fatigue, treatment with erythropoietin or red blood cell transfusion may be considered. The potential benefit of erythropoietin should be weighed against recent concerns that it may be associated with faster tumor progression, thrombosis, and increased mortality in adults [38,39].

Stimulants

Methylphenidate (MPH) improves fatigue in adults who have cancer and HIV regardless of the underlying cause of fatigue [40–42]. In one open-label study of adults who had cancer-related fatigue receiving MPH, participants had significantly less fatigue when compared with their baseline ($P < .001$) [41]. More recently, Bruera and colleagues [43] reported that MPH was not better than placebo in improving fatigue scores. The lack of a difference between MPH and placebo was ascribed to a therapeutic effect of frequent supportive contacts from research nurses, however. One case series reports success in treating opioid-related fatigue in children who have cancer with MPH [44]. MPH relieves other symptoms related to fatigue, such as mental clouding, pain, and depressed mood [41,42]. MPH improves cognition in childhood survivors of cancer [45]. MPH has been extensively used in children who have attention-deficit/hyperactivity disorder (ADHD), including those who have coexisting depressed mood [46]. MPH has been reported to cause anorexia in children. Giving the first dose of MPH after breakfast reduces this problem.

Modafinil, another stimulant, has been used to treat adults who have fatigue and multiple sclerosis or those who have opioid-related sedation. It is well tolerated by children when used as treatment for ADHD; however, no published studies have evaluated it in children who have a life-threatening illness and fatigue.

Other pharmacologic treatments

Corticosteroids, megestrol acetate, adenosine triphosphate infusions, and carnitine have all been described as therapies for fatigue; however, there are no data for their use in pediatrics.

Return to the case study

B.H.'s experience of fatigue is similar to that faced by many pediatric patients who have life-threatening illness. It is a symptom unlike any that she has experienced before, has physical and cognitive components, and is not responsive to rest. It pervades multiple domains of her life, preventing her from partaking in the things that provide pleasure and meaning in her life, and it distresses her greatly.

B.H.'s illness and its treatment include several factors that may contribute to her fatigue, some of which are modifiable. Potential contributing factors include multiple chemotherapy regimens; opioid therapy; antiemetics, including a benzodiazepine, metoclopramide, and an antihistamine; and unrelieved pain. On initial questioning she seemed to sleep well; however, further exploration of her sleep habits revealed that uncontrolled pain did in fact disrupt her sleep. Despite her frustration and sadness, she did not seem anxious or depressed. Her physical examination, with decreased muscle mass, suggested that deconditioning may also be contributing to her difficulty with activities of daily living. In her case, anemia, thyroid, or other organ dysfunction did not seem to be contributing to her fatigue.

It was discussed with B.H. that multiple factors were likely causing her fatigue, it was not a result of lack of effort on her part, and it was a treatable condition. She agreed to several changes, including (1) modification of her antiemetic regimen to include less sedating medications, (2) converting the oxycodone to a long-acting formulation that would last through the night, (3) implementing a routine consisting of her taking her dog for a walk on the beach three times a week and riding a stationary bike on other days, (4) limiting daytime naps when possible, and (5) a trial of methylphenidate 10 mg after breakfast and at noon. With this plan B.H. was able to complete her exams. Although she did not return to school, she was able to enjoy time with her family and friends, and coach a local girls' soccer team before she ulitmately succumbed to progressive disease.

Future directions

The opportunities to improve the recognition, assessment and treatment of fatigue in children who have life-threatening illness are abundant. Fatigue has yet to receive the clinical and research attention that other symptoms have gained. Assessment methods for children at a variety of developmental stages and capabilities, including nonverbal children, are needed. Studies to better characterize fatigue as experienced by children and how it impacts the child's family are needed as well. Longitudinal studies will provide a picture of fatigue throughout the illness trajectory. Determination of the factors contributing to fatigue will allow the identification of children at risk for severe and lasting fatigue and the development of targeted interventions to ameliorate fatigue. Finally, education for patients, families, and clinicians is needed to enhance recognition and understanding of this symptom. Given the prevalence and impact of fatigue, advances in the management of this symptom are sure to alleviate a significant source of suffering in children who have life-threatening illness.

Summary

- Fatigue associated with life-threatening illness is an entity distinguishable from the day-to-day fatigue experienced by healthy people. It may cause significant distress, impair functioning and quality of life, and interfere with the goals of palliative care.
- Despite its prevalence and impact, fatigue is frequently underrecognized and underappreciated.
- Fatigue is frequently multifactorial, but targeting contributing factors can improve fatigue.
- Even when no particular contributing factor is identified, nonspecific interventions may ameliorate fatigue.

Dyspnea
Oscar H. Mayer, MD

Dyspnea is a broad complaint that is used to describe the feeling of breathlessness that can occur when the respiratory system is unable to meet the body's need for oxygen uptake or carbon dioxide removal [47]. It has also aptly been described as a neuromechanical dissociation, or a mismatch between the neural stimulus to breathe and the mechanical output [48]. Beyond that, the extent or severity of dyspnea is also modified and expressed by the patient based on his or her own interpretation of what is being felt. Although it is difficult to disguise dyspnea, it is easy to embellish as it occurs with anxiety.

Typically treating dyspnea is focused on diagnosing and aggressively treating the underlying cause. This approach is applicable in most situations, especially when recovery and improvement is a practical goal. In cases in which a more palliative approach is supported, treating dyspnea often focuses more on symptom relief and maximizing quality of life. The approach taken is predicated on the clinical situation and the goals of the patient and family. For that reason it is important to have a full understanding of the causes and pathophysiology of dyspnea so that symptoms are recognized properly and interventions can be tailored to individual situations and family preferences.

Pathophysiology

Dyspnea can occur under completely normal circumstances, such as after brisk activity of exercise. In this situation it is transient and improves promptly after a period of rest when the acid–base, oxygen, and carbon dioxide abnormalities normalize. In disease states, this condition can be prolonged and unremitting, and may in and of itself cause substantial discomfort. Because respiratory failure is a common outcome in terminal disease and because dyspnea is a common component of worsening respiratory failure, in palliative care it is extremely important to recognize and treat dyspnea intensively.

Dyspnea is a broad complaint that that is challenging to diagnose and treat because of its subjectivity and occurrence with many diseases. As a mismatch between the neural stimulus to breathe and the mechanical output, dyspnea really is an imbalance between the metabolic needs of the body (producing the stimulus) and the ability of the respiratory system (mechanical output) to meet them. Although this imbalance can occur because of increased metabolic need, it can also occur when the respiratory system is compromised by decreased surface area for gas exchange, fatigue, or decreased ventilatory capacity or efficiency. The ventilatory measuring stick, per se, or output of the respiratory system is the minute ventilation, which is the product of the respiratory rate and tidal volume.

For example, a patient who has a severe infection with a resultant metabolic acidosis and more carbon dioxide production has a respiratory compensation to increase either respiratory rate or tidal volume. With a normally functioning respiratory system the increased needs should be met; however, if the metabolic acidosis is too high or the respiratory system, including parenchyma and muscles, begins to fatigue or fail, dyspnea will occur as long as the imbalance is present.

The opposite example is of a person who has normal metabolic function but a loss of surface area for gas exchange or an inability to breathe with a normal minute ventilation, or primary respiratory failure. This situation is common in parenchymal failure, such as with cystic fibrosis, pneumonia, or interstitial disease, or in failure caused by fatigue, such as with neuromuscular disease.

In conditions of infiltration of the lungs with either cells (as in infection or neoplasia) or fluid, the compliance of the lungs decreases or it takes more energy to move the lungs during inspiration. This situation makes it much more likely that the patient will fatigue and become dyspneic.

The simple way to treat dyspnea, therefore, is a combination of reducing the metabolic demand and supporting the respiratory system; however, it is much more easily said than done. After identifying the presence of dyspnea, identifying the cause, whether it is an increased metabolic demand, decreased respiratory capacity, or a combination, can be challenging. Furthermore, in a palliative care realm where there are often limits on the extent of medical intervention the patient and family are willing to accept, treatment can be an even larger challenge.

Metabolic demand

The metabolic demand of the body is a combination of the basal energy needs of the body and the additional burden from inefficient activity or deconditioning, organ system dysfunction, and systemic infection and inflammation. Addressing each of these issues is important. For a deconditioned patient, there is a greater lactic acid production with exercise or activity than for someone who has better conditioning [47]. Although challenging the muscles by putting them under a controlled stress is important in rehabilitation, for someone in a palliative care mode this can cause unnecessary stress and discomfort. Instead, reducing the workload may be more appropriate, such as ceasing ambulation.

Treating organ system dysfunction or systemic infection and inflammation can certainly reduce metabolic demand and may balance it better with the respiratory capacity, such as by treating organ system failure, inflammation, or infection. However, such intensive measures may not be consistent with a patient's or family's goals towards the end of life. In this case augmenting the respiratory system capacity or pharmacologically treating symptoms may be more useful.

Respiratory system failure

There are two broad categories of respiratory failure: failure caused by lung parenchymal dysfunction and that caused by muscle fatigue or failure, so-called "pump" failure. It is important to distinguish between these two categories, because the treatment options for each can vary widely in a palliative and nonpalliative mode.

Lung parenchymal failure can occur because of progressive airway obstruction from interstitial or bronchial inflammation and secretions progressively filling the airways and preventing airflow. This situation can cause ventilation–perfusion mismatch or an increased diffusion barrier, which is common in cardiac, pulmonary, or inflammatory disease, or as a side effect of chemotherapy or radiation. Parenchymal failure can also occur because of external compression by pleural fluid or pleural-based lesions or infiltration of the interstitium by metastases or cellular or noncellular inflammation. This process decreases the surface area for diffusion and can narrow airway caliber and make airway obstruction more likely, causing a relative barrier to diffusion and ventilation–perfusion mismatching, both of which can cause hypoxemia often without hypercarbia.

Muscle fatigue and failure can be either primary or secondary. Patients who have neuromuscular disease not only have weak musculature but also have a lowered fatigue threshold and a prolonged recovery time after fatigue. In these patients respiratory muscle failure is a substantial cause of morbidity and mortality. Separately, patients who have normal underlying muscle function who are burdened by increased load on the respiratory system or whose muscles are weakened by systemic disease also may develop respiratory failure. This failure presents as hypercarbia with hypoxemia.

In both parenchymal and muscle failure hypoxemia occurs; hypercarbia should only occur with the hypoventilation of respiratory failure. For that reason treatment of the two conditions is different.

Treatment

Palliative treatment of dyspnea or respiratory failure can be divided into three general categories: supporting respiration mechanically, supporting gas exchange, and providing therapy to decrease the perception of dyspnea.

Noninvasive positive pressure ventilation has been used in both acute and chronic respiratory failure. Although it can be used in acute respiratory failure in the hospital as a step before intubation or as part of weaning from invasive mechanical ventilation, it can also be used effectively at home. The system involves two main components. The first is an interface, typically a nasal interface, either going over the bottom of the nose or into both nares. The second component is a ventilator to provide the pressure assistance during breathing.

Noninvasive positive pressure ventilation (NIPPV) can be used in several ways. It can be used to assist fatigued muscles by providing pressure assistance during a breath to make it easier to breathe properly to maintain minute ventilation. To the extent that this does not occur hypercapnic respiratory failure occurs. In addition, this pressure assistance allows a patient to take a deeper breath and may help overcome the feeling of dyspnea.

Although NIPPV can be used to support respiration mechanically, it can also be used effectively to augment gas exchange. In conditions with low lung volumes the surface area for gas exchange is smaller and the caliber of the airways is narrower and more likely to obstruct with mucus, causing diffusion abnormality and ventilation–perfusion mismatch. Here continuous positive airway pressure (CPAP) can be used to increase lung volume and surface area for diffusion and a higher airway caliber. If the pressure needed to do this becomes too high, then bilevel positive airway pressure can be useful because it releases the distending pressure after inspiration to make it easier to exhale.

Although NIPPV is the treatment of choice for dyspnea related to hypercapnic respiratory failure and can relieve increased work of breathing in hypoxemia without hypercapnia, supplemental oxygen can also be used effectively in non-hypercapnic states; this option may be preferable for children who cannot tolerate wearing NIPPV apparatus. In increased gradient to diffusion and ventilation–perfusion mismatch, supplemental oxygen can correct the hypoxemia. Reversing hypoxemia with supplemental oxygen pulmonary vasodilates and prevents the intracranial vasodilation that occurs with hypoxemia and can cause headaches. This process can be a simple and relatively nonthreatening intervention that should be well tolerated by a wide variety of patients; it can be an effective way of relieving dyspnea [47].

It is important, however, to be selective in when to use supplemental oxygen. In hypercapnia from chronic respiratory failure the hypercarbic drive to breathe may be blunted because of an increased "set point" for carbon dioxide in the blood. This means that although a $PaCO_2$ may have climbed to 60 mm Hg and remained there, with renal compensation the acute respiratory acidosis is corrected. The respiratory drive center in the medulla accepts the higher CO_2 and only responds to increased respiration if it increases further. In this situation then the primary drive to breathe is hypoxemia, and with the use of supplemental oxygen this drive is removed and the patient may become hypopneic or apneic. In an end-of-life situation in which hypopnea or apnea may be less of a concern, it may be important to a family to have an unobstructed view of their child's face, in which case it may make more sense to use supplemental oxygen instead of a larger NIPPV nasal or oronasal interface.

Finally, there are several pharmacologic and nonpharmacologic means of treating dyspnea.

There are case reports of using nebulized analgesics, although the results are variable and they are not universally accepted [48–56]. The most common is nebulized morphine at doses between 2.5 mg and 20 mg titrated to effect. It is hypothesized that the receptors in the lungs involved in the sensation of dyspnea are the J-type stretch receptors, and that the output from these receptors is attenuated by opioids. One advantage of nebulized analgesia is that it is topical as opposed to systemic therapy and should minimize the opioid sedative effect. In addition the benefit should be likened to how well the medication can be delivered and may be compromised in progressive obstructive lung disease, although nebulized analgesia has been used in end-stage obstructive lung disease [52,57].

Outside of nebulized morphine there are also reports in the literature of using nebulized fentanyl and lidocaine [52,58]. Although nebulized lidocaine would avoid the sedative effect of opioids, if absorbed systemically it can affect the cardiac rhythm and may also anesthetize the pharynx to the point that swallowing can be compromised and may put the patient at risk for aspiration.

If nebulized opioids are not effective in controlling dyspnea, then promptly switching to systemic delivery (enteral, parenteral, or subcutaneous) is important. In a patient who has dyspnea and significant pain, or in a patient who has dyspnea at the end of life needing particularly rapid relief from dyspnea, systemic delivery should be used. There is no evidence that any particular opioid is superior to another for dyspnea, although morphine, fentanyl, or hydromorphone are most commonly used, due to experience with them for this indication, flexibility in route of administration, and rapid onset of action. The dose of systemic opioid required to relieve dyspnea is often relatively small, even when a patient is not opioid-naïve. A common practice for opioid-naïve patients is to start by giving .025 mg/kg of morphine intravenously (or the equivalent amount of a different opioid). This is about 25% of a starting dose of .1 mg/kg, the typical starting dose for pain. In a patient already receiving opioids, an increase of 25% in the baseline dose may effectively control dyspnea. The dose given for dyspnea is then titrated as indicated to provide relief, with no set upper limit of dosing.

There is no role for systemic steroid use in dyspnea, outside of treating a steroid-sensitive underlying process, such as inflammatory lung disease of the airways, interstitium, or pleura. Although there is empiric evidence for using systemic steroids for inflammation associated with brain tumors there is no evidence to support its use in other situations [59–62]. Furthermore, using systemic steroids without a clear rationale puts a patient at risk for further problems, such as steroid-induced myopathy and further respiratory dysfunction.

Dyspnea can cause anxiety and anxiety can worsen the sensation of dyspnea by causing the patient to become tachypneic and to breathe in a physiologically inefficient manner. Although systemic opioids often can also be anxiolytic, benzodiazepines have been shown to be more useful as adjunctive treatment to opioids, as opposed to working effectively on their own [63].

Supportive therapies are often recommended in conjunction with pharmacologic therapies. Both cold air to the face and chest wall vibration have been shown to be useful in reducing dyspnea. In fact, blowing air may be as effective as supplemental oxygen. There are also suggestions in the literature that relaxation therapy or counseling can be useful in reducing dyspnea by patient report and validated dyspnea assessment tools [64]. To that end some large hospitals have developed clinics specializing in relaxation therapy [65]. Other suggestions, such as positioning, limitation of activities, a cooler room temperature, and elimination of respiratory irritants, such as cleaning fluids and tobacco, are often anecdotally helpful [66]. Even the most vociferous advocates of nonpharmacologic therapy acknowledge that it is most useful when used as an adjunct to pharmacologic therapy [67–69].

Cases

Case 1

A 12-year-old female has refractory neuroblastoma encasing the aorta and trachea and extending into the left pleural space. The patient has had standard and experimental chemotherapy, but the tumor has not responded and continues to grow slowly. The patient's exertional capacity is severely limited, and until recently she enjoyed going to school and participating in social activities. On physical examination the patient is breathing shallowly, with a rate of 30 breaths per minute and increased accessory muscle activity. The room air oxyhemoglobin saturation is 91%.

Clinical significance

The pattern of breathing is consistent with restrictive lung disease, and the patient has mild hypoxemia, which with the tachypnea shows severely abnormal gas exchange. This way of breathing is labor intensive, with obstruction and restriction and no optimal respiratory pattern. In this situation the major concerns are external compression of the lung and potentially of the aorta and trachea or main bronchi. The compression of the lung gradually decreases lung volume, gradually increases the barrier to diffusion of oxygen, and makes peripheral airway obstruction more likely; in addition the compression of the trachea creates a fixed obstruction that limits inspiration and expiration. The compression of the aorta increases aortic pressure and may cause left-sided heart failure. This process can then cause pulmonary hypertension and may lead to interstitial and alveolar edema, which can further compromise gas exchange.

Treatment options

The only potentially reversible abnormality in this case is the hypoxemia. The air hunger the patient likely feels could be helped with high-flow supplemental oxygen or CPAP to maximize inspiratory flow. The likelihood of relieving dyspnea in this case is extremely small because of the fixed compression of the trachea and lungs. In this situation, a trial of nebulized morphine to blunt the sensation of dyspnea might be a reasonable intervention, although data to support this intervention are very limited. If this does not provide symptom relief for the patient, systemic opioids with or without a benzodiazepine to relieve anxiety could be used. In addition, a discussion with the family about supportive therapies, such as positioning, limitation of activities, increased air circulation, elimination of respiratory irritants such as tobacco, and relaxation techniques, should occur.

Case 2

A 15-year-old male who has trisomy 22 has acute respiratory failure because of another aspiration pneumonia. He is breathing 24 times per minute and has a room air oxyhemoglobin saturation of 85%, which increases to 95% on 3 Lpm of oxygen by nasal cannula. His parents do not want to escalate his respiratory support beyond supplemental oxygen, but are comfortable with his having antibiotic therapy for acute infection. They wish for have him stay at home and are concerned about his comfort.

Clinical significance

This patient has bronchopneumonia and has secretions filling his smaller airways. In this situation the mechanism of hypoxemia is ventilation–perfusion mismatching, which can occur without hypercarbia. Although the patient may develop hypercarbia and respiratory muscle fatigue and failure, this would occur in the later stages of the infection.

Treatment options

In this situation supplemental oxygen is a reasonable intervention and should correct the gas exchange abnormality. Although NIPPV may help prevent or delay respiratory muscle fatigue and can be helpful in airway clearance, it is not consistent with the family's goals. If this patient were to become more dyspneic and progress to the point of requiring ventilatory support, nebulized morphine could be considered. Depressing respiratory sensation suppresses the patient's cough, however, and makes recovery from the pneumonia unlikely. The use of systemic opioids followed by a benzodiazepine should be considered if symptoms are not relieved with nebulized morphine. In addition, a discussion with the family about supportive therapies, such as positioning, modification of activities, increased air circulation, elimination of respiratory irritants such as tobacco, and relaxation techniques, should occur.

Case 3

A 4-year-old female who has spinal muscular atrophy type 1(SMA-1) is on NIPPV during awake hours and has contracted respiratory syncytial virus. The patient's parents have elected not to place a tracheostomy tube, but would consider intubation if it there is a good chance that their daughter could recover and breathe on her own again. The patient is now on continuous NIPPV and has a baseline oxyhemoglobin saturation that is greater than 95% that often drops down to between 85% and 90%, but improves after airway clearance therapy. The patient is breathing asynchronously on NIPPV a little more than normal.

Clinical significance

This patient has chronic respiratory failure because of her underlying neuromuscular disease and has acute respiratory failure on top of it because of respiratory syncytial virus. Although the patient is on continuous NIPPV now she is showing signs of respiratory distress and instability (thoracoabdominal asynchrony and intermittent hypoxemia). Although patients who have SMA-1 at this age have thoracoabdominal asynchrony at baseline, it can certainly become worse with other changes, such as increased lower airway secretions or fatigue from an underlying infection, both of which are happening here.

Treatment options

The patient is now on continuous NIPPV with the same ventilator pressures as at baseline. Just as applying positive pressure to someone who has peripheral airway obstruction can increase lung volume and airway caliber, to improve airway clearance and decrease respiratory muscle fatigue, increasing the ventilator rate and pressures above baseline levels can be useful in a patient already on NIPPV support. The option of intubation and invasive ventilation in this setting is reasonable to consider as long as the family had the opportunity to discuss plans, in the event she does not improve as hoped with intubation. If that were to happen, one option would be to extubate to NIPPV again with additional supplemental oxygen in an attempt to maintain normal oxyhemoglobin saturations. If the patient continues to worsen, systemic opioids to relieve the sensation of dyspnea may be helpful.

Conclusion

Dyspnea can be defined relatively simply as the sensation of breathlessness. The challenge in treating it, however, is that it can come from various different abnormalities so understanding the underlying disorder and the acute abnormality are critical. With that understanding several different treatments can be offered to treat the underlying cause of the dyspnea or palliate the symptom itself.

References

[1] Stone P, Hardy J, Broadley K, et al. Fatigue in advanced cancer: a prospective controlled cross-sectional study. Br J Cancer 1999;79(9–10):1479–86.
[2] Vozelgang NJ, Breitbart W, Cella D, et al. Patient, caregiver, and oncologist perceptions of cancer-related fatigue: results of a tripart assessment survey. The Fatigue Coalition. Semin Hematol 1997;34(3 Suppl 2):4–12.
[3] Ng K, von Gunten CF. Symptoms and attitudes of 100 consecutive patients admitted to an acute hospice/palliative care unit. J Pain Symptom Manage 1998;16(5):307–16.
[4] Goldman A, Hewitt M, Collins GS, et al. Symptoms in children/young people with progressive malignant disease: United Kingdom Children's Cancer Study Group/Paediatric Oncology Nurses Forum survey. Pediatrics 2006;117(6):e1179–86.
[5] Jalmsell L, Kreicbergs U, Onelov E, et al. Symptoms affecting children with malignancies during the last month of life: a nationwide follow-up. Pediatrics 2006;117(4):1314–20.
[6] Wolfe J, Grier HE, Klar N, et al. Symptoms and suffering at the end of life in children with cancer. N Engl J Med 2000;342(5):326–33.
[7] Curt GA, Breitbart W, Cella D, et al. Impact of cancer-related fatigue on the lives of patients: new findings from the Fatigue Coalition. Oncologist 2000;5(5):353–60.
[8] Gibson F, Mulhall AB, Richardson A, et al. A phenomenologic study of fatigue in adolescents receiving treatment for cancer. Oncol Nurs Forum 2005;32(3):651–60.
[9] Bourdeanu L, Loseth DB, Funk M. Management of opioid-induced sedation in patients with cancer. Clin J Oncol Nurs 2005;9(6):705–11.
[10] Shaiova L. The management of opioid-related sedation. Curr Pain Headache Rep 2005;9(4): 239–42.
[11] Iop A, Manfredi AM, Bonura S. Fatigue in cancer patients receiving chemotherapy: an analysis of published studies. Ann Oncol 2004;15(5):712–20.
[12] Stasi R, Abriani L, Beccaglia P, et al. Cancer-related fatigue: evolving concepts in evaluation and treatment. Cancer 2003;98(9):1786–801.

[13] Cancer-related fatigue. National comprehensive cancer network clinical practice guidelines in oncology. Available at: www.nccn.org. Accessed in 2007.

[14] Malik UR, Makower DF, Wadler S. Interferon-mediated fatigue. Cancer 2001;92(6 Suppl): 1664–8.

[15] Stromgren AS, Groenvold M, Pedersen L, et al. Does the medical record cover the symptoms experienced by cancer patients receiving palliative care? A comparison of the record and patient self-rating. J Pain Symptom Manage 2001;21(3):189–96.

[16] Stone P, Richardson A, Ream E, et al. Cancer-related fatigue: inevitable, unimportant and untreatable? Results of a multi-centre patient survey. Cancer Fatigue Forum. Ann Oncol 2000;11(8):971–5.

[17] Temel J, Pirl WF, Recklitis C, et al. Feasibility and validity of a one-item fatigue screen in a thoracic oncology clinic. J Thorac Oncol 2006;1(5):454–9.

[18] Hockenberry MJ, Hinds PS, Barrera P, et al. Three instruments to assess fatigue in children with cancer: the child, parent and staff perspectives. J Pain Symptom Manage 2003;25(4): 319–28.

[19] Varni JW, Burwinkle TM, Katz ER, et al. The PedsQL in pediatric cancer: reliability and validity of the Pediatric Quality of Life Inventory Generic Core Scales, Multidimensional Fatigue Scale, and Cancer Module. Cancer 2002;94(7):2090–106.

[20] Hinds PS, Hockenberry-Eaton M, Gilger E, et al. Comparing patient, parent, and staff descriptions of fatigue in pediatric oncology patients. Cancer Nurs 1999;22(4):277–88, quiz 88–89.

[21] Irvine D, Vincent L, Graydon JE, et al. The prevalence and correlates of fatigue in patients receiving treatment with chemotherapy and radiotherapy. A comparison with the fatigue experienced by healthy individuals. Cancer Nurs 1994;17(5):367–78.

[22] Akechi T, Kugaya A, Okamura H, et al. Fatigue and its associated factors in ambulatory cancer patients: a preliminary study. J Pain Symptom Manage 1999;17(1):42–8.

[23] Tsai LY, Li IF, Lai YH, et al. Fatigue and its associated factors in hospice cancer patients in Taiwan. Cancer Nurs 2007;30(1):24–30.

[24] Holzner B, Kemmler G, Greil R, et al. The impact of hemoglobin levels on fatigue and quality of life in cancer patients. Ann Oncol 2002;13(6):965–73.

[25] Munch TN, Zhang T, Willey J, et al. The association between anemia and fatigue in patients with advanced cancer receiving palliative care. J Palliat Med 2005;8(6):1144–9.

[26] Gutstein HB. The biologic basis of fatigue. Cancer 2001;92(6 Suppl):1678–83.

[27] Bruera E, Brenneis C, Michaud M, et al. Muscle electrophysiology in patients with advanced breast cancer. J Natl Cancer Inst 1988;80(4):282–5.

[28] Shafqat A, Einhorn LH, Hanna N, et al. Screening studies for fatigue and laboratory correlates in cancer patients undergoing treatment. Ann Oncol 2005;16(9):1545–50.

[29] Strasser F, Palmer JL, Schover LR, et al. The impact of hypogonadism and autonomic dysfunction on fatigue, emotional function, and sexual desire in male patients with advanced cancer: a pilot study. Cancer 2006;107(12):2949–57.

[30] Stone P, Hardy J, Huddart R, et al. Fatigue in patients with prostate cancer receiving hormone therapy. Eur J Cancer 2000;36(9):1134–41.

[31] Hugel H, Ellershaw JE, Cook L, et al. The prevalence, key causes and management of insomnia in palliative care patients. J Pain Symptom Manage 2004;27(4):316–21.

[32] Fernandes R, Stone P, Andrews P, et al. Comparison between fatigue, sleep disturbance, and circadian rhythm in cancer inpatients and healthy volunteers: evaluation of diagnostic criteria for cancer-related fatigue. J Pain Symptom Manage 2006;32(3):245–54.

[33] Mock V, Dow KH, Meares CJ, et al. Effects of exercise on fatigue, physical functioning, and emotional distress during radiation therapy for breast cancer. Oncol Nurs Forum 1997; 24(6):991–1000.

[34] Forester B, Kornfeld DS, Fleiss JL, et al. Group psychotherapy during radiotherapy: effects on emotional and physical distress. Am J Psychiatry 1993;150(11):1700–6.

[35] Information for healthcare professionals. Erythropoiesis stimulating agents (ESA) [Aranesp (darbepoetin), Epogen (epoetin alfa), and Procrit (epoetin alfa)]. In: Alert US FDA, editor.

Available at: http://www.fda.gov/cder/drug/InfoSheets/HCP/RHE2007HCP.htm. Accessed May 11, 2007.

[36] Demetri GD, Kris M, Wade J, et al. Quality-of-life benefit in chemotherapy patients treated with epoetin alfa is independent of disease response or tumor type: results from a prospective community oncology study. Procrit Study Group. J Clin Oncol 1998;16(10):3412–25.

[37] Razzouk BI, Hord JD, Hockenberry M, et al. Double-blind, placebo-controlled study of quality of life, hematologic end points, and safety of weekly epoetin alfa in children with cancer receiving myelosuppressive chemotherapy. J Clin Oncol 2006;24(22):3583–9.

[38] Leyland-Jones B, Semiglazov V, Pawlicki M, et al. Maintaining normal hemoglobin levels with epoetin alfa in mainly nonanemic patients with metastatic breast cancer receiving first-line chemotherapy: a survival study. J Clin Oncol 2005;23(25):5960–72.

[39] Wright JR, Ung YC, Julian JA, et al. Randomized, double-blind, placebo-controlled trial of erythropoietin in non-small-cell lung cancer with disease-related anemia. J Clin Oncol 2007; 25(9):1027–32.

[40] Breitbart W, Rosenfeld B, Kaim M, et al. A randomized, double-blind, placebo-controlled trial of psychostimulants for the treatment of fatigue in ambulatory patients with human immunodeficiency virus disease. Arch Intern Med 2001;161(3):411–20.

[41] Bruera E, Driver L, Barnes EA, et al. Patient-controlled methylphenidate for the management of fatigue in patients with advanced cancer: a preliminary report. J Clin Oncol 2003; 21(23):4439–43.

[42] Bruera E, Miller MJ, Macmillan K, et al. Neuropsychological effects of methylphenidate in patients receiving a continuous infusion of narcotics for cancer pain. Pain 1992;48(2): 163–6.

[43] Bruera E, Valero V, Driver L, et al. Patient-controlled methylphenidate for cancer fatigue: a double-blind, randomized, placebo-controlled trial. J Clin Oncol 2006;24(13):2073–8.

[44] Yee JD, Berde CB. Dextroamphetamine or methylphenidate as adjuvants to opioid analgesia for adolescents with cancer. J Pain Symptom Manage 1994;9(2):122–5.

[45] Thompson SJ, Leigh L, Christensen R, et al. Immediate neurocognitive effects of methylphenidate on learning-impaired survivors of childhood cancer. J Clin Oncol 2001;19(6):1802–8.

[46] Greenhill LL, Pliszka S, Dulcan MK, et al. Summary of the practice parameter for the use of stimulant medications in the treatment of children, adolescents, and adults. J Am Acad Child Adolesc Psychiatry 2001;40(11):1352–5.

[47] Society AT. Dyspnea. Mechanisms, assessment, and management: a consensus statement. American Thoracic Society. Am J Respir Crit Care Med 1999;159(1):321–40.

[48] Enck RE. The role of nebulized morphine in managing dyspnea. Am J Hosp Palliat Care 1999;16(1):373–4.

[49] Baydur A. Nebulized morphine: a convenient and safe alternative to dyspnea relief? Chest 2004;125(2):363–5.

[50] Brown SJ, Eichner SF, Jones JR. Nebulized morphine for relief of dyspnea due to chronic lung disease. Ann Pharmacother 2005;39(6):1088–92.

[51] Bruera E, Sala R, Spruyt O, et al. Nebulized versus subcutaneous morphine for patients with cancer dyspnea: a preliminary study. J Pain Symptom Manage 2005;29(6):613–8.

[52] Cohen SP, Dawson TC. Nebulized morphine as a treatment for dyspnea in a child with cystic fibrosis. Pediatrics 2002;110(3):e38.

[53] Howe JL. Nebulized morphine for hospice patients. Am J Hosp Palliat Care 1995;12(5):6.

[54] Sarhill N, Walsh D, Khawam E, et al. Nebulized hydromorphone for dyspnea in hospice care of advanced cancer. Am J Hosp Palliat Care 2000;17(6):389–91.

[55] Westphal CG, Campbell ML. Nebulized morphine for terminal dyspnea. Am J Nurs 2002; (Suppl):11–5.

[56] Zeppetella G. Nebulized and intranasal fentanyl in the management of cancer-related breakthrough pain. Palliat Med 2000;14(1):57–8.

[57] Lord E. Nebulized morphine: one intervention for end-stage chronic obstructive pulmonary disease (COPD). AARN News Lett 1997;53(10):10–1.

[58] Wilcock A, Corcoran R, Tattersfield AE. Safety and efficacy of nebulized lignocaine in patients with cancer and breathlessness. Palliat Med 1994;8(1):35–8.

[59] Galicich JH, French LA, Melby JC. Use of dexamethasone in treatment of cerebral edema associated with brain tumors. J Lancet 1961;81:46–53.

[60] Koehler PJ. Use of corticosteroids in neuro-oncology. Anticancer Drugs 1995;6(1):19–33.

[61] Kofman S, Garvin JS, Nagamani D, et al. Treatment of cerebral metastases from breast carcinoma with prednisolone. J Am Med Assoc 1957;163(16):1473–6.

[62] Wen PY, Marks PW. Medical management of patients with brain tumors. Curr Opin Oncol 2002;14(3):299–307.

[63] Thomas JR, von Gunten CF. Clinical management of dyspnoea. Lancet Oncol 2002;3(4): 223–8.

[64] Ripamonti C, Bruera E. Dyspnea: pathophysiology and assessment. J Pain Symptom Manage 1997;13(4):220–32.

[65] Hately J, Laurence V, Scott A, et al. Breathlessness clinics within specialist palliative care settings can improve the quality of life and functional capacity of patients with lung cancer. Palliat Med 2003;17(5):410–7.

[66] Tyler LS. Dyspnea in palliative care patients. In: Lipman A, Jackson KC II, Tyler LS, editors. Evidence based symptom control in palliative care. Binghamton (NY): Haworth Press, Inc; 2000. p. 109–28.

[67] Bardia A, Barton DL, Prokop LJ, et al. Efficacy of complementary and alternative medicine therapies in relieving cancer pain: a systematic review. J Clin Oncol 2006;24(34):5457–64.

[68] Ernst E. Complementary and alternative medicine. Lancet 2001;357(9258):802–3.

[69] Gallo-Silver L, Pollack B. Behavioral interventions for lung cancer-related breathlessness. Cancer Pract 2000;8(6):268–73.

PEDIATRIC CLINICS
OF NORTH AMERICA

Pediatr Clin N Am 54 (2007) 757–771

Do Not Attempt Resuscitation Orders in Pediatrics

Wynne Morrison, MD[a],*,
Ivor Berkowitz, MBBCh[b]

[a]*Department of Anesthesiology and Critical Care, The Children's Hospital of Philadelphia,
University of Pennsylvania School of Medicine, 34th Street and Civic Center Boulevard,
Room 7C20, Philadelphia, PA 19104, USA*
[b]*Division of Pediatric Anesthesiology and Critical Care Medicine, Johns Hopkins School
of Medicine, 600 North Wolfe Street, Blalock 904, Baltimore, MD 21287, USA*

Reports of the first "do-not-resuscitate" (DNR) orders appeared in the medical literature in 1976 [1]. Since that time, these orders are increasing in frequency [2], such that they have "become a part of the ritual of death in our society, so commonplace that nearly all physicians have written one" [3]. It is no coincidence that the proliferation of such orders has coincided with the era of tremendous advances in life-sustaining technology, because although such interventions can sometimes lead to wondrous cures, they can also become merely death-prolonging. Cardiopulmonary resuscitation (CPR) is unique in medicine in that an order is necessary to forego an intervention. Because of the emergent nature of cardiopulmonary arrest, there is a presumption that resuscitation is desired unless explicitly refused.

Do-not-attempt-resuscitation (DNAR) orders are also becoming more common in pediatrics [4], particularly as programs for hospice and palliative care in children develop [5]. The proportion of childhood deaths in which a DNAR order is in place varies from 16% to 74% [6–20], depending on the country, location of death (eg, intensive care unit [ICU] versus home), and diagnoses included in the population studied.

Case

Katie is a 9-year-old girl who was diagnosed with a brain tumor 8 months ago. Surgical resection of the tumor was attempted at the time of diagnosis, but the entire mass could not be removed. She has since been undergoing

---

* Corresponding author.
E-mail address: morrisonw@email.chop.edu (W. Morrison).

doi:10.1016/j.pcl.2007.06.005 *pediatric.theclinics.com*

chemotherapy and radiation and has been able to attend school, except for two brief hospitalizations. On the day of admission, she had the sudden onset of confusion and difficulty in standing, followed by a brief seizure. Her parents rushed her to the hospital, where neuroimaging showed an acute hemorrhage in and around the tumor causing mild midline shift and ipsilateral ventricular compression. She is now in the ICU. She is still lethargic but responds to voice and stimulation. The ICU team and her primary neuro-oncologist meet to discuss her prognosis and whether a DNAR order is appropriate. They also consider how to approach this conversation with the family.

Terminology

DNAR ("do not attempt resuscitation") is becoming a more commonly used term, as opposed to the term *DNR* ("do not resuscitate"). DNAR presupposes that there is no guarantee that resuscitation attempts are going to be successful. This shift in terminology arose partly in response to the realization that the general public had a falsely optimistic perception of the success rate of resuscitation. This misunderstanding may be attributable to frequent media portrayals of successful CPR [21]. The term *DNAR* is not, however, specific enough to stand alone. It could mean "no chest compressions or defibrillation in the event of cardiac arrest" or could be intended more broadly, such as "no CPR, no intubation, no vasoactive infusions, provide comfort measures only." DNI is also sometimes used as an abbreviation for "do not intubate." To avoid confusions during transitions in care, the interventions that are to be attempted need to be spelled out in detail in the patient care orders and in communications among the health care team. The requirement for such explicit statements does not imply, however, that a patient or family should be presented with a checklist or "menu" of interventions for which to check off "yes" or "no." In family conversations, it is more appropriate to focus on the overall goals of care, and the clinician can then determine which specific interventions further these mutually acceptable goals. Acceptable goals, depending on the circumstances, could include prolonging life (indefinitely or until a specific event), treating symptoms, avoiding invasive interventions, or choosing a location of death (home versus hospital). In Katie's case, because her quality of life has been fairly good up until this point, it might be a reasonable decision to pursue an intervention as aggressive as a neurosurgical procedure, if feasible, to attempt to return her to her baseline status yet still have a DNAR order should she progress to the point of a cardiac arrest.

There has been a recent call to modify the standard terminology further and replace the term *DNR* or *DNAR* with the term *allow natural death* (AND) [22,23]. Rather than emphasizing that something is being withheld, AND focuses on the benefits of allowing a natural process to take place. Although it initially seems to be a mere semantic trick, some medical centers that have changed the terminology have anecdotally reported easier conversations with patients and families about code status. In Katie's case, if the medical team decides to recommend a DNAR order to the family, they could use such language to emphasize what is going to continue (eg, pain control, symptom relief, family support) when discussing what they think it best not to do (invasive death-prolonging interventions). Emphasizing what can and should be done to continue to improve care and quality of remaining time for a patient who is DNAR is a core tenet of palliative care.

Withholding versus withdrawing

There is consensus in the literature that there is no ethical distinction between never beginning a certain therapy (withholding) and discontinuing it once it has been instituted (withdrawing) [24–27]. This fact makes time-limited trials of some interventions an option when the prognosis is uncertain or a therapy is of questionable benefit, because it is still possible to discontinue aggressive measures at a later point if it becomes clear that they are not achieving the desired goals. Yet, even though both methods are ethically acceptable, for many families (and health care providers as well), there may be a different personal impact between withholding and withdrawing. Families are often more comfortable agreeing not to escalate interventions rather than to discontinue therapies that are already in place. Open discussions of these options may facilitate decision making.

Standards of decision making for pediatric patients

Ethicists and the courts have long agreed that a competent adult patient has the right to refuse any unwanted therapy, including resuscitation, as long as he understands the clinical situation and consequences of refused therapy [3,27,28]. Although they are not perfect, mechanisms also exist, such as advance directives or living wills, to allow an adult to state her wishes or appoint a decision maker for future circumstances in which she might be incompetent or unable to communicate. Young children are rarely able to comprehend a complex medical decision and long-term risks or benefits fully; thus, such decisions are typically made for them by their parents or guardians [29]. Why do we let parents decide for their children? Several ethical decision-making standards exist. The substituted judgment standard refers to surrogates basing a decision on what a patient would choose on his own if able to do so [30]. This standard is usually not the basis for decision making in pediatrics, because children typically have never had decision-making capacity and we therefore cannot determine what they would have wanted. Sometimes, as a way of focusing their decision making on what is right for their child rather than on their own wishes, it can be helpful to ask a family: "What do you think he would want us to do if he could tell us?"

The usual standard applied in pediatrics is the best interests standard [30,31]. Rather than attempting to determine what the child's wishes would be, the decision maker weighs the benefits and burdens of each option to decide what is best for the child. Often, such decisions are reached after conversations between the family and the health care team, wherein both contribute their opinions about what might be in the child's best interests. The health care team brings to the conversation knowledge about the medical condition, prognosis, interventions, and prior experiences with similar patients, whereas the family brings to the conversation their knowledge of the child as a person; the values of the family, culture, and community as a whole; and, sometimes, better knowledge of how the child's illness has responded to prior therapies. Some authors argue that parents or guardians should be allowed to choose any ethically, legally, and medically acceptable option in the care of their child, considering the needs of the family as a whole rather than being required to find a single "best" option for the one individual [32,33]. Although some maintain that DNAR orders are inappropriate in children because we are unable to rely on their own competent or prior wishes [34], this opinion is an extreme one that is not consistent with the reality experienced by clinicians and families each day.

Older children and adolescents present a special circumstance, because although they are not yet at an age of legal decision-making authority, they are often able to consider the implications of specific medical decisions rationally. In such cases, the "assent" (as opposed to "consent") of the child should be sought [31,35,36]. Although it would be wrong to let an adolescent choose a therapeutic option that is obviously counter to her best interests, one should encourage children, whenever age and developmentally appropriate [37], to participate in discussions and decision making regarding their health. Children who have had a long experience with an illness may have particularly strong opinions regarding whether to pursue aggressive or experimental therapies. They may even be able to participate in discussions about DNAR status. In some cases, a minor child may even be granted status as a legal decision maker, when he is judged to be an emancipated or mature minor [38,39]. Emancipated typically refers to an adolescent who is living completely independently from her parents or is, for some other reason (eg, marriage, parenthood), treated as an adult. A mature minor is legally judged to be adequately mature, with comprehension of the disease treatment and its consequences, to qualify for legal decision-making capacity regarding medical therapy in a particular circumstance (see example in the legal cases elsewhere in this article). States vary in how and when older adolescents can meet such legal thresholds. It is often ethically appropriate, however, to consider an older child's wishes even when not legally required. In our case, Katie is at an age at which her assent might be required by an institution before participating in a nontherapeutic research protocol; however, considering the complexity of the situation and her mental status changes, the team is likely to be making decisions entirely with her parents while informing her of what is happening in her immediate surroundings.

Legal cases in pediatrics

Most states have DNAR statutes, and regulatory authorities require that hospitals have DNAR policies [3]. The American Medical Association has also developed guidelines for writing DNAR orders and for patient and family discussions [40]. The process itself is not always straightforward and conflict-free, however. Most cases that come to legal attention involve disagreements between patients or families and physicians. A brief summary of some "classic" cases in pediatric end-of-life decision making follows. Although these cases are illustrative of the legal process and outcome, care should be taken not to assume that case law from one jurisdiction can be applied in another or that statutes or subsequent cases would not change legal opinion.

In re: Baby K

Baby K was an anencephalic infant born in 1992 who was intubated in the delivery room and whose mother subsequently refused to allow a DNAR order to be written or the ventilator to be withheld during periods of decompensation [27,41]. Attempts to transfer the patient to another hospital that would be willing to provide care were not successful. The infant was eventually transferred to a long-term care facility. After three readmissions during which full support was provided, the hospital, in conjunction with the infant's father, sought legal permission not to ventilate or provide other aggressive treatment with the next decompensation. The Federal Court of Appeals sided with the lower court in determining that under Federal legislation (the Emergency Medical Treatment and Active Labor Act [EMTALA] statutes), the hospital was obligated to provide stabilizing treatment as part of emergency care. No opinion was rendered about ongoing "nonemergent" care, and the court did not comment on what was or was not considered appropriate standard of care for infants with anencephaly.

Miller v Hospital Corporation of America

Sidney Miller was born at approximately 23 weeks of gestation, weighing 629 g. Her parents requested no resuscitation in the delivery room, based on information about her prognosis they had been given by physicians at the hospital. The parents were later informed that hospital policy required assessment of any infant born weighing greater than 500 g for potential resuscitation (no such written policy existed), and she was intubated in the delivery room. Over the next few months in the neonatal intensive care unit (NICU), the parents never asked to have support withdrawn but later sued the hospital, claiming that they had not given consent for the resuscitation and that Sidney was now living with severe disabilities. The parents were awarded a multimillion-dollar verdict at the initial trial, but this verdict was overturned on appeal when the Texas Supreme Court determined that a physician could act without consent to provide life-sustaining measures in an emergency situation and that assessments about whether to proceed in cases of extreme prematurity could not be made until the time of birth [42].

State v Messenger

In another case involving a premature birth, a physician-father himself disconnected his unstable 25-week premature son from a ventilator shortly after delivery [43]. Differing interpretations of conversations between the family, neonatologist, and physician's assistant had led to the infant's being resuscitated in the delivery room when the parents had requested no resuscitation if he was truly at 25 weeks of gestation. The medical examiner ruled the case a "homicide," and the father was charged with manslaughter but acquitted.

Benny Agrelo

There are also rare court cases involving adolescents who disagreed with the medical care they were receiving. Benny Agrelo was a 15-year-old boy who had undergone two liver transplants. When his liver failure recurred, he refused a third transplant and refused to take his immunosuppressive medications because of side effects [44]. His parents initially disagreed with him but later came to accept his decision. When his physicians realized his parents were not going to insist on treatment, the hospital had him forcefully removed from his home and hospitalized against his will. In the hospital, he refused to cooperate with care or blood tests, and a judge eventually ruled that he could refuse therapy. He died a few months later.

Baby Doe regulations

In the early 1980s, in response to a publicized case of an infant with trisomy 21 whose parents chose to forego surgery to relieve duodenal atresia and allowed the child to die, the administration of President Ronald Reagan interpreted prior legislation to state that nontreatment of neonates on the basis of disability or potential disability was a violation of their civil rights, except in cases of irreversible coma or when treatment merely prolonged dying [45]. These initial regulations were struck down by the US Supreme Court, which emphasized the privacy right of parents to decide in their child's best interests. Later, a similar set of rules was incorporated into legislation tying compliance to state child abuse and neglect funding but imposing no other penalties. In Montalvo v Borkovec, a Wisconsin court referred to the Baby Doe rules when it stated that parents should not be allowed to choose no resuscitation for an extremely premature infant in the delivery room [46]. This decision has not been further tested.

Most of the cases summarized here illustrate that the courts are loath to override families, particularly parents, as the appropriate decision makers for their loved ones. Cases involving adult patients have shown a similar trend. In the landmark case, In re: Wanglie [27], the courts decided that the husband of 53 years was the appropriate decision maker for an elderly woman in a persistent vegetative state on a ventilator. The hospital had sought to have a guardian appointed, arguing that ongoing support was futile; the court simply decided that her spouse was an appropriate representative, making no judgment about futility in the case. Even in Europe, where there is much less emphasis on patient autonomy than in the United States [47], the European Court of Human Rights supported a family who objected to their developmentally disabled son being made DNAR against their wishes [48]. The Baby Doe rules are an exception in attempting to remove decision-making authority from families (and physicians), and it is yet to be seen what the legal implications are on a national level.

Futility

The concept of futility is sometimes cited as a reason for initiating a unilateral DNAR order (ie, a DNAR order with which the patient or family does not have to be in agreement). This argument is based on the principle that no medical professional should be obligated to provide medically ineffective therapy. In fact, it is conceivably cruel to ask a patient or family to struggle with decisions about resuscitation status if medical circumstances are such that CPR would have no chance of being effective [49]. Although the premise is sound, the near impossibility of determining what is truly futile therapy makes such arguments difficult to apply.

A distinction should be made between various definitions of futility. Physiologic futility refers to therapy that is going to be medically ineffective at achieving the stated goal [27,41,50,51]. For example, surgery would be futile therapy for widely metastatic cancer, or continued CPR after an hour of asystole would be unsuccessful at restoring circulation. In such cases, the physician is justified in making a medical decision to stop a useless therapy, or not to offer it in the first place. Some have even argued that patients in the ICU on high-dose vasoactive infusions and maximal ventilatory support are undergoing a "continuous code" [52] and that escalation to bolus medication doses or chest compressions makes no sense.

Yet, in many cases in which physicians claim that CPR is futile, they do not mean that it stands no chance of achieving a return of a heartbeat; they usually mean that it stands little chance of restoring an acceptable quality of life or leading to long-term survival. Quantitative futility refers to a definition of futility based on the odds of success, with a less than 1% chance of the hoped for outcome often cited as a cutoff point [53]. Qualitative futility defines futility not merely in terms of survival (or return of heartbeat) but rather in terms of quality of life. Such an example would be the argument that continued mechanical ventilation for a severely brain-injured patient who was unlikely to ever regain consciousness was "futile." It is obviously not futile in terms of supporting breathing, which is successfully being achieved, but rather at achieving goals thought to be worthwhile by the person making the statement. The latter two definitions of futility involve value judgments, although, admittedly, values shared by many. Yet, there might be some who think a 1% chance worth taking, and for others, perhaps for religious reasons [3], continued life no matter what the quality may be of value.

Many have argued [51,54–56], and some institutions have mandated [41], that the concept of futility should not be used as a means of overriding a patient's wishes [57]. Although many states have statutes including language that physicians are not obligated to provide ineffective therapy [41], most do not define it. The fairly recently enacted Texas Advance Directives Act outlines a "procedural" approach to futility disputes [58,59]. Rather than the nearly impossible task of attempting to define futile therapy, the statute delineates a process for physicians who believe that a patient or family is demanding ineffective therapy. The process includes review of the case by an institutional committee, notification of the patient/family of the review process, a mandated 10-day waiting period after a determination is made that therapy is ineffective before life-sustaining measures can be withdrawn, and a requirement to explore options for transfer of care. There is debate about whether such an approach is successful [60], and recent controversial cases have led some to argue that a 10-day waiting period is far too short for families to explore other options.

When physicians are quite certain that a therapy is going to be ineffective, an acceptable approach is to inform the family of what therapies or interventions are medically inappropriate. In Katie's case, her physician might say: "If the bleeding in her brain becomes so severe that her heart stops, CPR would only get a heartbeat back temporarily, if at all, and I think it's best not to do it." A family's "informed approval" of such a decision is adequate, as long as they are aware that it is being made. Such an approach should be reserved only for cases with a near-certain outcome rather than being based on value judgments. It also recognizes that it is unfair and potentially burdensome to ask a family to make a choice when no real choices exist. Conversely, a unilateral DNAR order over strong objections is only likely to cause problems. "Slow codes" or "Hollywood codes" are inappropriate [3].

Specific situations

Out-of-hospital do-not-attempt-resuscitation orders

Many states have legislated a process for out-of-hospital DNAR orders so that paramedics have a standard form to offer them reassurance and protection from liability when they forgo resuscitation in the field [61]. Not all these laws, however, apply to children [62]. In some cases, emergency responders have ignored home DNAR orders when the order is unclear or they are otherwise unwilling to comply [63]. Advance preparation for a child with a DNAR order at home might include notification of the local emergency responders and making sure that there is official paperwork immediately on hand in the home. A family should also be told to access alternative resources, such as hospice, rather than activating emergency medical services (EMS). In the unfortunate event that aggressive measures are mistakenly instituted by emergency responders, undesired interventions can be discontinued once the medical situation and family's wishes are clarified at the site of more definitive care. Such a situation is, however, often emotionally difficult for the family and health care team.

School

Some children with a terminal illness or complex medical condition may have a DNAR order and also wish to attend school. Doing so may help them to maintain as normal a life as possible. Schools often have significant concerns about honoring DNAR orders. These include fear of making a mistake, fear of liability, and concerns for the effect a dying child would have on other students. Few school districts have written policies about DNAR orders, and those that do often prohibit them [64]. Proactive meetings of the family and physician with school officials can help to ensure that resuscitation wishes are honored [62]. Families should keep children home at times when instability can be anticipated [65]. Bereavement support may be necessary for other students and teachers no matter where the death occurs. The school also needs a plan for whom to call and how to get appropriate help, so that the staff is prepared to handle an emergency. If Katie's family had decided to put a DNAR order in place fairly early, when they knew that her tumor was not completely resected, she should still have had a right to attend school.

Perioperative period

Occasionally, children who have DNAR orders require surgical intervention, whether for a palliative procedure to improve their quality of life or for an intercurrent medical problem unrelated to their life-limiting illness. Managing complications from the surgical procedure or anesthetic might require intubation, vasoactive medications, or even CPR. In many cases, it is appropriate to rescind a DNAR order temporarily for an operative procedure. Yet, in other cases, a procedure may be purely palliative, and any resuscitation, even for a cardiac arrest precipitated by an anesthetic, would be counter to the patient's and family's wishes. Every case is different and requires advance discussion with the patient and family. Solutions could vary depending on the preprocedure quality of life of the patient, indication for surgery, risks involved, and patient's stage of illness [66]. A thorough understanding of the patient's or family's goals of care by the anesthesiologist, surgeon, and postoperative care team is more important than developing a list of what interventions are or are not going to be applied. Such an understanding allows for interpretation of changing circumstances as a result of unexpected intraoperative or postoperative events.

If Katie has a DNAR order written during this hospitalization but survives to discharge and develops appendicitis 2 months later, her parents and physicians might decide to pursue an appendectomy if her quality of life at the time is reasonable and death is not imminent. They might rescind the DNAR order completely for the procedure and perioperative period, or possibly agree to limited interventions for a reversible event. Yet, they might not want heroic measures used for a severe decompensation. Whatever the decision, the family, surgeon, and anesthesiologist all need to be informed and comfortable with the plan before proceeding. If a DNAR order is rescinded in the perioperative period, the timing of its reinstitution must be determined by discussion between the parents and physicians.

Iatrogenic arrest

Many physicians believe that an iatrogenic cardiac arrest is a special situation during which a DNAR order should be overridden [67]. This may be attributable to the physician feeling responsible for causing the arrest, particularly if it is the result of an error, or perhaps because she believes the cause is easily reversible (eg, a pneumothorax leading to cardiac arrest during a central line attempt). In addition, the physician may believe that the patient or family had not anticipated the medical complication when the DNAR order was requested. Overriding a DNAR order in these circumstances may actually be counter to the goals of the patient and family [68], however, and the situation may not be as easily stabilized as hoped. In pediatrics, because parents are almost always readily available, if there is any doubt about the goals of care, temporary life-sustaining measures can begin while a quick discussion is held to clarify wishes.

Hospice

In the past, many hospices have required a DNAR order as a precondition for admission. Although it is now rarely a mandate, it can still be a difficult balance to treat pain adequately and decide whether or not to activate EMS for a patient on home hospice who is not DNAR. Yet, because the scope of palliative care has been extended to include earlier support of patients with life-threatening illness who are not imminently dying, patients receiving hospice or palliative care services might increasingly wish to undergo attempted resuscitation in the hopes that their life can be extended [69]. It is also relatively common for a family of a child with an acknowledged terminal illness still to be emotionally unable to agree to a DNAR order. Many of these patients can still benefit from hospice services. If a family is well informed about the consequences of not having a DNAR order (eg, it may mean that the patient has to come to an ICU and have invasive interventions rather than being home at the time of death), most clinicians choose to respect this decision.

Discussions and resolving conflicts

Discussions about options at the end of life are best approached by striving for mutual understanding, clarifying goals, and alliance building rather than by pressing for a rapid decision about specific interventions [70]. Working on building a relationship with a family while giving them time to understand and process a situation often helps to avoid conflicts. It is also extraordinarily helpful to have health care providers involved who know the patient and family well. In Katie's case, it would probably be helpful to have the primary neuro-oncologist lead most discussions rather than the intensivist, who the family may have just met. Involving her primary care pediatrician as well might be helpful and reassuring to the family. Physicians should also not hesitate to make a recommendation when they believe that a certain choice (eg, a DNAR order) would be most appropriate. Doing so can be a way to inform the family that such an option is indeed a legal, moral, and compassionate option. Such a recommendation can also allow a family to accept the decision without feeling that they are somehow "giving up" on their child [71]. Phrases like "Do you want everything done?" should be avoided because they may imply that the alternative is doing nothing. Rather, emphasis should be placed on the care that is going to continue no matter what choices are made. A patient and family should also be reassured that a DNAR order does not signify abandonment by the medical team. Doctors and nurses are still going to continue to care for the patient, with a shift in goals of care toward comfort and optimizing the quality of the remaining time. Sometimes, it can also help a family to be reminded that they are trying to help the team figure out what their child would want if the child could tell us rather than sharing only their own wishes, which might be survival of the child at all costs. Acknowledging in all conversations that the family knows the child better than anyone on the medical team and assuring them that their values and wishes are going to be respected can allow them to speak more freely and develop trust with the team. Giving them positive feedback for difficult but loving decisions that they have made and their devotion to their child can also help to support them.

There are times when conflicts arise between members of the health care team and the parents. For example, clinicians may believe that the suffering of the child is too great and that they are violating their professional integrity by deferring to the parents' wishes [72]. In such cases, health care providers should feel that they can openly express their concerns to a family.

Pressuring a family to change their mind, however, may be unlikely to move them and only encourage entrenched positions on the part of the family and team, wherein neither is willing to alter their stance. Few families object when the health care team appropriately proposes that they are going to do all they can to keep the child comfortable, no matter what the goals. In particularly difficult cases, consultation with the hospital's ethics committee may be helpful. In the extremely rare circumstance that physicians truly feel they are unable to participate in a plan of care demanded by a family, transfer of care to another provider should be sought. If a team is struggling because a family insists on CPR when the odds of success are miniscule, the staff can at least reassure themselves that the child is unlikely to be conscious or suffering during the event. A realization that the family members are the ones who have to live with whatever decisions are made can also help the team to cope.

Summary

Incredible advances in medical technology over the past few decades have brought amazing cures to many. Concomitantly, there arises the need to decide when it is appropriate to use these technologies, and it is at this point that the skills of relationship building, listening, and empathic concern become indispensable. Physicians have always had the privilege and responsibility of being present with patients and families at incredibly difficult times in their lives, and this is going to continue to be the case no matter how many ventilators, pumps, or tubes come between us.

References

[1] Rabkin MT, Gillerman G, Rice NR. Orders not to resuscitate. N Engl J Med 1976;295(7): 364–6.
[2] Prendergast TJ, Luce JM. Increasing incidence of withholding and withdrawal of life support from the critically ill. Am J Respir Crit Care Med 1997;155(1):15–20.
[3] Burns JP, Edwards J, Johnson J, et al. Do-not-resuscitate order after 25 years. Crit Care Med 2003;31(5):1543–50.
[4] Kipper DJ, Piva JP, Garcia PC, et al. Evolution of the medical practices and modes of death on pediatric intensive care units in southern Brazil. Pediatr Crit Care Med 2005; 6(3):258–63.
[5] Feudtner C, Connor S. Epidemiology and health services research. In: Carter BS, Levetown M, editors. Palliative care for infants, children, and adolescents. Baltimore (MD): The Johns Hopkins University Press; 2004. p. 3–22.
[6] Wall SN, Partridge JC. Death in the intensive care nursery: physician practice of withdrawing and withholding life support. Pediatrics 1997;99(1):64–70.
[7] van der Heide A, van der Maas PJ, van der Wal G, et al. Medical end-of-life decisions made for neonates and infants in the Netherlands. Lancet 1997;350(9073):251–5.
[8] Vernon DD, Dean JM, Timmons OD, et al. Modes of death in the pediatric intensive care unit: withdrawal and limitation of supportive care. Crit Care Med 1993;21(11):1798–802.

[9] Balfour-Lynn IM, Tasker RC. At the coalface—medical ethics in practice. Futility and death in paediatric medical intensive care. J Med Ethics 1996;22(5):279–81.

[10] Ackerman AD. Death in the pediatric intensive care unit. Crit Care Med 1993;21(11): 1803–5.

[11] Roy R, Aladangady N, Costeloe K, et al. Decision making and modes of death in a tertiary neonatal unit. Arch Dis Child Fetal Neonatal Ed 2004;89(6):F527–30.

[12] Postovsky S, Levenzon A, Ofir R, et al. "Do not resuscitate" orders among children with solid tumors at the end of life. Pediatr Hematol Oncol 2004;21(7):661–8.

[13] Garros D, Rosychuk RJ, Cox PN. Circumstances surrounding end of life in a pediatric intensive care unit. Pediatrics 2003;112(5):e317–79.

[14] Althabe M, Cardigni G, Vassallo JC, et al. Dying in the intensive care unit: collaborative multicenter study about forgoing life-sustaining treatment in Argentine pediatric intensive care units. Pediatr Crit Care Med 2003;4(2):164–9.

[15] Devictor DJ, Nguyen DT. Forgoing life-sustaining treatments: how the decision is made in French pediatric intensive care units. Crit Care Med 2001;29(7):1356–9.

[16] Keenan HT, Diekema DS, O'Rourke PP, et al. Attitudes toward limitation of support in a pediatric intensive care unit. Crit Care Med 2000;28(5):1590–4.

[17] van der Wal ME, Renfurm LN, van Vught AJ, et al. Circumstances of dying in hospitalized children. Eur J Pediatr 1999;158(7):560–5.

[18] Ryan CA, Byrne P, Kuhn S, et al. No resuscitation and withdrawal of therapy in a neonatal and a pediatric intensive care unit in Canada. J Pediatr 1993;123(4):534–8.

[19] Lantos JD, Berger AC, Zucker AR. Do-not-resuscitate orders in a children's hospital. Crit Care Med 1993;21(1):52–5.

[20] Mink RB, Pollack MM. Resuscitation and withdrawal of therapy in pediatric intensive care. Pediatrics 1992;89(5):961–3.

[21] Diem SJ, Lantos JD, Tulsky JA. Cardiopulmonary resuscitation on television. Miracles and misinformation. N Engl J Med 1996;334(24):1578–82.

[22] Knox C, Vereb JA. Allow natural death: a more humane approach to discussing end-of-life directives. J Emerg Nurs 2005;31(6):560–1.

[23] Cohen RW. A tale of two conversations. Hastings Cent Rep 2004;34(3):49.

[24] American Academy of Pediatrics Committee on Bioethics: guidelines on foregoing life-sustaining medical treatment. Pediatrics 1994;93(3):532–6.

[25] Truog RD, Cist AF, Brackett SE, et al. Recommendations for end-of-life care in the intensive care unit: the Ethics Committee of the Society of Critical Care Medicine. Crit Care Med 2001;29(12):2332–48.

[26] Solomon MZ, Sellers DE, Heller KS, et al. New and lingering controversies in pediatric end-of-life care. Pediatrics 2005;116(4):872–83.

[27] Menikoff J. Law and bioethics: an introduction. Washington (DC): Georgetown University Press; 2001. p. 256, 308–11, 356–73.

[28] Uniform Health-Care Decisions Act. Issues Law Med 2006;22(1):83–97.

[29] United States. President's Commission for the Study of Ethical Problems in Medicine and Biomedical and Behavioral Research. Deciding to forego life-sustaining treatment: a report on the ethical, medical, and legal issues in treatment decisions. Washington (DC): President's Commission for the Study of Ethical Problems in Medicine and Biomedical and Behavioral Research: For sale by the Supt. of Docs., U.S.G.P.O.; 1983.

[30] Beauchamp TL, Childress JF. Principles of biomedical ethics. 5th edition. New York: Oxford University Press; 2001. p. 99–103.

[31] Zawistowski CA, Frader JE. Ethical problems in pediatric critical care: consent. Crit Care Med 2003;31(5 Suppl):S407–10.

[32] Ross LF. Children, families, and health care decision making. New York: Oxford University Press; 1998. p. 39–56.

[33] Kopelman LM. Rejecting the Baby Doe rules and defending a "negative" analysis of the best interests standard. J Med Philos 2005;30(4):331–52.

[34] Krautkramer CJ. Pediatric resuscitation: questioning DNAR legitimacy and offering an alternative decision-making model. Am J Bioeth 2005;5(1):86–8 [author reply W19–21].

[35] Kunin H. Ethical issues in pediatric life-threatening illness: dilemmas of consent, assent, and communication. Ethics Behav 1997;7(1):43–57.

[36] Informed consent, parental permission, and assent in pediatric practice. Committee on Bioethics, American Academy of Pediatrics. Pediatrics 1995;95(2):314–7.

[37] McCabe MA. Involving children and adolescents in medical decision making: developmental and clinical considerations. J Pediatr Psychol 1996;21(4):505–16.

[38] Frader J. Younger yet wiser: courts allow mature minors medical autonomy. Bull Park Ridge Cent 2000;(16):3–4.

[39] Baren JM. Ethical dilemmas in the care of minors in the emergency department. Emerg Med Clin North Am 2006;24(3):619–31.

[40] Guidelines for the appropriate use of do-not-resuscitate orders. Council on Ethical and Judicial Affairs, American Medical Association. JAMA 1991;265(14):1868–71.

[41] Cantor MD, Braddock CH 3rd, Derse AR, et al. Do-not-resuscitate orders and medical futility. Arch Intern Med 2003;163(22):2689–94.

[42] Annas GJ. Extremely preterm birth and parental authority to refuse treatment—the case of Sidney Miller. N Engl J Med 2004;351(20):2118–23.

[43] Clark FI. Making sense of state v Messenger. Pediatrics 1996;97(4):579–83.

[44] Behind a boy's decision to forgo treatment. NY Times (Print). June 13, 1994:A12.

[45] Kopelman LM. Are the 21-year-old Baby Doe rules misunderstood or mistaken? Pediatrics 2005;115(3):797–802.

[46] Clark F. Baby Doe rules have been interpreted and applied by an appellate court. Pediatrics 2005;116(2):513–4 [author reply 514–15].

[47] Mohr M, Bahr J, Kettler D, et al. Ethics and law in resuscitation. Resuscitation 2002;54(1): 99–102.

[48] Elias-Jones AC, Samanta J. The implications of the David Glass case for future clinical practice in the UK. Arch Dis Child 2005;90(8):822–5.

[49] Baskett PJ, Steen PA, Bossaert L. European Resuscitation Council guidelines for resuscitation 2005. Section 8. The ethics of resuscitation and end-of-life decisions. Resuscitation 2005; 67(Suppl 1):S171–80.

[50] Miles SH. Medical futility. Law Med Health Care 1992;20(4):310–5.

[51] Consensus statement of the Society of Critical Care Medicine's Ethics Committee regarding futile and other possibly inadvisable treatments. Crit Care Med 1997;25(5):887–91.

[52] Stern SG, Orlowski JP. DNR or CPR—the choice is ours. Crit Care Med 1992;20(9): 1263–72.

[53] Schneiderman LJ, Jecker NS, Jonsen AR. Medical futility: its meaning and ethical implications. Ann Intern Med 1990;112(12):949–54.

[54] Youngner SJ. Who defines futility? JAMA 1988;260(14):2094–5.

[55] Lantos JD, Singer PA, Walker RM, et al. The illusion of futility in clinical practice. Am J Med 1989;87(1):81–4.

[56] Truog RD, Brett AS, Frader J. The problem with futility. N Engl J Med 1992;326(23): 1560–4.

[57] Dunphy K. Futilitarianism: knowing how much is enough in end-of-life health care. Palliat Med 2000;14(4):313–22.

[58] Medical futility in end-of-life care: report of the Council on Ethical and Judicial Affairs. JAMA 1999;281(10):937–41.

[59] Fine RL, Mayo TW. Resolution of futility by due process: early experience with the Texas Advance Directives Act. Ann Intern Med 2003;138(9):743–6.

[60] Truog RD, Mitchell C. Futility—from hospital policies to state laws. Am J Bioeth 2006;6(5): 19–21.

[61] Iserson KV. Foregoing prehospital care: should ambulance staff always resuscitate? J Med Ethics 1991;17(1):19–24.

[62] Do not resuscitate orders in schools. Committee on School Health and Committee on Bioethics. American Academy of Pediatrics. Pediatrics 2000;105(4 Pt 1):878–9.

[63] Guru V, Verbeek PR, Morrison LJ. Response of paramedics to terminally ill patients with cardiac arrest: an ethical dilemma. CMAJ 1999;161(10):1251–4.

[64] Kimberly MB, Forte AL, Carroll JM, et al. Pediatric do-not-attempt-resuscitation orders and public schools: a national assessment of policies and laws. Am J Bioeth 2005;5(1):59–65.

[65] Weise KL. The spectrum of our obligations: DNR in public schools. Am J Bioeth 2005;5(1): 81–3 [author reply W19–21].

[66] Fallat ME, Deshpande JK. Do-not-resuscitate orders for pediatric patients who require anesthesia and surgery. Pediatrics 2004;114(6):1686–92.

[67] Casarett DJ, Stocking CB, Siegler M. Would physicians override a do-not-resuscitate order when a cardiac arrest is iatrogenic? J Gen Intern Med 1999;14(1):35–8.

[68] Casarett D, Ross LF. Overriding a patient's refusal of treatment after an iatrogenic complication. N Engl J Med 1997;336(26):1908–10.

[69] Willard C. Cardiopulmonary resuscitation for palliative care patients: a discussion of ethical issues. Palliat Med 2000;14(4):308–12.

[70] Lo B, Ruston D, Kates LW, et al. Discussing religious and spiritual issues at the end of life: a practical guide for physicians. JAMA 2002;287(6):749–54.

[71] Way J, Back AL, Curtis JR. Withdrawing life support and resolution of conflict with families. BMJ 2002;325(7376):1342–5.

[72] Feudtner C. Tolerance and integrity. Arch Pediatr Adolesc Med 2005;159(1):8–9.

PEDIATRIC CLINICS

OF NORTH AMERICA

Pediatr Clin N Am 54 (2007) 773–785

Withdrawal of Mechanical Ventilation in Pediatric and Neonatal Intensive Care Units

David Munson, MD[a,b,*]

[a]Division of Neonatology, The Children's Hospital of Philadelphia,
University of Pennsylvania School of Medicine, 34th Street & Civic Center Boulevard,
Room 2442, Philadelphia, PA 19104, USA
[b]The Pediatric Advanced Care Team, The Children's Hospital of Philadelphia, 9th Floor,
Philadelphia, PA 19104, USA

In pediatrics we are gifted with good outcomes. We enjoy high survival rates in our intensive care units and oncology programs thanks to the resilient nature of children and the advances in pediatric science. Unfortunately our medical interventions are not always successful. Pediatric patients may become too sick to respond to our ministrations, may suffer from an incurable disorder, or may be faced with a future of severe suffering or terrible quality of life. Although it is difficult for pediatricians to face the limits of medical technology, we are obligated to provide exceptional care at these limits. Thorough and compassionate care at the end of life includes learning how to discontinue life-sustaining treatments when they no longer provide a means to a good outcome.

A body of literature in medical ethics has established that there is no ethical difference between discontinuing an intervention (withdrawal) and not starting one (withholding). Further, it is well established legally that a medical team and the family can discontinue overly burdensome treatment [1–3]. Palliative care principles have made inroads into intensive care units, and some surveys of practice and physician attitudes toward withdrawing life-sustaining treatment have been published [4,5]. Although there is little empiric research into the most effective way to withdraw ventilator support, there is now a body of literature that describes application of basic

* Division of Neonatology, The Children's Hospital of Philadelphia, University of Pennsylvania School of Medicine, 34th Street & Civic Center Boulevard, Room 2442, Philadelphia, PA 19104.

E-mail address: munson@email.chop.edu

pediatric.theclinics.com

principles and theory to guide compassionate end-of-life care in an intensive care setting [6,7]. This article is aimed at providing a practical approach to the withdrawal of life-sustaining treatment, and more specifically mechanical ventilation. Although every situation is unique, some general principles can guide a medical team through a process that seeks to help a family in their grief and achieve a more comfortable and peaceful death for the pediatric or neonatal patient.

Case

It had been a long 6 months. Born at 24 weeks and less than 500 g, the odds had always been stacked against Jonathan. He had survived surgery for necrotizing enterocolitis, laser therapy for retinopathy of prematurity, and several severe exacerbations of his bronchopulmonary dysplasia. Jonathan's parents had always been aware of the high risk for death and struggled throughout his life with the balance of short-term suffering and the possibility of a good quality of life later on. At 5 months of age, he had significant bronchopulmonary dysplasia and associated pulmonary hypertension. Despite this, he was maintained on stable, if high, ventilator support and was growing well on nasoduodenal feeds. After extensive discussions about the possibility of significant developmental problems and the complications associated with long-term ventilation, the family and medical team decided to proceed with a tracheostomy and surgical placement of a feeding tube.

The day before the planned surgery, Jonathan became sick again. He needed to go back on high-frequency ventilation, 100% oxygen, and inhaled nitric oxide. Even with all of these therapies, his oxygen saturations were difficult to keep above 90%. After several days of attempting to discover treatable causes for the decompensation, the medical team sat down with the family again to discuss the gravity of the situation and explore the most loving choices for Jonathan. Review of a recent MRI demonstrated significant periventricular leukomalacia. The team reviewed the likely future. The most likely outcome was that he would not survive this current event or the planned surgical interventions. If he did survive, he was likely to have profound developmental problems. After several days of deep soul searching and no improvement in Jonathan's clinical condition, the family and the medical team agreed that withdrawal of mechanical ventilation was the best course of action. He had become difficult to sedate over the prior 2 weeks, requiring high-dose infusions of morphine and midazolam and escalating doses of methadone. Consequently several challenges faced the team in planning for withdrawal of the ventilator.

A communication toolbox

Family experience and satisfaction with hospitalization depends on the quality of family–staff communication, relationships, and the extent to which families and staff members are engaged in partnership. If bad news is communicated poorly, it can result in confusion, long-lasting distress, and resentment. If done well, it can promote understanding, acceptance, and adjustment. Families remember the words and manner of clinicians long after they have forgotten the medications, procedures, and details of treatment [8]. Nowhere is this more critical than in conversations around the withdrawal of life-sustaining therapy.

McDonagh and colleagues [9] published a study evaluating communication with families in the context of a family meeting. An increased proportion of time during which the family spoke and the physician listened was related to increased satisfaction, improved impressions of the physician, less conflict, and a greater sense that the family's needs were being met. Clinicians need to remember to keep the message they are delivering concise. They need to allow silence and time for parents to process the information and they need to elicit the parents' thoughts and values.

For critically ill patients, efforts should be made from early in the admission to explore the family's hopes, fears, values, and goals. Clinicians can have these conversations in the context of hoping for the best while preparing for the worst. Invite multiple perspectives and promote dialog early in the admission. Creating a relationship and a true understanding of how the family views their child's illness facilitates conversations about difficult choices should the need arise.

Although learning to engage in conversations with families around this difficult issue is best achieved through experience, it is helpful to prepare by having mental resources on which to draw. By developing a group of phrases and ideas with which the clinician feels comfortable, he or she can more comfortably focus on direct communication. These phrases and ideas can be conceptualized as a "communication toolbox" (Box 1).

Convey empathy

Parents consistently report that they appreciate compassion, tenderness, and emotional availability from the physician who is conveying bad news [10]. Consequently, the clinician should demonstrate her concern for the patient and family through words and body language. When a family is hurting, it is a normal human response to want to tell them "it will all be OK." In fact, it is the emotional connection that drives this desire that the clinician should harness to convey empathy. We are sincerely sorry for the pain the family is experiencing, but it is not exactly an apology that we are wishing to communicate. The key here is sincerity. It is perfectly acceptable to say, "I am so sorry that things have become so bad," but it is easy to get into a trap of saying "I am sorry" over and over again. A useful substitute is the phrase "I wish." By declaring that you wish things were different, you make it clear that you are aligned with the family and that you care. By saying "I wish the EEG had shown some improvement, but I am afraid there is no change," you have conveyed empathy while giving accurate information [11].

Box 1. A communication toolbox

Convey empathy. Use "I wish things were different" instead of
  "I am sorry." Be open to a real connection with the family.
Speak directly. Do not use euphemisms. Ask about a family's
  hopes and fears.
Focus on compassion. The fundamental question is how best
  to love this patient.
Wait quietly. Use the power of silence to convey empathy,
  reinforce your presence, and to allow time for processing.
Review the goals. Sometimes the two goals of medicine come
  into conflict—adding time versus adding quality. Be clear
  which medical interventions are consistent with stated goals.
Guide parents through the process. Explore with them how they
  might participate in the care of their child. What will help them
  create meaning and memories?
Address spirituality. Most families rely on spirituality for coping
  to some degree. Offer to assist in providing resources and
  support spiritual practices.

Speak directly

When discussing withdrawal of life-sustaining therapies, talk about death
and dying without using euphemisms [10,12]. Ask the parents what they fear
the most. Asking about seemingly forbidden topics can relieve a family of
secret anxiety. Do not fear addressing a family's anxiety directly. "Many
parents feel like they are leading to the death of their child by agreeing to
stop the ventilator; are you struggling with this?" [6] Affirming that such
concerns are common can help. It also may provide an opportunity to
address the goals that lead to the decision. It is the disease or injury that
has put the patient into the situation, not anyone's decision.

Focus on compassion

Frame the conversation in a way that respects the parents' love for their
child. When discussing goals of therapy at the end of life, the real question is
how best to love the patient. A decision to withdraw life-sustaining technology can be an extraordinary act of love and courage. Compliment the parent's devotion to their child. Speaking about loving decisions keeps the
conversation within the mental framework of parenting. It gives the parents
permission to talk about end-of-life issues without feeling like they are abandoning their core identity as the patient's mother or father.

Wait quietly

In addition to using words to convey empathy, remember the power of silence. When a family is processing newly acquired bad news, simply sitting with them makes it clear that you are there to support them. The clinician should wait for body language in the family members that they are ready to receive more information before continuing the meeting. Until they are ready, the family members will not hear the next piece of information. The most important questions often arise after a long period of silence [13]. In addition, your presence relieves a family of the fear of abandonment, and also sends the message that you are committed to giving the family as much time as they need.

Review the goals

Tell parents about the two goals of medicine. The first is to add time to life. The second is to add quality to life. Usually we can pursue both goals without conflict, but sometimes the burdens of technology become so great and the chance of recovery so small that the goal of simply adding time comes into conflict with improving quality or minimizing suffering. Ensure that families understand the rationale for initiating certain therapies. It should be clear that the medical team will not initiate therapies that will cause suffering without the hope of improving the condition [14,15].

Guide parents through the process

The time around removing ventilator support is profoundly personal and intimate. Every family has a different path toward grieving. Clinicians need to explore with the family the options they have to participate in the care of their child or baby and the opportunities for creating memories. In the neonatal intensive care unit (NICU), the severity of illness may have prevented the parents from ever having the opportunity to hold their baby. They may wish to hold him while he is still on the ventilator to have adequate time for this experience before the baby dies. For older patients, the parents may desire to climb into the bed for some final time of holding their child. A family may wish to give their infant a bath and dress him or her in baby clothes for the first time. In general, any opportunity to facilitate the parents being just that – parents—without having to focus on the monitors, tubes, and machines interfering should be made available [14,16]. Help families understand what options they have to participate in the care of their child.

Families need to be prepared for what they will see and hear. They need to know about color changes, gasping breaths, and the unpredictability of the time to death from the time of withdrawal of support. As discussed later, the medical team needs to be clear about what symptoms are anticipated and how they will be managed. The family should be educated about these plans. This education reassures the family that the team will continue to aggressively care for their child and empowers them to know which symptoms require treatment and which are simply changes in physiology or reflexes anticipated during the process of dying [7,14,16].

Address spirituality

For many families incorporating a spiritual practice or ritual is critical. In the NICU, many families want their baby baptized before he or she dies. Other families benefit from the presence of the hospital chaplain, or may arrange for their own spiritual advisor to be present. There is an opportunity here to empower the parents to feel that they are actively caring for their child by engaging in religious ceremony important to them. Prayer, faith, access to clergy, and a perception of something transcendent in the relationship between the parents and child were common themes of support in a survey of parents whose children had died [17].

Medical management

In every case, it is critical to anticipate symptoms that the patient may experience during the process of dying. In pediatric critical care and neonatal intensive care, the most common problem is respiratory distress after withdrawal of ventilator support.

It is important to distinguish respiratory distress—manifested as increased work of breathing, a sense of shortness of breath, or other signs of air hunger—from agonal respirations. These terminal breaths occur sporadically with long periods of apnea in between. The patient is invariably unconscious at this point in the process. Such a breathing pattern is reflexive, and consequently should not be a source of discomfort for the patient. Families need to be informed of this and reassured. In addition, the clinician should avoid the term "agonal respirations" and instead simply describe the reflexive deep breaths that they may see.

Goals of intervention

Withdrawal of mechanical ventilation is a unique act in palliative care with significant ethical challenges. One major concern is precipitating air hunger and respiratory distress [6]. Physicians in intensive care are obligated to adequately control symptoms of discomfort in their patients at the end of life. The discomfort of air hunger and respiratory distress should be no different and warrants special attention.

Historically, there has been hesitation among critical care physicians to use narcotics during the withdrawal of mechanical ventilation. Because a known side effect is respiratory depression, physicians worry about hastening a patient's death or directly contributing to their demise [18]. There are two critical concepts that guide the use of pain medications and sedatives during end-of-life care. The first is the concept of "double effect," and the second is awareness of literature demonstrating that critically ill patients who receive narcotics and benzodiazepines do not die more quickly.

A physician's intent is the critical component in understanding the idea of the double effect [19]. If we accept that an infant or child should not have to experience pain or discomfort at the end of life, then choosing medications with the goal of achieving adequate pain relief or sedation is appropriate. Narcotics, such as morphine, fentanyl, or hydromorphone have good pain-relieving properties but often are not adequate on their own to deal with the symptoms of air hunger and respiratory distress. It should therefore be the goal of the team to achieve moderate to deep sedation in the patient from whom mechanical ventilation is going to be withdrawn [6]. Respiratory depression is a known side effect of narcotics and sedatives, but it is just that—a side effect [19]. The medical team crosses into difficult ethical and legal territory if they choose such large doses of a medication that it is clear that their intent is to suppress respiratory drive and commit euthanasia.

Interestingly, there is evidence from retrospective reviews in adult critical care and in the neonatology literature that use of narcotics and sedatives in this way does not shorten time to death [20]. In an adult study, use of benzodiazepines was associated with an increased time to death from the moment of withdrawal [18]. Because of these findings and a general moral imperative to treat suffering, it is our obligation to treat symptoms of discomfort at the end of life. There is simply no reason not to aggressively pursue adequate sedation when withdrawing an infant or child from mechanical ventilation.

Choosing a medication regimen

The medical team needs to think carefully about the medication plan. The plan needs to include starting doses, when they plan to administer them (generally before extubation), and how they plan to titrate the dose (Box 2). The team should also be explicit about what signs and symptoms they will be treating. This plan needs to be clear to all members of the team, and the general concepts should be discussed with the family also.

Morphine is the most commonly used narcotic and has several advantages. In addition to pain relief it elicits a sense of euphoria. It has vasodilatory properties that result from histamine release. These properties may have benefit in reducing venous return and consequently relieving cardiogenic pulmonary vascular congestion, which may in itself decrease respiratory distress in some patients. It has a reasonable half life of 1 to 2 hours, especially compared with some synthetic opioids, such as fentanyl. The synthetic opiates also tend to induce a marked and rapid tolerance. Meperidine should be avoided because its metabolic byproduct can cause seizures and

---

Box 2. Selecting medications

Goal: In general when withdrawing mechanical ventilation, ensuring comfort requires sedation in addition to pain relief. The rule of double effect and recent clinical trials support our moral obligation to treat suffering at the end of life.

Narcotics
- Morphine is the most commonly used analgesic. Dosing is 0.1 to 0.2 mg/kg for an opiate-naïve patient, but should be titrated to effect with no real maximum.
- Hydromorphone is a semisynthetic narcotic that may be useful in older patients who have a morphine allergy.
- Fentanyl has a shorter half life, making it less ideal for use during end-of-life care.
- Meperidine should be avoided because of its centrally active metabolite.

Benzodiazepines
- Midazolam is a short-acting sedative that can be effective in achieving sedation. Usual dosing is 0.1 to 0.2 mg/kg, but also should be titrated to effect. If multiple doses are expected, strongly consider starting an infusion.
- Lorazepam has a longer half life, but should not be used in neonates.

For patients who are difficult to sedate, plan ahead
- Propofol has anesthetic and sedative properties and can be titrated to a specific level of sedation.
- Pentobarbital can also be effective in patients who are already resistant to benzodiazepines.

---

agitation. Hydromorphone is a semisynthetic agent that may be valuable in patients who have previously had a negative reaction to morphine [7].

Narcotics alone are often insufficient in the management of air hunger and respiratory distress at the end of life. A medication regimen needs to be selected that can relieve all signs of discomfort, including grimacing, agitation, anxiety, and physiologic signs of distress. Fundamentally, the goal is to treat symptoms that indicate suffering, not just pain, and it is usually necessary to achieve moderate to deep sedation to meet this goal when discontinuing mechanical ventilation [6,21]. As stated by the American Academy of Pediatrics, "dying with dignity and without pain or distress is the primary goal" [15]. Benzodiazepines, such as lorazepam or midazolam, should be added and titrated to effect. They have specific anxiolytic effects in addition to sedative effects, giving them usefulness in the setting of withdrawing ventilatory support. Lorazepam has a longer half life, but should be avoided in neonates because of the benzyl alcohol preservative. Midazolam is equally effective, but strong consideration should be given to starting an infusion because its clinical effect may be short following rapid redistribution. It also has the advantage of minimal pain on administration through a peripheral vein because it is water soluble [7].

Occasionally, patients have required significant escalation of narcotics and benzodiazepines over the days or weeks before the decision to withdraw life-sustaining treatments. Most patients respond to further increases in doses, but the team should consider having alternative drugs available if adequate sedation and relief of respiratory distress cannot be achieved. Barbiturates, such as pentobarbital, can be titrated carefully to achieve sedation. Starting doses of pentobarbital for infants and children should generally be around 0.5 to 2 mg/kg and titrated to effect. Like fentanyl, pentobarbital can induce a rapid tolerance, so clinicians should be prepared to escalate doses if needed. Propofol is an intravenous anesthetic that may prove an attractive alternative in pediatric intensive care units (PICUs). It is given by continuous infusion with a typical starting dose in pediatrics of 0.5 mg/kg/hour. It can be titrated from there to achieve the desired level of sedation [21].

Regardless of the medications selected, it is generally important to anticipate the acute symptoms that are expected when the patient is extubated. In general, the first doses should be given before extubation and an adequate level of sedation should be achieved to avoid having the patient experience significant air hunger at all. Responding to air hunger after extubation is frequently inadequate, and it is simply unnecessary for an infant or child at the end of life to experience such discomfort.

Guidance about dosing is difficult given the varied degrees of opiate and sedative exposure and tolerance in infants and children in intensive care. Starting doses of morphine in the range of 0.1 to 0.2 mg/kg should suffice for opiate-naïve patients. For patients on longstanding infusions, the medical team should be prepared to substantially increase the doses given. For practical purposes, there is no maximum dose of morphine or benzodiazepines.

It should be noted that paralytics are distinctly absent from the above list of medications. Paralytic agents prevent the medical team from adequately assessing a patient's level of sedation or pain. They have no analgesic or sedative properties of their own, and consequently have no role in end-of-life care. Furthermore, because they directly prevent respiration, it is difficult to argue that they do not play a direct role in the patient's demise once the ventilator is removed. There may be rare circumstances when a patient is so clearly moribund that delaying extubation long enough for paralysis to wear off is not in the best interest of the patient or family. It should be emphasized, however, that these circumstances are rare and that one must pay exceptional attention to ensuring adequate sedation in those circumstances [22].

Withdrawing the ventilator

There is no substantial research in pediatrics or neonatology to guide us on the proper way to discontinue mechanical ventilation. We can explore the options available and then determine which choices fit the particular circumstances best. There are essentially two approaches. The first has been termed "terminal extubation" and describes removing the endotracheal tube without weaning ventilatory support [7]. The second approach has been termed "terminal weaning." With this approach, the clinician gradually decreases ventilator support before extubating [7,23]. In either case, clinicians should abandon this terminology because it is confusing, but should fully understand the advantages and disadvantages of the two approaches. In most cases some combination of the two approaches is most appropriate.

Gradually weaning ventilator support has several advantages. Weaning the oxygen, pressures, and rate should provoke some signs of respiratory distress in the patient. This signal gives the clinician the opportunity to ensure that pharmacologic sedation is adequate. Second, while taking the time to titrate the medications as the ventilator support is decreased, the subsequent hypoxemia and hypercarbia may contribute to the level of sedation. Advocates of true terminal weaning avoid extubating the patient at all to avoid any sudden changes in physiology or any contribution of upper airway obstruction to respiratory distress. The clinicians should, however, be meticulous in avoiding the concept that they are weaning the ventilator. The clinical use of the term weaning is fairly specific for improving status. When describing the plans to the family, simply explain that the amount of support given by the ventilator will be decreased so that the sedation can be titrated [7]. There are also circumstances in which the mode of ventilation might be changed to facilitate time with the patient before withdrawal. In the NICU especially it may be impossible to hold an infant while the baby is on the oscillator. Changing the baby to conventional mode of ventilation may facilitate time holding the baby before he is extubated.

The disadvantage of the above approach is that it could result in prolongation of the dying process. Descriptions of terminal weaning in the literature demonstrate variations in duration of the procedure from minutes to days [23–25]. In this author's opinion, decreasing ventilatory support is best done over a short period of time in an effort to evaluate and adjust the level of sedation. Adequate time may be provided to titrate medications to treat symptoms without prolonging the dying process. Once it is assured that adequate sedation has been achieved, extubation can be performed with minimal risk for increasing the patient's suffering.

The advantage of extubation without adjustment in the ventilator rests mainly with the avoidance of prolonging the death [7]. There may also be situations in which once a family has made a decision, delaying extubation only serves to heighten anxiety and anticipation in the family. In the end, choosing an approach rests primarily on ensuring the patient's comfort and meeting the needs of the family. Preparations to ensure adequate sedation and discussions about how the family would like to participate in their child's care at the end of life are more important than the details of removing the ventilator.

Choosing a location

Some NICUs and PICUs have created special rooms specifically designed for this purpose. They have low lighting, the ability to provide music, are large enough to accommodate several members of the family, and have comfortable seating for the family [16,26]. They should be equipped with the necessary connections for a ventilator so that the patient can be settled in the room before weaning ventilator support. In other situations, a family or child may be particularly bonded with the staff of their primary unit. It is not uncommon for a family to desire spending their child's final hours back on the oncology floor. If this wish is expressed, efforts should be made to meet the family's needs [16]. If these options are not available, then the medical team should work to ensure a private and peaceful setting within the patient's current care space. In the NICU this may require setting up screens and bringing in chairs to the primary care area. Visitation policies should be loosened so that the family can have as many people as they need to support them.

Supporting the family

It is critical that the family not feel abandoned at this important time. Many families do desire privacy, and this should be respected. The medical and nursing team must make their presence and care felt, however. They need to assess the child frequently and determine if the family has any needs. Sitting with a family in silence shows support and empathy. If the patient appears comfortable, the team should say so and reassure the family about changes in breathing patterns and appearance. End-of-life care needs to be conceptualized as aggressive care in the sense that the team is just as committed to ensuring comfort and family support as they were to heroic interventions. If the family does want privacy, the team needs a simple and rapid mechanism in place to respond if the patient needs something [16].

The case

Jonathon was placed on a conventional ventilator and moved to a family sleep room equipped with connections for the ventilator. The family sat with him on the ventilator. The team gradually weaned the supplemental oxygen and supporting pressures. His infusions were increased. He appeared to have some agitation with the increased work of breathing, however, so a small dose of pentobarbital was given. He appeared adequately sedated thereafter, although he continued to have some increased work of breathing. When the parents felt ready, he was extubated. The parents held him and rocked him. They had a compact disc of their favorite lullabies playing. He was dressed in clothes that they had been saving for when he might go home. Jonathon died 40 minutes after extubation. He appeared peaceful throughout the process. His parents were profoundly sad, but grateful for the time they had with Jonathon in their life.

Summary

In some ways, withdrawing life-sustaining technologies requires all of the resources and concepts that the field of palliative care has to offer. By learning some fundamental principles of medical management at the time of withdrawal, however, and by mastering a few communication techniques, pediatricians, neonatologists, and pediatric intensivists can dramatically improve the care provided to their patients at the end of life. Many neonatal intensive care units, including ours, have developed palliative care guidelines to assist clinicians in providing the best end-of-life care possible [14,27]. Although we may argue in pediatrics if there is ever such a thing as a good death, we should all strive to ensure one that is free of suffering and one that supports the family in moving down a path of healthy grief and recovery.

References

[1] Ethical and moral guidelines for the initiation, continuation, and withdrawal of intensive care. American College of Chest Physicians/ Society of Critical Care Medicine Consensus Panel. Chest 1990;97(4):949–58.

[2] The initiation or withdrawal of treatment for high-risk newborns. American Academy of Pediatrics Committee on Fetus and Newborn. Pediatrics 1995;96(2 Pt 1):362–3.

[3] American Academy of Pediatrics Committee on Bioethics: Guidelines on foregoing life-sustaining medical treatment. Pediatrics 1994;93(3):532–6.

[4] Burns JP, Mitchell C, Outwater KM, et al. End-of-life care in the pediatric intensive care unit after the forgoing of life-sustaining treatment. Crit Care Med 2000;28(8):3060–6.

[5] Wall SN, Partridge JC. Death in the intensive care nursery: physician practice of withdrawing and withholding life support. Pediatrics 1997;99(1):64–70.

[6] Rubenfeld GD. Principles and practice of withdrawing life-sustaining treatments. Crit Care Clin 2004;20(3):435–51.

[7] Truog RD, Cist AF, Brackett SE, et al. Recommendations for end-of-life care in the intensive care unit: The Ethics Committee of the Society of Critical Care Medicine. Crit Care Med 2001;29(12):2332–48.

[8] Fallowfield L, Jenkins V. Communicating sad, bad, and difficult news in medicine. Lancet 2004;363(9405):312–9.

[9] McDonagh JR, Elliott TB, Engelberg RA, et al. Family satisfaction with family conferences about end-of-life care in the intensive care unit: increased proportion of family speech is associated with increased satisfaction. Crit Care Med 2004;32(7):1484–8.

[10] Krahn GL, Hallum A, Kime C. Are there good ways to give "bad news?". Pediatrics 1993; 91(3):578–82.

[11] Quill TE, Arnold RM, Platt F. "I wish things were different": expressing wishes in response to loss, futility, and unrealistic hopes. Ann Intern Med 2001;135(7):551–5.

[12] Ptacek JT, Eberhardt TL. Breaking bad news. A review of the literature. JAMA 1996;276(6): 496–502.

[13] Curtis JR. Communicating about end-of-life care with patients and families in the intensive care unit. Crit Care Clin 2004;20(3):363–80.

[14] Catlin A, Carter B. Creation of a neonatal end-of-life palliative care protocol. J Perinatol 2002;22(3):184–95.

[15] American Academy of Pediatrics. Committee on Bioethics and Committee on Hospital Care. Palliative care for children. Pediatrics 2000;106(2 Pt 1):351–7.

[16] Garros D. [A "good" death in pediatric ICU: is it possible?]. J Pediatr (Rio J) 2003;79(Suppl 2): S243–54 [in Portuguese].

[17] Robinson MR, Thiel MM, Backus MM, et al. Matters of spirituality at the end of life in the pediatric intensive care unit. Pediatrics 2006;118(3):e719–29.

[18] Chan JD, Treece PD, Engelberg RA, et al. Narcotic and benzodiazepine use after withdrawal of life support: association with time to death? Chest 2004;126(1):286–93.

[19] Sulmasy DP, Pellegrino ED. The rule of double effect: clearing up the double talk. Arch Intern Med 1999;159(6):545–50.

[20] Partridge JC, Wall SN. Analgesia for dying infants whose life support is withdrawn or withheld. Pediatrics 1997;99(1):76–9.

[21] Burns JP, Mitchell C, Griffith JL, et al. End-of-life care in the pediatric intensive care unit: attitudes and practices of pediatric critical care physicians and nurses. Crit Care Med 2001; 29(3):658–64.

[22] Truog RD, Burns JP, Mitchell C, et al. Pharmacologic paralysis and withdrawal of mechanical ventilation at the end of life. N Engl J Med 2000;342(7):508–11.

[23] Gianakos D. Terminal weaning. Chest 1995;108(5):1405–6.

[24] Gilligan T, Raffin TA. Rapid withdrawal of support. Chest 1995;108(5):1407–8.

[25] Campbell ML, Bizek KS, Thill M. Patient responses during rapid terminal weaning from mechanical ventilation: a prospective study. Crit Care Med 1999;27(1):73–7.

[26] Levetown M. Palliative care in the intensive care unit. New Horiz 1998;6(4):383–97.

[27] Carter BS, Bhatia J. Comfort/palliative care guidelines for neonatal practice: development and implementation in an academic medical center. J Perinatol 2001;21(5):279–83.

ELSEVIER
SAUNDERS

PEDIATRIC CLINICS
OF NORTH AMERICA

Pediatr Clin N Am 54 (2007) 787–798

Palliative Care for the Family Carrying a Fetus with a Life-Limiting Diagnosis

David Munson, MD[a,b,c,*],
Steven R. Leuthner, MD, MA[d]

[a]Division of Neonatology, The Children's Hospital of Philadelphia,
The University of Pennsylvania School of Medicine, 34th Street & Civic Center Boulevard,
Room 2442, Philadelphia, PA 19104, USA
[b]The Pediatric Advanced Care Team, The Children's Hospital of Philadelphia, 9th floor,
34th Street and Civic Center Boulevard, Philadelphia, PA 19104, USA
[c]The Medical College of Wisconsin, Children's Corporate Center, Suite C410,
999 North 92nd St, Wauwatosa, WI 53226, USA
[d]Fetal Concerns Program, Children's Hospital of Wisconsin,
PO Box 1997 Milwaukee, WI 53201, USA

The prenatal diagnosis of a lethal condition creates a crisis in the lives of the prospective parents and family of an affected fetus. The family is subject to shock, anger, disbelief, and despair similar to parents of children who face a life-limiting diagnosis. Although there may be debate about viewing a fetus as an individual, it is clear that families receiving the news of a lethal condition in their fetus need help. The construct of palliative care with its focus on emotional, spiritual, social, and symptom support can provide a model for caring for these families [1–6]. Some of the decisions that a family of an affected fetus faces are unique to the prenatal situation, but a palliative care model nonetheless can be applied.

In spite of improvements in technology in obstetrics and neonatal intensive care, the neonatal mortality rate remains at 4.7 per 1000 live births in 2003 and the infant mortality rate is 6.9 per 1000 live births. Congenital malformations are the leading cause of death in 20% of these cases [7]. Although a lethal diagnosis overall is rare, it is clear from these data that clinicians and families are faced with these circumstances thousands of times a year. In addition, many families who receive a lethal diagnosis in their fetus in the first trimester choose to terminate the pregnancy. All of these

* Corresponding author. Division of Neonatology, The Children's Hospital of Philadelphia, University of Pennsylvania School of Medicine, 34th Street & Civic Center Boulevard, Room 2442, Philadelphia, PA 19104.

  E-mail address: munson@email.chop.edu (D. Munson).

families are faced with difficult emotions and choices and could benefit from proper clinical guidance and support.

Perinatal hospice has been proposed as an alternative to termination of a pregnancy [8]. Calhoun and colleagues reported a substantially lower rate of termination at their institution where they have an active perinatal hospice program compared with national estimates. Breeze and colleagues [5] reported 40% of families offered palliative care made a decision not to terminate. The proposed explanation surrounds how a perinatal hospice program alters the way the choice between termination and carrying to term may be presented. Without a perinatal hospice program, families may be presented the choice of termination or carrying to term in incomplete terms. As Calhoun states, "A bare presentation of these options may leave parents with the perceived choice of futilely watching their infant die...versus actively doing something to end this new and emotionally wrenching dilemma" [9]. Describing in more detail what kind of support will be provided to the families and infants through the remainder of gestation and delivery may help them make an empowered choice of what is best for the baby and family.

Palliative care in newborns has been supported in three general situations: (1) congenital anomalies incompatible with life, (2) newborns born at the limits of viability, and (3) infants who have overwhelming illness not responding to life-sustaining intervention. It seems a logical extension to consider a palliative care approach when a lethal diagnosis is made prenatally. There is a significant challenge in decision making that is related to the degree of certainty of the diagnosis and the certainty of lethality [4]. Palliative care principles can be used to guide supportive conversations. If one likely outcome is perinatal death, preparing for that outcome, along with the other possible outcomes, is critical to a family's experience of the remainder of the pregnancy and in setting the stage for a normal grieving process.

The general tenets of palliative care can form the basis of compassionate care for families in this situation (Box 1). Clear communication, an exploration of values, the role of spirituality, and what role the parents want to play in creating meaning and memories all should be explored. The purpose of this article is to lay out a framework for engaging families in these discussions and to help clinicians and families make decisions that can begin the process of emotional healing and grieving. There is little research available that has assessed the specifics of this approach. Rather than shy away from giving any guidance in the absence of data, however, this article offers specific advice about commonly encountered problems. It is our hope to increase the comfort level of obstetricians, pediatricians, and neonatologists in helping these families.

Case

It was with complete shock that Mrs. Brown learned her fetus had trisomy 18. The decision to undergo an amniocentesis had seemed fairly routine. It

---

Box 1. Tenets of palliative care, modified from the World Health Organization

1. Affirm life while accepting death as a normal process.
2. Intend to neither hasten nor postpone death.
3. Offer a support system to help a families cope during a patient's illness and in their own bereavement.
4. Interventions are aimed at comfort and quality of life.
5. Consider values beyond the physical needs of a dying individual.
6. Apply palliative care early in the course of illness in conjunction with other therapies intended to prolong life
7. Pediatric palliative care begins when illness is diagnosed and continues regardless of whether or not a child receives treatment directed at the disease

---

Adapted from World Health Organization definition of palliative care. Available at: www.who.int. Accessed June 5, 2007.

---

simply was a test to make sure everything was going well, not to discover something had gone terribly wrong. She and her husband agonized about what to do. They were advised to terminate because this was a lethal diagnosis, and they felt a tremendous pressure to "do something." But Mrs. Brown already has felt the fetus moving, and she carried a tremendous sense of attachment. She could not help but want to meet her baby. After much discussion with their family, Mrs. and Mr. Brown decided to carry the baby to term or at least to try, because they knew there was a significant chance the fetus might not survive even that long.

Things became only more complicated as they learned about the challenges facing their unborn daughter. They learned at their level 2 ultrasound that she had a large ventricular septal defect and a large meningomyelocele. They met with a geneticist, maternal fetal medicine specialist, and neonatologist. They struggled to make sense of the information. They were told that all babies who had meningomyelocele were born by cesarean section to improve the level of spinal function. This advice did not seem to fit with the idea that the baby most likely would die within the first few days of life.

As they struggled with all of the information they had been given and with the sadness that frequently overtook them, they were struck by the difficulties of continuing with their normal life. Well-meaning strangers met Mrs. Brown with the usual ebullient, "You must be so excited! When are you due?" At routine prenatal visits, she felt awkward waiting with all of the other women who were there to complete the unfolding of their normal pregnancies.

Eventually, the Browns found an obstetrician and a neonatologist who seemed interested in helping them devise a birth plan that met their needs.

They supported the family in their choices, including a vaginal delivery and postnatal interventions aimed at maximizing comfort and time with the parents. The Browns wanted nothing more than a chance to meet their daughter and to hold her. The neonatologist agreed to a limited resuscitation to assist her through the transition period only. There was to be no endotracheal intubation or cardiovascular resuscitation. They all agreed that if their daughter did survive the initial days of her life that the team would assist them in finding resources to care for her at home. All other interventions, such as closing the myelomeningocele, would be discussed in the context of whether or not it would add quality to their baby's life. They knew that they would have only a limited time to spend with their daughter and looked to whatever time she would spend with them as a gift.

The decision to carry on

Often, families are advised to terminate a pregnancy when a major congenital abnormality is found. Sometimes the options are expressed as terminate or "do nothing." It often is with the best intentions that medical professionals give this advice. There has been a general view that carrying an affected fetus to term unnecessarily prolongs an emotionally difficult time. It has been known for decades, however, that women who terminate a wanted pregnancy, after receiving a severe diagnosis in their fetus, experience an acute grief reaction comparable to that experienced by women who have had a spontaneous pregnancy loss or even the loss of a neonate after birth [10]. It is, therefore, not clear that termination achieves the goal of optimizing the grief process for families. Every family grieves differently. For some, terminating a pregnancy is the right decision. Others may benefit from an alternative approach. A perinatal palliative care program could provide support to families who make either of these decisions.

The first step in using a fetal palliative care approach is to create a safe place for discussion without assumptions. In helping a family decide whether or not termination, induction of labor, or carrying to term is right for them, an open dialog needs to occur. This dialog needs to address specifics about this pregnancy and also the family's philosophic, theologic, and even political feelings about termination. Families take these decisions seriously and struggle as this decision suddenly moves from the political to the personal. What does this pregnancy mean to them? What does this diagnosis or prognosis mean to them? What are the challenges they will face if they choose to terminate the pregnancy? What are the challenges they will face if they choose to continue the pregnancy? What might it look like if they deliver the baby near term? What can they expect after birth?

Painting a clearer picture for a confused family can enable them to make a choice that makes sense for them. For many, termination is the swiftest road to healing, and these families need to be supported and given access to resources to help them through their grief. For others, creating a birth plan may offer a chance to create needed meaning and memories. Because it is unclear which approach facilitates healthier emotional recovery, both options should be made available.

Support during the pregnancy

As illustrated in the fictional case described previously, it can be difficult to cope with normal interactions while carrying a fetus with a potentially life-limiting medical condition. In the United States, perfect strangers feel at liberty to offer congratulations or comments when they encounter a pregnant woman in public. Such encounters can be magnified in particular situations. The prospective parents already may have one or more children. Gatherings for their friends' birthday parties may be a concentrated experience of pregnancy-oriented discussions. Clinicians should acknowledge these difficulties. Even the business of routine pregnancy care may be challenging for families. Some obstetricians accommodate these families by offering after-hours visits or make them the first clinic visit of the day to avoid a crowded waiting room. Similar efforts can be made around follow-up ultrasounds or other tests [1]. Many families want to prepare for the delivery but feel uncomfortable joining a group birthing class. Private birth classes could be offered, or perhaps a family would benefit from the support of a doula [2]. Finally, some families may reach a point at which they feel their mental health is stretched and they cannot take the pregnancy much further. Early induction of labor for maternal mental health reasons can be considered just as induction for other physical maternal health reasons [11].

It is important to make special note about the concept of facilitating attachment. Many clinicians talk about an affected fetus in dispassionate tones and focus exclusively on the diagnosis and the associated risks. Inherent in the warnings that a fetus will not survive is a benevolent attempt to protect the family from growing too close to the baby. By preventing a strong bond, clinicians believe they can lessen the pain of the loss. This may be the driving force behind the recommendation to terminate a pregnancy. Unfortunately, this is not how grief works. In 1984, White and colleagues noted that "to establish normal grieving the bereaved must accept the reality of the person who has died" [12]. The way to facilitate healthy grieving is to help create meaningful memories and enhance the sense of reality of the person who is at risk for dying. The families at the focus of this article are at particular risk for an exaggerated grief response precisely because there is limited time for bonding with their offspring. They will not have long to stare at their child to imprint the image or absorb the baby's scent and feel. Precisely because of this lack of time, some women see the time of continued pregnancy as extending the time they have with their child [13]. We are biologically driven to bond with our children. This process begins in utero [14]. Our goal should be to facilitate the formation of that bond (Box 2).

Box 2. Tips for prenatal care

Prenatal care should include a focus on facilitating attachment,
    creating memories, and helping families cope with experiences
    that accentuate grief:
1. Ask the parents if they have chosen a name and if you may
    refer to the fetus by it. Families find this affirming and it
    demonstrates respect for their view of the expected baby as
    a whole person, not just a diagnosis.
2. View any needed follow-up ultrasounds not only as
    monitoring and diagnostic studies but also as opportunities
    for a prospective family to interact with their unborn child.
3. Try to minimize waits in crowded waiting rooms by offering
    off-hour visits or making the family the first visit of the day.
4. Explore private options for birthing classes, such as a doula or
    a private Lamaze class.
5. Assist the family in connecting with any needed resources.
    If the baby might survive the immediate postnatal period,
    investigating hospice support services ahead of time may be
    helpful. If a family thinks they would benefit from
    counseling or grief specific counseling, help identify local
    resources.
6. "In all this, there is no substitute for real compassion..." [12].
    Listen to the family's experiences with a sympathetic ear. We
    cannot stop normal encounters that may be hurtful, but we
    can help ease the hurt by listening and reassuring.

It follows that when a family chooses to continue a pregnancy, they are interested in using the time for bonding and memory building with their as-yet unborn child. Caring clinicians honor this choice when they treat a fetus as a real and complete future child rather than as an unfortunate event [1]. There are a few ways this process can be facilitated prenatally. Clinicians should ask families if they have chosen a name, and if so can they refer to the baby by that name. Families find this to be affirming and reassuring. This action conveys to families that they will be real parents of a real baby rather than the unfortunate observers of a terrible event. Families also may benefit from follow-up ultrasounds. This chance to "see" their baby is one more piece of reality and memory building [1]. This can be important especially if a fetus is at high risk for in utero demise. For these families, they may not have the chance to meet their baby alive. The fetal movements and images are all they have to construct their memories.

Intrapartum care

Intrapartum care should be well thought out ahead of time. The involved clinicians should spend time with families to generate a birth plan (Box 3). Such a plan can begin by asking a family to create a wish list. It can and should include medical and nonmedical goals and questions.

Clinicians need to explore what kinds of medical interventions they consider open for negotiation during the delivery. Although there certainly are cases where clinicians feel pushed to make an intervention that they typically would not feel comfortable doing, most families who elect to carry to term in this situation are seeking reasonable and well thought-out options. One area of potential conflict is in the selection of a mode of delivery.

A standard recommendation for method of delivery has been to avoid cesarean section when a fetus has a lethal diagnosis. Because there is no beneficence-based obligation to the fetus, who will die regardless of the mode of delivery, then the risks to the mother of a cesarean section should be the driving force in this decision. It has, however, been argued eloquently that in some cases, a woman may have a powerful desire to meet her infant alive. The risk for a stillbirth after carrying an infant to term is experienced as an extreme emotional burden and an expectant mother may be willing to accept the risk to herself for any limited time with her infant alive [15].

Pediatricians or neonatologists who consult with families are faced with similar challenges. Families seeking comfort care may be clear that they do not want an endotracheal tube placed for mechanical ventilation. They may, however, want the infant to receive a few minutes of positive pressure ventilation in the hope that initial respiratory difficulties are related to problems with transitioning rather than a consequence of an underlying disease. Such a request may seem counter to the usual conception of an advanced Do Not Attempt Resuscitation plan. In some cases, however, the reassurance that every possible chance was given to their infant will make a huge difference in a family's grieving process.

A frank and open discussion about the medical options available at birth forms the beginnings of a birth plan. The details of the planned resuscitation should be discussed carefully in the context of meeting a family's goals. Most elements of routine newborn care likely are optional. For example, if death truly is imminent, the application of eye ointment serves no purpose. Similarly, a vitamin K shot or the state newborn screen becomes only an uncomfortable experience for the baby with no benefit and would be inconsistent with truly "comfort care only." If the baby is likely to survive the immediate postnatal period, then these interventions might fit better with parental goals.

Consider what symptoms the baby may experience. An infant who has severe pulmonary hypoplasia might exhibit respiratory distress and signs of air hunger. Options for management of these symptoms could include giving sublingual morphine, placement of a nasogastric tube to administer

Box 3. Creating a birth plan

Encourage families to create a wish list. This should include any ideas they might have of what could make the birth experience and immediate postnatal period meaningful and memorable. They should then use the wish list in conversations with their obstetrician or midwife and consulting neonatologist or pediatrician to create a birth plan. The ultimate birth plan may not be able to accommodate all the wishes depending on medical limitations, but the involved clinicians should make every effort to accommodate wishes or explain limitations.

1. Mode of delivery. In most cases, spontaneous vaginal delivery without monitoring is appropriate. Occasional families may benefit from a scheduled delivery or cesarean section. If clinicians are uncomfortable offering this and cannot dissuade a family, they should assist the family in finding another obstetrician.
2. Resuscitation. A pediatrician or neonatologist should explain all of the steps in routine resuscitation. They then should discuss which pieces fit with a family's goals and which do not.
3. Symptom management. Anticipate the kinds of symptoms an infant may experience. If there is a chance of significant air hunger or pain, discuss the different options from sublingual morphine, to nasogastric tube placement, to placement of an intravenous line for more direct medication administration.
4. Spiritual considerations. Does the family want a baptism or other religious ceremony? Do they want to bring their local spiritual leader or do they want support from a hospital chaplain?
5. Pictures or video. The family should consider if they want to take pictures or videos themselves or if they want to have external help with this. There are professional photographers available in many communities who volunteer their time to help create memories for families facing the death of their infant.
6. Mementos. Most nurseries offer additional mementos, such as handprints, molds of hands or feet, collection of locks of hair, and so forth. Ask the families to consider these possibilities, and know what your local institution offers.
7. Participation in care. Are there certain activities that a family might find meaningful, such as giving an infant a bath or dressing her? Are there other family members, including older siblings, who should have a chance to hold her?

medications, or placement of an intravenous line or umbilical line for the administration of intravenous medications. The correct approach depends on balancing the perceived risks (such as delay in getting an infant into a parent's arms, the pain of a needle stick, and so forth) and benefits and must fit with parents' overall goals of care.

In addition to a discussion about medical interventions, involved clinicians should assist families in planning for memory building and participation in the baby's care. Are the prospective parents interested in photographs? If so, do they want a member of the family responsible for taking pictures or do they want to seek outside help? There are professional photographers who volunteer their time for this kind of service. A program called Now I Lay Me Down to Sleep [16] can be helpful in identifying local resources for this.

Nurseries generally offer additional mementos that prospective parents might want to have or help create. Hand or foot molds commonly are available. Parents also might want to collect a lock of hair. Footprints or handprints can be made easily. Nurses also should plan on helping families participate in the care of their baby if there are any activities that the families want to pursue. They may want to bathe or dress the baby. Some families have specific desires of whom they wish to hold the baby and in what order. They may want to include older siblings in some of these activities.

A birth plan also should incorporate any spiritual ceremonies that families want to occur. If they want a baptism, are they content to have a hospital chaplain involved, or do they want to make arrangements for someone from their local organization to participate? Discussing whether or not a ritual needs to be done before a baby dies is important to make necessary arrangements to achieve the goal. Openly reviewing the possibilities of fetal demise before or during labor or a baby being born alive but living for a short time or the possibility of survival to discharge all may influence what may be arranged.

As families explore their wish list with the involved clinicians, a true birth plan will emerge. This plan needs to be shared with all of the clinicians who might attend the delivery and the nursing staff who will care for the mother and baby. Some areas of the country have active perinatal hospice organizations. They may be able to supply a hospice nurse to be present and assist in the planning and execution of the details.

It is important to discuss the details of a delivery plan with as many of the clinicians as possible who could be involved at the delivery. A multidisciplinary meeting between obstetrics and neonatology is the ideal setting. All of these cases are emotionally challenging and may challenge the ethical constructs of some of the clinicians. It is critical to make sure everyone who might be involved is comfortable with the plan. If individuals are not willing to participate in the plan as outlined, arrangements should be made for them to opt out. For example, if one neonatologist in a group insists that he or she would feel obligated to resuscitate an infant with the disease process described, then a backup physician could be made available for the delivery. Conflicts need to be anticipated and dealt with in advance. A well-laid plan is for naught if parents perceive genuine discomfort and lack of support from a clinical team. If the conflict is too great to resolve, it may be in a family's best interest to seek delivery plans with a different clinical group or at an alternative institution.

Other pathways

In spite of advances in diagnostic technology, the ability to prognosticate with certainty remains limited. It is important to discuss all possible pathways with a family before delivery. For example, an infant who has severe hydrocephalus may have enough brainstem dysfunction so as not to survive the immediate perinatal period. The prospective parents would benefit tremendously from the palliative care approach laid out previously. Physicians would be remiss, however, to also not help a family plan for the possibility of a normal respiratory drive. A family might choose to take their infant home with hospice for a period of time, anticipating that he may yet succumb to his abnormal neurologic status. The same family may decide later that they want an infant to have a ventriculoperitoneal shunt to optimize the baby's potential function and improve comfort. Another family might decide that if the baby breathes well in the first hours that they then are committed to aggressive intervention from that moment on. To the extent that various pathways can be anticipated, the clinicians involved should help families anticipate what to expect and plan for the different decision points. It is not be possible to plan for every eventuality nor is it critical to arrive at a decision for all of the "what ifs." Simply knowing in advance can arm a family with the information they need to explore their hopes and goals of care.

As the possibilities for experimental fetal inteventions are developed, they may be offered at a time in the pregnancy where it is deemed a compassionate-use basis because a fetus is dying. This seems to be when palliative care concepts can go hand in hand with aggressive experimental procedures. As these procedures come with a high risk for fetal death, potential maternal complications (including pregnancy loss), and just a sliver of hope, having palliative care as a backup plan offers families support if a procedure does not work. Some families may be referred to or search out a fetal program only to find out that the fetus has a lethal condition and there is no applicable fetal intervention. Palliative care principles should be incorporated into any center performing fetal interventions.

After the infant's death

Consideration of further diagnostic information, such as parental testing, placental tissue for cytogenetics, cord blood or skin biopsy for fibroblast culture for cytogenetic testing, radiographs, postmortem examination by a geneticist, and autopsy should be considered, often planned ahead but performed after the death of the baby. Encouraging autopsy is important particularly as it adds new information at least 10% to 40% of the time [17]. This information may confirm or enhance the prenatal diagnosis and subsequently supports parents' decision to provide palliative care for their child. The decision for autopsy may alleviate guilt and helps families feel altruistic in giving back to the medical community and perhaps other future families. It can aid in predicting recurrence risk and the decision of whether or not to seek a subsequent pregnancy or further diagnostic testing for any other children [11]. Parents holding their baby's body for any length of time after death has minimal to nonexistent impact on postmortem pathology studies [18]. Although a skin biopsy should be done within the first few hours after death, other evaluations can be delayed for hours or a day without significant consequence to their being informative. Discussions with the local pathologist are recommended.

Bereavement follow-up begins by supporting families in making burial and memorial service arrangements and, whenever possible, staff should be supported in personally attending services. Follow-up with families during their maternal postpartum examination again can show that an infant's life was meaningful to others. A scheduled appointment to review autopsy or genetic results, typically a few months post death, offers another opportunity to meet with a family. During either of these visits, an assessment of parental coping, grief and depression, and a review of the events of the pregnancy, delivery, time with the baby, and memorial service can be performed. Families often enjoy the opportunity to retell their story to an audience that is accepting of people talking about the death of a child. They may have questions about how to discuss the events with their neighbors, employers, friends, family, or other support systems, and this gives an opportunity to guide them in how to ask for help from these sources.

Bereavement follow-up also might include continued contact with families by phone at scheduled times throughout the year after a baby is born and on anniversary dates, such as the due date, birth date, or day of death. Having some available service for families to find further support in dealing with their grief is critical. Many hospitals have specific bereavement ceremonies and programs that may may serve patients in this function.

Summary

Palliative care constructs for families who have a fetus at risk for dying are every bit as meaningful, and should be as clinically and socially acceptable, as the provision of continued life-extending endeavors. Prenatal diagnosis of a lethal anomaly is a monumental moment in a family's life. It requires extensive team counseling and planning about complex neonatal and obstetric medical management. The construct of palliative care with its focus on emotional, spiritual, social, and symptom support can provide a model for caring for these families.

References

[1] Hoeldtke NJ, Calhoun BC. Perinatal hospice. Am J Obstet Gynecol 2001;185(3):525–9.
[2] Sumner LH, Kavanaugh K, Moro T. Extending palliative care into pregnancy and the immediate newborn period: state of the practice of perinatal palliative care. J Perinat Neonatal Nurs 2006;20(1):113–6.
[3] Leuthner SR. Palliative care of the infant with lethal anomalies. Pediatr Clin North Am 2004; 51(3):747–59, xi.
[4] Leuthner SR. Fetal palliative care. Clin Perinatol 2004;31(3):649–65.
[5] Breeze AC, Lees CC, Kumar A, et al. Palliative care for prenatally diagnosed lethal fetal abnormality. Arch Dis Child Fetal Neonatal Ed 2007;92(1):F56–8.
[6] Leuthner SR, Lamberg-Jones E. The Fetal Concerns Program: a Model for Perinatal Palliative Care. The American Journal of Maternal Child Nursing, 2007;32(5):272–8.
[7] Hoyert DL, Mathews TJ, Menacker F, et al. Annual summary of vital statistics: 2004. Pediatrics 2006;117(1):168–83.
[8] Calhoun BC, Reitman JS, Hoeldtke NJ. Perinatal hospice: a response to partial birth abortion for infants with congenital defects. Issues Law Med 1997;13(2):125–43.
[9] Calhoun BC, Napolitano P, Terry M, et al. Perinatal hospice. Comprehensive care for the family of the fetus with a lethal condition. J Reprod Med 2003;48(5):343–8.
[10] Lloyd J, Laurence KM. Sequelae and support after termination of pregnancy for fetal malformation. Br Med J (Clin Res Ed) 1985;290(6472):907–9.
[11] Sankar VH, Phadke SR. Clinical utility of fetal autopsy and comparison with prenatal ultrasound findings. J Perinatol 2006;26(4):224–9.
[12] White MP, Reynolds B, Evans TJ. Handling of death in special care nurseries and parental grief. Br Med J (Clin Res Ed) 1984;289(6438):167–9.
[13] Leuthner SR, Bolger M, Frommelt M, et al. The impact of abnormal fetal echocardiography on expectant parents' experience of pregnancy: a pilot study. J Psychosom Obstet Gynaecol 2003;24(2):121–9.
[14] Thearle MJ, Gregory H. Evolution of bereavement counselling in sudden infant death syndrome, neonatal death and stillbirth. J Paediatr Child Health 1992;28(3):204–9.
[15] Spinnato JA, Cook VD, Cook CR, et al. Aggressive intrapartum management of lethal fetal anomalies: beyond fetal beneficence. Obstet Gynecol 1995;85(1):89–92.
[16] Now I Lay Me Down to Sleep. Available at: www.nowilaymedowntosleep.org. Accessed August 7, 2007.
[17] Craft H, Brazy JE. Autopsy. High yield in neonatal population. Am J Dis Child 1986; 140(12):1260–2.
[18] Pregnancy Loss and Infant Death Alliance (PLIDA) position statement. Available at: www.plida.org. Accessed June 5, 2007.

PEDIATRIC CLINICS

OF NORTH AMERICA

ELSEVIER
SAUNDERS

Pediatr Clin N Am 54 (2007) 799–812

Providing Care in Chronic Disease: The Ever-Changing Balance of Integrating Palliative and Restorative Medicine

Jeffrey C. Klick, MD[a,b,*], Allison Ballantine, MD[a,b]

[a]Department of Pediatrics, University of Pennsylvania School of Medicine,
3600 Market Street, Suite 240, Philadelphia, PA 19104, USA
[b]Division of General Pediatrics and the Pediatric Advanced Care Team,
The Children's Hospital of Philadelphia, 2nd Floor Main Hospital, Room 2415,
34th and Civic Center Blvd., Philadelphia, PA 19104, USA

Chronically ill children who have life-limiting diagnoses are a unique and challenging population in palliative care. Although many chronic diseases, such as muscular dystrophy or spinal muscular atrophy, are associated with a shortened life span and fit well into the paradigm of palliative care, this article focuses on other diseases, similarly life-limiting, that may not follow as clear an illness trajectory. They tend to follow an undulating, unpredictable course and include disorders as diverse as certain metabolic diseases, genetic syndromes, and congenital anomalies, along with conditions associated with neurologic devastation [1–4].

Through the course of their life, many children who have these diseases experience life-threatening events and then recover some or all of their baseline function. They may then have a period of time of relatively high functioning with a good quality of life only to be followed by another downturn. These ups and downs have a dramatic affect on the well-being of the child, the functioning of the family unit, the ability of the family to make difficult decisions, and the ability of the medical professionals to provide consistent medical care [5–7]. Each child endures a unique set of experiences because of the fluctuating course of the illness that makes integrating restorative and palliative care essential and constant re-evaluation of care imperative.

* Corresponding author. Division of General Pediatrics and the Pediatric Advanced Care Team, The Children's Hospital of Philadelphia, 2nd Floor Main Hospital, Room 2415, 34th and Civic Center Blvd., Philadelphia, PA 19104.
E-mail address: klick@email.chop.edu (J.C. Klick).

0031-3955/07/$ - see front matter © 2007 Elsevier Inc. All rights reserved.
doi:10.1016/j.pcl.2007.07.003
pediatric.theclinics.com

No set pattern of palliative or restorative care is always a perfect fit for these children. Each child's clinical condition changes, and at any given time the child and family may need psychosocial support or symptom management that they will not need when the situation is better. A child may seem to be actively dying and still recover to have years of good life. A family may decide to limit care and later decide that they want "everything" done. The provider's job is to educate, support, and advise and to find an ever-changing balance of restorative and palliative interventions that help maximize potential for quality of life and help limit physical and emotional suffering throughout the child's life.

The chronicity and unpredictability of the disease course present unique challenges to integrating restorative and palliative care and highlight the need for repeated re-evaluation of the child's illness and the family's perspective on illness severity and quality of life. This article outlines the main barriers to incorporating palliative care into the care of chronically ill children who have life-limiting diseases and presents some specific techniques to help the medical professional overcome some of these barriers.

Course of illness: the roller coaster of life with a chronic illness

> Jane was born a full-term infant who had no apparent medical problems. At 6 months of life, she suffered a massively destructive stroke from an isolated arteriovenous malformation, leaving her neurologically devastated. As a result of her severe brain injury she suffered from poorly controlled seizures, chronic aspiration, and hypertonicity.
>
> Over the next several years, Jane was readmitted to the hospital repeatedly for various acute illnesses. Although the underlying cause of the illness was always the neurologic sequelae from the stroke, the acute setbacks were secondary to septic episodes, viral illnesses, respiratory decompensation (from aspiration or upper respiratory infections), status epilepticus, or episodes of severe agitation with no clear cause. In all, she was admitted more than 20 times over a 2-year period of time. Often these admissions lasted for a week or two, or even longer.

Predicting the outcome of a given episode of acute illness in a patient who has severe, complex medical issues is often difficult [2]. A seemingly minor viral illness may spiral downward to respiratory failure, or a small bed sore can evolve into a decubitus ulcer followed by an episode of life-threatening sepsis. Although none of these specific events is foreseeable, anticipating the overall medical trajectory of a patient's life may be possible. Understanding the comprehensive picture of a child's medical life helps the provider to recognize the effect the illness experience has on the child and family. In turn, families may be better at recognizing evolving symptoms, better prepared for future setbacks, and better able to make decisions when the clinical situation changes.

In the case of Jane, the medical team and the family were in agreement that although Jane would likely rebound from many acute illnesses, given

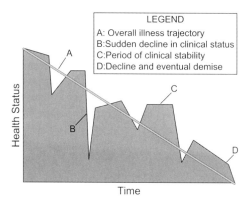

Fig. 1. Course of illness.

her overall frailty and multiple vulnerabilities, she could potentially die of any one of them. Providers need to understand the effect this undulating course has on the child and family to develop a medical care plan that combines acute medical management with supportive palliative care. Fig. 1 illustrates a general picture of the long-term course of illness for these children.

This diagram depicts the medical health of the child over time. Patients who have chronic, life-limiting illnesses experience acute decompensations, recoveries, and periods of relative stability, usually superimposed on a general downward trajectory. In many situations, the functional ability of the child over time mirrors this course also. The child has many setbacks, and although some of these setbacks include a complete recovery, others may result in a decline in functional ability.

Uncertain prognosis: what will the future bring?

During later hospitalizations, the family often reported that one of the hardest things about taking care of Jane was the unknown. Throughout her life, even very subtle symptoms could lead to a life-threatening illness. It was impossible to know how long she would be hospitalized, what interventions would be required during her stays, or if she would even survive the acute illness.

Uncertain prognoses are common in palliative care, and chronic deteriorative illnesses are especially challenging in this regard. The unpredictable drop-offs and plateaus of chronic illness make it difficult to offer the family a timeline or concrete predictions about the child's illness. Predictions based on population studies of children who have similar diseases are so often off the mark that they may lead to further uncertainty for the family [2].

The impact of this uncertainty needs to be recognized when providers talk with families about goals, hopes, or limits of care. Some families who seem to be at peace with the concept that their child has a life-limiting condition may have tremendous difficulty when trying to make decisions about care within the context of so much medical uncertainty. As a result, attempting to focus exclusively on the end-of-life aspects of palliative care may not meet the needs of the family or the child and may be met with some resistance [5,8,9].

In discussing medical expectations with the family, admitting uncertainty and outlining the likely fluctuations in acute illnesses and challenges that the child and family will face serves to frame events as they occur and invite ongoing dialogue as the child's condition evolves over time. Being frank about the life-limiting nature of their child's illness and the severity of acute illnesses is essential to integrating good palliative care with restorative care. It is equally important to validate the uncertainty.

Burden of past successes: "she always seems to prove us wrong"

> On admission, Jane often appeared very ill. Sometimes, there was real concern that she would die soon. The medical team and the family had many discussions regarding her expected course of illness and the limitations of care. Each time, the family was receptive to conversations, sometimes limiting interventions. She always seemed to recover, however, despite their worst fears. The family reported that she returned to baseline most times, and what functional setbacks she did suffer did not significantly affect her overall quality of life. "That's just Jane; she always seems to prove us wrong," her mother would say.

The one constant for these children is the repetition of episodes of severe illness. Some may be life-threatening, appropriately prompting discussions of limitations of care. Unexpected recoveries are both gratifying and disconcerting for the providers and family. These "resurrection episodes" offer the family hope for the future health of their child, but also bring added uncertainty and often an increased mistrust of medical prognostication [5,10]. These episodes can be unsettling for providers also, causing them to doubt their own perceptions of the patient's condition. Even so, when being open with families about the difficulty of predicting the future and admitting when predictions are wrong, providers build a relationship of honesty and increased comfort with uncertainty in which difficult conversations can occur.

Hope of the future: the promise of medicine

> At the time of discharge, as the team was preparing to inform Jane's home nursing company of her impending return to home, her mother was

uncharacteristically reticent, but said she would not be needing nursing right away. Eventually she admitted to the team that she was taking Jane to another state for a trial of hyperbaric oxygen therapy, which she hoped would help her brain recover some amount of function.

The hope of medical advances, or the perceived promise of medical and alternative therapies, can make advance care planning difficult [2,5,7]. Many families feel obligated to pursue all potential therapies that might improve their child's disease course, insisting that they would be giving up on their child if they limited care [11]. Under these circumstances, the family may pursue unproven therapies, hoping for some level of restoration.

This situation can be difficult for the medical providers and other family members who may believe there is little to be gained from such therapies. Many medical providers report experiencing discomfort around providing care that they feel may be causing prolonged suffering or discomfort for the patient [2].

The challenge for the provider in this circumstance is to strike the fine balance between supporting the family and assuring that they are not being misled. In most situations, families act out of a sense of duty to their child and a sense of hope for the child's restoration. For many families, this hope can balance some of their grief and serves as a coping mechanism in taking care of a child who has a severe chronic illness [12,13]. Finally, providers need to remember that when these children do die, the families are often left wondering if they did all they could. In some circumstances it may therefore be appropriate for the provider to accept such efforts as part of the patient's care plan while openly discussing and trying to avert undue suffering or discomfort.

Perceived quality of life: quality is in the eye of the beholder

When Jane was hospitalized with an acute illness she often appeared uncomfortable, with much posturing and moaning. She seemed unaware of her environment and perceived only painful stimuli. This situation was disconcerting to her mother, but she believed she was able to comfort Jane and that such episodes were transient.

Jane's mother would often tell stories and bring in pictures of her experiences at home. She said Jane loved to be with her brother, and though they were unable to play together they both seemed to "light up" when they were in the same room. Although she conceded that Jane did have periods of discomfort or agitation at home, she reported that she was often relaxed and comfortable, smiling and vocalizing with what seemed to her like squeals of happiness.

Medical professionals, especially those who are based in acute care settings, have limited opportunity to assess a child's true functional ability and quality of life. During acute illnesses, these providers see children at their worst [14,15]. Because many medical providers base their opinions on interactions with the family during acute illnesses, gaining insight into the child's baseline well-being can be difficult. The family's perspective, which extends over periods of illness and relative good health, may be one of higher overall quality of life [16].

Over time, most families do develop an understanding of the severity of their child's illness that is in line with that of the medical providers. They may focus on their child's abilities and apparent successes (eg, a hypertonic infant who "rolls over") in ways that the medical team may have difficulty accepting, however [2,17–22]. In this situation, many providers feel obligated to attempt to emphasize the severity of the child's illness or bleak outlook for restoration or recovery. Although honesty about a child's condition is imperative, providers should attempt to comprehend the family's perspective of the child's condition, recognizing that choosing not to focus on a bleak future may be one of their coping mechanisms.

Providers also need to recognize that the family's perception of their child's experience of the world affects their goals for care. Through this understanding, providers are better able to discuss potential interventions and their implications. Although the medical team may be reluctant to agree to an intervention they see as increasing suffering or complexity of care, the family may sometimes feel that suffering is an acceptable tradeoff for potential improvement that may result.

Challenges for families: the work of care

> When Jane had been admitted for the ninth time in as many months, the inpatient care team convened a meeting to discuss the medical and social aspects of her care at home. Many of the staff were worried about her mother. Although she was extremely capable and provided excellent care to Jane, the team was concerned that the stresses of her role and relationship to Jane had undermined her ability to maintain balance in her life, and that she was close to "breaking down."

Research on the care of chronically ill children has demonstrated that the family is under tremendous stress, and may have limited ability to access resources essential for coping. Parents of chronically ill children perform a multitude of complex tasks, both manual (eg, tube feeds) and cerebral (eg, coordinating appointments or juggling shift nursing schedules). They are also called on to maintain a high degree of vigilance, monitoring closely for any sign or symptom that might herald a decompensation [12,23–25].

This focus on the child as patient can result in a dramatic reconfiguration of the parents' role. The child's needs can engulf the parents' existence, shutting out other supports and creating a sense of isolation. In a sense, the family's life becomes medicalized [5,12,16,23–25].

Underpinning this reconfiguration of the parents' role is the chronic sorrow connected with caring for children who have chronic illnesses. Initially described by Simon Olshansky as grieving without finality, the concept of chronic sorrow encompasses the losses that the parents face with each deterioration; the losses that come when milestones are not achieved, such as walking or getting a driver's license; and the sadness that comes with anticipating an early death. Families often live in a constant state of fear, mourning, grief, and transitory hope.

In addition to the emotional cost of living with a chronically ill or dying child, parents are often forced to change their life circumstances—quit jobs, move to be closer to hospital—to accommodate their child's care. When their child dies, they lose a lifestyle in addition to their child [2,5,12,23–26]. These life changes can lead to extreme difficulty making decisions and "moving on" after their child dies.

Guidelines: an approach to integrating care

> Jane died before her third birthday. Before her death she had become very ill with increasingly frequent seizures and even more limited interaction with her surroundings. In meeting with the family, in similar fashion to many earlier meetings, the team discussed goals of care. This time the family believed that her underlying condition had significantly deteriorated and that she was suffering. Although they never gave up hope that she would recover, they decided to focus on her comfort.
>
> From that point until her death a few weeks later, the team provided aggressive symptom management for agitation, dyspnea, and seizures. In addition, they encouraged the family to spend the rest of her life focusing on time together and less on her medical concerns. This approach required frequent phone calls and visits with the family to support the medical decision making of the hospice providers and family.
>
> Discussions continued with the family as they questioned their decision from time to time. Each time, after some patient listening from the care providers, the family decided they had made a loving decision for their child and that they truly enjoyed the peaceful time at the end of Jane's life.

The ultimate goal of incorporating palliative care is to maximize potential, minimize suffering, and support the child and family in all phases of life. The inherent uncertainty of prognosis for these children makes it difficult to apply an "either–or" model of palliative and restorative care [7,27]. The focus of care for these children should be integrating the two models throughout the child's life [5,8,9].

The remainder of this article outlines guidelines for integrating palliative and restorative care. The main themes include consistent communication in times of crisis and stability, teamwork with the family in decision making, and continual re-evaluation throughout the child's life.

Step 1: Know yourself

Some medical professionals who care for children who have chronic life-limiting illnesses question whether invasive procedures and medications are in the best interest of the child, whether the benefit of restorative care is worth the suffering [2,5,7]. Some even wonder if prolonging the life of a child in this condition is in the best interest of the child and family.

In contrast, some medical providers are influenced by health care and ethics policies and popular culture to lean toward not limiting care. Further, laws in place to protect children sometimes obstruct providers' choices about withholding life-sustaining therapies or limiting procedures [2,28–30].

To provide the best possible care to the child and family, providers must consciously assess their own positions. Past negative experiences with suffering patients, strong feelings about allocation of medical resources, and religious beliefs are some of the factors that may influence their approaches. Understanding how beliefs and morals affect advice to families helps providers remain open minded, support the family's decisions, and relieve some of the burden of guilt when a difficult decision is made.

Step 2: Know the family and build a team

Providers need to understand that the family often has beliefs and backgrounds different from their own that lead to different quality-of-life values and decisions. The medical profession regularly challenges families to make leaps of faith regarding decisions about their child's health (eg, initiation of therapeutic medications) but sometimes finds it difficult to accept a family's version of what constitutes a good quality of life. Taking the time to understand these values helps build trust with the family and the sense of teamwork necessary for difficult discussions over time [1,2,8,31–33].

Step 3: Family meetings

The framework for a family meeting regarding decision making and goal setting is outlined in the communication article by Feudtner found elsewhere in this issue. The inherently undulating course and unpredictability of life-limiting chronic disease make all decision making a moving target. Medical providers should encourage the family to revisit their goals frequently, during times of both stability and decline.

Step 4: Goal setting

When discussing goals of care it is helpful to identify overarching themes. One approach is to focus on what the family does want for their child, as opposed to specific decisions associated with limiting care, such as resuscitation or intubation. When a family states "we just want him to be happy and comfortable" or "we just want him to be here for his next birthday," they are laying out concrete goals that can frame future decision making. All interventions can then be weighed against this overall goal [2].

Periods of stability can be ideal times to explore goals. These goals can then serve as a guideline for the most difficult conversations that must take place when a child is ill. The provider may be able to say, "Last time we talked you mentioned that your main goal was for your child to be comfortable." The family members may change their minds, but this framework provides a starting place, particularly in stressful, acute situations [2].

Deciding what the family does want for their child helps make the specific questions easier. By not starting with a laundry list of decisions, difficult discussions feel more organized and the fears associated with the acute illness are limited. In other words, it may be easier to limit resuscitation and intubation if those interventions do not meet the overall goal of comfort and limiting interventions already agreed on. For many families, it is much more difficult to limit interventions when they only see that it will end their child's life sooner. It is easier when they can see that it will accomplish the stated goal of keeping the child more comfortable.

Step 5: Advance care planning

Box 1 offers an algorithm for advance care planning [2]. These steps may proceed over several meetings because the process can be daunting for the family and the provider. In situations in which discussion seems to have

---

Box 1. Steps in advance care planning

Step 1—Identify. Identify the decision makers and the primary supports who will be affected by decisions. Limit those identified as unimportant in decision making.

Step 2—Listen. Allow the family to describe their understanding of the situation. This situation may involve the underlying disease and course of illness, an acute illness or setback, or a difficult decision.

Step 3—Clarify. Clarify any important misunderstandings that the family may have. Provide them with your best guess as to what may occur in the near future and before the next meeting.

Step 4—Goals. Discuss goals of care. Focus on what they hope for their child.

Step 5—Limits. Discuss the limits of care. Identify which limitations are consistent with or inconsistent with their goals of care.

Step 6—Summarize. Briefly summarize the major decisions from the meeting and how they are consistent with the goals of care.

Step 7—Invite. Set a meeting time for next discussion and leave with an invitation for open communication.

slowed down, the meeting should be brought to a close and a time set to resume the conversation. At that time, the discussion should return to step 1. The discussion can then progress quickly until it returns to where it ended at the last meeting.

Step 6: Coordinate care

Many families complain that bridging perceived communication gaps between medical providers is difficult. Their children often see multiple subspecialists. Coordinating care plans and scheduling visits often fall to the parents [2,12,13,25]. Poor communication often leads to significant medical error or iatrogenic complications of their children's medical management [34]. Providers can help reduce errors and relieve some of the family's burden by working to coordinate care.

Often families report that coming to a doctor's visit takes a lot out of their child. The stress of these visits should not be underestimated. Limiting nonessential provider visits and coordinating the important ones help keep the child at home and prevent undue stress.

Care plan and medication diary

When multiple medical providers are involved, care plans change multiple times. For example, a neurologist may want to increase a medicine based on seizure activity, whereas a gastroenterologist may want to decrease it because of the medication's side effects. It is often left to the parents to communicate these changes to other medical providers. Ideally, medical providers should communicate with each other. As an alternative, a care plan and medication diary can help providers communicate with each other and the family. By listing all changes and a brief reason for the change, providers can dramatically improve day-to-day communication and help prevent competing care plans and medical errors.

Step 7: Symptom management

Attention to symptom management is essential to limiting suffering. Although therapies managing symptoms are essentially the same, evaluating them can be challenging. Often a seemingly minor or straightforward symptom can herald a more complex problem. Difficulties managing symptoms may suggest an undiagnosed and unexpected underlying cause for the symptom.

For example, a child who has severe neurologic disability may present with extreme agitation. The agitation may be secondary to the natural course of illness, pain attributable to secondary injury (a dislocated hip, bed sore, or hair tourniquet), constipation, reflux, changes in medications, or numerous other possibilities. Although treating the agitation may involve starting or increasing a sedative, the agitation may persist or get worse if the underlying cause is not found. Discovering the cause sometimes requires time and multiple laboratory and radiographic studies. When the cause cannot be found or requires invasive procedures to diagnose, often a trial of presumptive treatment is required.

Providers should schedule frequent contact with parents—in person or by phone—to reassess the therapy to make sure the current medical plan remains effective. Even minor changes in medications can alter the tenuous balance of symptom management and unwanted side effects. For example, adding Carafate for reflux-induced agitation may change the absorption of a seizure medication, leading to increased seizure activity.

Symptom diaries

Symptom diaries can facilitate teamwork with the family. The family should keep a detailed log of any changes in their child's activity and anything temporally associated with a concerning symptom. This diary improves the family's ability to give a good history and the provider's ability to re-evaluate the efficacy of therapy.

Step 8: Re-evaluate and revisit

Because circumstances and health status change over time for the child and the family, decisions about care change also. The undulating nature of disease calls for an equally shifting approach to care. Providers must frequently revisit the child's state of health, the medical team's care plans, and the family's decisions.

Summary

About one year after Jane's death, her mother met with some of Jane's medical care providers. She reported that only after Jane's death was she truly able to grasp how ill and disabled Jane was. She was then able to see the ups and downs of Jane's life and the profound effect it had on her family. She repeatedly thanked the care providers for the compassion they showed Jane and her family. She recognized that their willingness to make themselves available, their constant re-evaluation of the medical plan, and their awareness of the family's perspective were important reasons that Jane had what quality of life she had along with a meaningful and peaceful death.

Caring for children who have a chronic life-limiting illness can be emotionally and physically challenging. Just as families may struggle with whether they are making the right decisions, care providers struggle with whether they are giving the right advice, predicting the medical course correctly, and making the correct medical decisions. Uncertainty is a constant for the family and the care provider. The willingness of the care provider to develop a relationship with the family that involves continuing communication and re-evaluation of the child's condition and the family's perspective can relieve some of emotional and physical suffering associated with a chronic disease and support the family in times of hope and grief.

Direction for future care

Caring for medically complex children by integrating restorative and palliative care is not a new concept. Much of the understanding of the experience of these children and their families is based on data extrapolated from other patient populations, however. Although this research gives us insights into caring for these children who have complex, chronic conditions, their experience is fundamentally different from that of other populations. More research is needed to provide better knowledge of how to support these children and their families more effectively.

We need more reliable measures of quality of life and symptom assessment for children who have chronic, life-limiting illnesses. We need better information regarding how families make decisions in times of stress. In addition, we need greater understanding of the physical and emotional work associated with the tasks of providing care. Finally, we need to learn more about the long-term outcomes for families with a child who has a chronic, life-limiting illness so we can predict areas of concern and intervene in ways that help these families cope with the challenges they face.

References

[1] Behrman R, Field MJ. When children die: improving palliative and end-of-life care for children and their families. Washington, DC: National Academy Press; 2002. p. 490.
[2] Himelstein BP, Hilden JM, Boldt AM, et al. Pediatric palliative care. N Engl J Med 2004; 350(17):1752–62.
[3] Arias E, MacDorman MF, Strobino DM, et al. Annual summary of vital statistics—2002. Pediatrics 2003;112(6 Pt 1):1215–30.
[4] Mortality data from the National Vital Statistics System. Available at: http://www.cdc.gov/nchs/about/major/dvs/mortdata.htm. Accessed March 29, 2004.
[5] Graham RJ, Robinson WM. Integrating palliative care into chronic care for children with severe neurodevelopmental disabilities. J Dev Behav Pediatr 2005;26(5):361–5.
[6] Ray LD. Parenting and childhood chronicity: making visible the invisible work. J Pediatr Nurs 2002;17(6):424–38.
[7] Selwyn PA, Forstein M. Overcoming the false dichotomy of curative vs palliative care for late-stage HIV/AIDS: "let me live the way I want to live, until I can't". JAMA 2003; 290(6):806–14.
[8] American Academy of Pediatrics. Committee on Bioethics and Committee on Hospital Care. Palliative care for children. Pediatrics 2000;106(2 Pt 1):351–7.

[9] A guide to the developement of the children's palliative care services. London: Association for Children with Life Threatening or Terminal Conditions and their Families, Royal College of Paediatrics and Child Health; 1997.

[10] Steele RG. Trajectory of certain death at an unknown time: children with neurodegenerative life-threatening illnesses. Can J Nurs Res 2000;32(3):49–67.

[11] Wolfe J, Klar N, Grier HE, et al. Understanding of prognosis among parents of children who died of cancer: impact on treatment goals and integration of palliative care. JAMA 2000;284(19):2469–75.

[12] Granvelle A. Caring for a child with a progressive illness during the complex chronic phase: parents' experience of facing adversity. J Adv Nurs 1997;25(4):738–45.

[13] Clements DB, Copeland LG, Loftus M. Critical times for families with a chronically ill child. Pediatr Nurs 1990;16(2):157–61, 224.

[14] Bradford R. Staff accuracy in predicting the concerns of parents of chronically ill children. Child Care Health Dev 1991;17(1):39–47.

[15] Coyne IT. Partnership in care: parents' views of participation in their hospitalized child's care. J Clin Nurs 1995;4(2):71–9.

[16] Kirk S. Families' experiences of caring at home for a technology-dependent child: a review of the literature. Child Care Health Dev 1998;24(2):101–14.

[17] Siperstein GN, Wolraich ML, Reed D. Physicians' prognoses about the quality of life for infants with intraventricular hemorrhage. J Dev Behav Pediatr 1991;12(3):148–53.

[18] Siperstein GN, Wolraich ML, Reed D. Professionals' prognoses for individuals with mental retardation: search for consensus within interdisciplinary settings. Am J Ment Retard 1994; 98(4):519–26.

[19] Wolraich ML, Siperstein GN, Reed D. Doctors' decisions and prognostications for infants with Down syndrome. Dev Med Child Neurol 1991;33(4):336–42.

[20] Siperstein GN, Wolraich ML, Reed D, et al. Medical decisions and prognostications of pediatricians for infants with meningomyelocele. J Pediatr 1988;113(5):835–40.

[21] Affleck GG. Physicians' attitudes toward discretionary medical treatment of Down's syndrome infants. Ment Retard 1980;18(2):79–81.

[22] Todres ID, Krane D, Howell MC, et al. Pediatricians' attitudes affecting decision-making in defective newborns. Pediatrics 1977;60(2):197–201.

[23] Young B, Dixon-Woods M, Findlay M, et al. Parenting in a crisis: conceptualising mothers of children with cancer. Soc Sci Med 2002;55(10):1835–47.

[24] Coffey JS. Parenting a child with chronic illness: a metasynthesis. Pediatr Nurs 2006;32(1): 51–9.

[25] Hewitt-Talor J. Caring for children with complex and continuing health needs. Nurs Stand 2005;19(42):41–7.

[26] Wheeler I. Parental bereavement: the crisis of meaning. Death Stud 2001;25(1): 51–66.

[27] Robinson W. Palliative care in cystic fibrosis. J Palliat Med 2000;3(2):187–92.

[28] Kunin H. Ethical issues in pediatric life-threatening illness: dilemmas of consent, assent, and communication. Ethics Behav 1997;7(1):43–57.

[29] Amendments to Child Abuse Prevention and Treatment Act. Public Law 98-457. US Statut Large, 1984. 98(Title I Sections 101a–312a): p. Unknown.

[30] Kopelman LM, Irons TG, Kopelman AE. Neonatologists judge the "Baby Doe" regulations. N Engl J Med 1988;318(11):677–83.

[31] Children's International Project on Palliative/Hospice Services (ChIPPS). A.P.W. A call for change: recommendations to improve the care of children living with life-threatening conditions. 2001. Available at: http://www.nhpco.org/files/public/ChIPPSCallforChange.pdf. Accessed March 29, 2004.

[32] Levetown M, editor. Compendium of pediatric palliative care: Children's International Project on Palliative/Hospice Services (ChIPPS). Alexandria (VA): National Hospice and Palliative Care Organization; 2000.

[33] Last Acts Palliative Care Task Force. Precepts of palliative care for children/adolescents and their families. Available at: http://www.lastacts.org/files/publications/pedprecept.pdf. Accessed March 29, 2004.
[34] Slonim AD, LaFleur BJ, Ahmed W, et al. Hospital-reported medical errors in children. Pediatrics 2003;111(3):617–21.

ELSEVIER
SAUNDERS

PEDIATRIC CLINICS
OF NORTH AMERICA

Pediatr Clin N Am 54 (2007) 813–827

Issues Related to Providing Quality Pediatric Palliative Care in the Community

Jean M. Carroll, RN, BSN[a,*],
Christy Torkildson, RN, MSN, PHN[b,c],
Jeannine S. Winsness, RN, MSN, CRNP[d]

[a]*The Pediatric Advanced Care Team, The Children's Hospital of Philadelphia,
34th Street and Civic Center Boulevard, Philadelphia, PA 19104, USA*
[b]*School of Nursing, University of California, San Francisco,
San Francisco, CA 94143, USA*
[c]*Research and Professional Relations, George Mark Children's House,
2121 George Mark Lane, San Leandro, CA 94578, USA*
[d]*Pediatric Palliative Care Consultants, LLC, 122 Washington Place,
Wayne, PA 19087, USA*

JR is a 12-year-old ex-preemie diagnosed with severe cerebral palsy, profound mental retardation, cortical blindness, moderate reactive airway disease, and multiple other complex chronic conditions associated with his history. He receives continuous overnight enteral nutrition by way of a gastric feeding tube and supplemental oxygen at night by way of nasal cannula. His family has been receiving 10 hours of shift nursing at night to support them in caring for JR at home. JR is an adopted child in a loving family consisting of a mother, a father, and a younger sibling.

Sometimes children die. However obvious the statement, it neglects the complex issues that often accompany the death of a child. The medical practitioner in the community is in a unique position to assist children and their families from the time of diagnosis with a life-threatening condition through to the end of life. The purpose of this article is to inform medical practitioners who care for children with complex, chronic, and life-limiting

---

This article is submitted as a partial requirement for completion of a Masters degree at the College of Nursing, Villanova University, Villanova, PA, under the supervision of Dr. Patricia Haynor, faculty advisor.

* Corresponding author.

E-mail address: carrollJ@email.chop.edu (J.M. Carroll).

doi:10.1016/j.pcl.2007.06.002

conditions about pediatric palliative care in the community. It is intended to serve as a guide to improve understanding about (1) the misconceptions and barriers surrounding the provision of care in the community for children with chronic, complex, and life-limiting conditions; (2) the availability of services for care in the community; (3) challenges concerning out-of-hospital do-not-attempt-resuscitation orders (DNAROs) for children; and (4) reimbursement issues that impact the provision of care.

These issues are addressed in the context of a brief history of the children's hospice movement that led to the development of guidelines for pediatric palliative care, and a brief review of the literature regarding how and where children die. Additionally, the authors provide practical resources to assist the medical practitioner in caring for these special children and their families and an overview of innovative models of care that currently exist.

Brief history of the children's hospice movement

A brief review of the children's hospice movement in England and North America reveals its value and its influence on the provision of pediatric hospice services today. Once Helen House opened in Oxford, England, in 1982, the movement spread quickly in the United Kingdom [1,2]. Today, more than 40 in-patient children's hospices exist in the United Kingdom, many of which also provide home hospice care in the community [3]. Although called hospice houses, these organizations follow a pediatric palliative care model [4]. Children and families are served by the hospice houses from the point of being diagnosed with a life-threatening condition that is likely to lead to death before adulthood. Intermittent respite and supportive care is the focus of the hospices in the United Kingdom. Although children do sometimes die in these facilities, death often occurs in the child's home with the support of the home care team.

Hospice-based home care programs are more common in the United States. The first pediatric hospice program in the United States, Edmarc Hospice for Children, was established in 1978 in the Tidewater region of Virginia. A 1983 survey indicated that only 4 (0.28%) of the approximately 1,400 home hospice agencies in the country served children [5]. According to a 2001 survey by the Children's International Project on Palliative/Hospice Services (ChiPPS), of the more than 3,000 hospice programs in the United States, 450 (15%) indicated that they were prepared to offer hospice services to children [6]. A brief review of the literature can bring a sharper perspective on the services that do exist for children with life-threatening illnesses.

Review of the literature

How children die, where children die, and when children die have become the focus of much discussion and interest nationally during the last 10 years

[7–9]. According to 2003 data from the National Center for Health Statistics, more than 50,000 children from birth to 19 years of age die each year, many of whom could benefit from hospice and palliative care [10]. It is estimated that close to 2 million children in the United States live with serious medical conditions [11–14].

A white paper produced by the ChiPPS Administrative/Policy Workgroup of the National Hospice and Palliative Care Organization estimates that palliative care would be an appropriate model of care for approximately 1.5 to 2 million children in the United States living with severity of illness ratings of major (S3) to extreme (S4) levels of disability, as designated by the National Association of Children's Hospitals and Related Institutions [6]. Feudtner and colleagues [13] described the hospital care received in the last year of life by children and young adults who died between 1990 and 1996 in Washington State. They found that the rate of hospital use increases as a child approaches death. Eighty-four percent of infants with chronic complex conditions were hospitalized at the time of death, and 50% of them were mechanically ventilated. Of the children and young adults with complex chronic conditions, 55% were hospitalized at the time of death and 19% had been mechanically ventilated during their terminal admission [13].

All general and subspecialty pediatricians, family physicians, pain specialists, and pediatric surgeons should become familiar and comfortable with the provision of palliative care to children, as emphasized in the American Academy of Pediatrics (AAP) position statement on pediatric palliative care [11]. The AAP's position statement specifically recommends the following:

- Palliative care and respite programs need to be developed and widely available to children with life-threatening or terminal conditions.
- Palliative care for children should be integrated into the care of children diagnosed with a life-threatening or terminal condition, regardless of outcome.
- Modifications need to be made to current regulatory and reimbursement limitations.
- All physicians caring for pediatric patients must become comfortable with the provision of palliative care.
- Physician education and certifying examinations must include training and testing on issues related to palliative care.
- More research needs to be done in the field of palliative care for children [15].

In 1993 the Children's Hospice International published Standards of Hospice Care for Children (Table 1). In 2004, the National Consensus Project (NCP) published guidelines for quality palliative care by outlining eight domains of care (Table 2). Together, these guidelines serve as the foundation for preferred standards in the field of hospice and palliative care. They were adopted by the National Quality Forum as the basis for the development of a National Framework and Preferred Practices for Palliative and Hospice Care Quality in 2006. The framework and guidelines can be used to identify

Table 1
Children's Hospice International published standards of hospice care for children

Access to care	Principle: Children with life-threatening illnesses and their families have special needs. Hospice services for children and their families offer developmentally appropriate palliative and supportive care to any child with a life-threatening condition in any appropriate setting. Children are admitted to hospice services without regard for diagnosis, gender, race, creed, handicap, age, or ability to pay.
Child and family as a unit of care	Principle: Hospice programs provide family-centered care to enhance the quality of life for the children and family as defined by each child-and family unit. It includes the child and family in the decision-making process about services and treatment choices to the fullest degree that is possible and desired.
Policies and procedures	Principle: The hospice program offers services that are accountable to and appropriate for the children and families it serves.
Interdisciplinary team services	Principle: Seriously ill children with life-threatening conditions and/or facing terminal stages of an illness and their families have a variety of needs that require a collaborative and cooperative effort from practitioners of many disciplines, working together as an interdisciplinary team of qualified professionals and volunteers.

From CHI. Standards of hospice care for children. Alexandria (VA): Children's Hospice International 1993; with permission.

and measure quality across settings, and are carefully referenced on evidence-based standards [10,16,17]. Although not specifically written for children, the guidelines include pediatrics (newborns to young adults). However, despite the current standards, guidelines, and position statement, misconceptions regarding pediatric end-of-life care persist, particularly those that lead to a reluctance to refer children to palliative care services [18–20].

Misconceptions about hospice home care services for children

It is often assumed that families routinely take their seriously ill children home to die. In fact, only 10% of American children who died between birth and 14 years of age, died at home, according to 2003 data retrieved from the National Center for Health Statistics [21]. Most children died in hospitals [21].

Another assumption is that physicians routinely refer dying children to home hospice care. The reality is that, too often, medical providers are either unaware of, or uncomfortable with, the specialized services that

Table 2
National Consensus Project for Quality Palliative Care clinical practice guidelines for quality palliative care

Domains of quality palliative care	Includes the following principles of palliative care
Domain 1 Structure and Processes of Care	Ages inclusive of perinatal through adult
Domain 2 Physical Aspects of Care	Patient and family-centered care
Domain 3 Psychological and Psychiatric Aspects of Care	Begins at the time of diagnosis and continues throughout care and into bereavement
Domain 4 Social Aspects of Care	Multidimensional, interdisciplinary, comprehensive care with expertise for children and their families
Domain 5 Spiritual, Religious and Existential Aspects of Care	Attention to relief of suffering
Domain 6 Cultural Aspects of Care	Communication skills are requisite
Domain 7 Care of the Imminently Dying Patient	Continuity across setting
Domain 8 Ethical and Legal Aspects of Care	Equitable access to care

Adapted from National Consensus Project for Quality Palliative Care. Clinical practice guidelines for quality palliative care. 2004. Available at: http://www.nationalconsensusproject. org. Accessed January 27, 2007.

pediatric hospice and palliative care programs can provide. In 1998, Children's Hospice International conducted a survey of hospice agencies and providers. In one section of the survey, respondents were asked to rate the significance of 11 barriers to their delivery of hospice services to children [12]. After "association of hospice with death" and "lack of clarity of when to refer," the third most significant barrier was "physician reluctance to refer."

It has also been assumed that dying children routinely have their distress effectively managed near the end of life. In truth, although major improvements have been made in educating providers to care for dying children, major inadequacies remain in training and preparing health care providers to meet the needs of dying children [22,23]. Wolfe and colleagues [24] explored the suffering of children with cancer at the end of life. The study included interviews with parents of 103 children who had undergone cancer treatment at the Children's Hospital and the Dana Farber Cancer Institute in Boston. Nearly 50% of the children died at home. According to parents, 89% of the children suffered "a lot" or a "great deal" from at least one symptom in the last month of life. Symptoms commonly included fatigue, pain, and dyspnea.

A general impression persists that specialized palliative and end-of-life care services are readily available to children in their homes and that children needing such services routinely receive them. In fact, the National Hospice and Palliative Care Organization Facts and Figures 2005 data noted that of the 4100 hospice and palliative care programs in the United

States that year, only 738 (18%) provided any pediatric services [25]. These figures do not indicate whether the hospice and palliative care programs have a history of experience with these kinds of care or have staff trained in pediatric care. A willingness to provide care cannot be equated with the ability to provide adequate care.

Finally, although the common misconception is that pediatric palliative care is readily reimbursed by insurers, expenses for pediatric palliative care services are often not readily reimbursed. Pediatric patients often meet with barriers to receiving hospice benefits that can force families to choose to forego any life-sustaining and life-prolonging therapies. For this reason, less than 10% of pediatric patients eligible for hospice care are enrolled to receive hospice benefits [26]. Individuals enrolled in the Center for Medicare and Medicaid have a hospice reimbursement benefit that is based on a per-visit model at a rate ranging from $125 to $190 per day, depending on geographic location. This rate is intended to cover all home nursing visits, medications, and any supportive services required [27].

To maximize the ability of the general practitioner to care successfully for dying children at home, it is important to understand the correlation between these misconceptions and the reality of care in the community. With continued education and training, the general practitioner should feel more comfortable with referring children for palliative and hospice care and with working with community-based agencies to provide optimal care for our most vulnerable population.

Services for children and their families at the end of life

> JR attends a full-time, school-based program for special-needs children in an urban public school district. While attending school, JR suffered a life-threatening respiratory event that prompted school personnel to call 911. He was transported to the local community hospital where he was intubated, placed on a ventilator, and stabilized for transfer to the tertiary children's hospital. While JR was in the pediatric intensive care unit, the intensivists consulted the hospital's palliative and supportive care team to meet with his parents to discuss goals of care. In this family meeting between the parents and the palliative care team, the parents decided that they did not want JR to have long-term ventilation requiring a tracheostomy.

Because children die in different settings (ie, at home, in the hospital, and sometimes at an in-patient community-based facility), children and the families who care for them should be given the resources to choose care that serves them best. Pediatric home hospice services may not be available, adequate, or appropriate for children throughout much of North America. Although coordinated and effective home hospice services are available and are often linked to a tertiary children's hospital in some areas, most hospice agencies, although expert in caring for dying adult patients, are limited in their experience with pediatric end-of-life care. Community medical practitioners are often experts in caring for children and their families during times of serious illness and death. How the general practitioner makes referrals and arranges services with hospice agencies, and what types of pediatric services are available, can be important issues in providing care.

In their book, *Shelter from the Storm*, Hilden and Tobin [28] explain that hospice services vary in the amount of experience their staff has had with dying children. Sumner writes that "adult focused programs and staff are typically unprepared to respond to the infrequent pediatric referrals and lack connections to pediatric providers to assist them in providing safe, appropriate hospice care" [29]. Maxwell finds that, of the palliative and hospice programs in the United States that admit children, 40% care for an average of three or fewer children per year [30]. Under these circumstances, the challenges of obtaining and maintaining expertise in caring for dying children and their families are formidable.

When discussing the option of pediatric hospice and palliative care or home care services with families, one should remember several key points: (1) the main goal of pediatric end-of-life care is to enhance a child's quality of life during his or her final journey; (2) home care nursing agencies that are not primarily hospice organizations may be a family's only option [28]; and (3) families often have misconceptions about what constitutes hospice care. The word hospice is often associated with the concepts "going home to die" or "giving up hope." Families need to be reassured that choosing hospice and palliative care services does not mean foregoing options such as returning to the hospital or continuing to receive care from their primary physician. Most pediatric programs admit children under a palliative care umbrella to minimize the barriers to traditional hospice care and do not always require parents to sign a do-not-resuscitate order [31].

Arranging hospice home care services

The medical practitioner becomes more than just a clinician when working with children and families to obtain services at home for end-of-life care. The roles of patient advocate, care coordinator, and educator become equally important in the effort to identify appropriate services and providers for the child and family. When arranging hospice home care services for dying children and their families, the practitioner should pursue the following steps:

1. Meet with the family to identify their goals and wishes for their child's care, exploring the limitations of treatment (ie, antibiotics, oxygen, nutrition and hydration, resuscitation, blood transfusions, and other treatment modalities).
2. Verify insurance plans and benefits; identify the available provider network for home hospice agencies.
3. Clarify the treatment plan with the third party payer in order to assure both authorization and reimbursement of services.

4. Make a referral to the home hospice agency that has been identified as best able to meet the child's and family's needs. When trying to determine an appropriate hospice and palliative care home-based agency, consider the following questions:
   - Has the agency had experience in caring for pediatric patients? If so, what has been its experience?
   - Does the agency have staff who have been trained in end-of-life care for children?
   - Are the staff available to have an introductory meeting with the child and family before initiating services?
   - Can the staff provide ongoing psychosocial bereavement services for parents and siblings after a child dies?
5. Provide a detailed treatment plan which includes medications for comfort in emergency situations at the end of life.

Hospice agencies that may be accomplished with managing adult symptoms and medications are frequently less comfortable with managing the pediatric patient. Therefore, the general practitioner needs to stay involved in the care of the child. Continuity of care may occur through regular communications with the agency staff and family. It may include the practitioner's constant availability to support the hospice caregiver in managing symptoms and prescribing medications for the pediatric patient. Because no one person can provide solutions for the myriad issues that arise related to pediatric end-of-life care, developing a collaborative relationship between community health care providers and general practitioners can yield more possible answers to problems when they do arise. Table 3 shows resources in pediatric palliative care available to practitioners.

Out-of-hospital do-not-attempt-resuscitation orders

JR was successfully extubated and discharged to home with noninvasive mask ventilation overnight. The hospital-based palliative care team subsequently facilitated a conversation among the parents, the local pediatrician, the local emergency medical service (EMS), and the school district to formalize JR's ongoing treatment plan. A cornerstone of this plan was the development of a formal out-of-hospital do-not-attempt-resuscitation document that identified the parent's wishes for JR's care in the case of a life-threatening event. The school district was willing to support the family's decisions regarding JR's treatment plan.

One problem that arises frequently concerns issues related to out-of-hospital DNAROs. Within the framework of pertinent laws, regulations, and precedents, one of the most difficult decisions that parents and legal guardians of children with complex chronic conditions or terminal illnesses are frequently called on to make concerns defining a DNARO for their children [32]. The intent of a DNARO is to limit aggressive life-sustaining

Table 3
Additional resources

Resource	Website
End-of-Life Nursing Education Consortium (ELNEC)	http://www.aacn.nche.edu/elnec/index.htm
Education in Palliative and End-of-Life Care (EPEC)	http://www.epec.net/EPEC/webpages/index.cfm
The Initiative for Pediatric Palliative Care (IPPC)	http://www.ippcweb.org/
City of Hope Pain & Palliative Care Resource Center (COHPPRC)	http://www.cityofhope.org/PRC/
Children's Hospice International (CHI)	http://www.chionline.org
The Association of Children's Hospices (U.K.)	http://www.childhospice.org.uk/
Children's Hospice and Palliative Care Organization	http://www.childrenshospice.org
Association for Children with Life-Threatening or Terminal Conditions and their Families (ACT)	http://www.act.org.uk
End-of-Life/Palliative Education Resource Center (EPERC)	http://www.eperc.mcw.edu/
American Academy of Hospice and Palliative Medicine (AAHPM)	http://www.aahpm.org/resources/
Hospice and Palliative Nurses Association (HPNA)	http://www.hpna.org
ChiPPS of the National Hospice and Palliative Care Organization	http://www.nhpco.org/pediatrics

This list is by no means exhaustive but a sampling of the resources available.

interventions that do not meet the child's and family's wishes. A DNARO is usually honored without reservation in the hospital or hospice setting, but often meets resistane for children outside the hospital in the community or school setting. Some members of the community may be concerned about their personal liability in the case of an out-of-hospital DNARO. Others may be concerned about the emotional impact of seeing a child die. In some instances, school personnel, children and parents in the school community, members of certain religious groups, and extended family members may see such a policy as "hastening death" and not valuing life.

Coordinating care for children with life-threatening illnesses in the community requires attention to issues related to out-of-hospital DNAROs. This issue can highlight conflicts between caring for the child in accordance with the family's wishes and meeting the regulations within the community, specifically those related to schools and EMS systems.

Historically, parents have the right to make choices about their children's care as long as their choices do not jeopardize the children's safety and well-being. Society accepts that parents are morally and legally the decision makers for their children. This position is supported ethically and legally [33]. Constitutional law states that "custody, care and nurture of the child resides first in the parents whose primary function and freedom include preparation for obligations that the state can neither supply nor hinder" (Prince v Massachusetts, 1994) [34]. However, the question of the "best interests" of the child must be balanced against the interests of others in the situation, such as the school community. Appreciating the context of the child's life, understanding what makes it meaningful, and respecting the relationships that are central to it are essential [35,36].

The Individuals with Disabilities Education Act mandates that an education, often in the classroom, is the right of all children despite medical or mental challenges, as long as it remains in their best interests and is not a danger to self or others [37]. The AAP Committees on Bioethics and School Health issued a position statement saying that "parents have a legal right to forego cardiopulmonary resuscitation and to ask the school to respect that decision" [38].

When a child with a complex chronic or terminal condition is returning to the school setting, it is important for the parents, the local pediatrician, EMS, and the school district to have a clear understanding of the goals of care. Rushton, Will, and Murray suggested in 1994 that the issue of whether to honor a DNARO is critical because the setting for decision making has moved, in many cases, from the hospital to the home and schools [35]. In a 2004 study of 80 public school districts, most school systems sampled had not addressed student DNAROs in their district policies or procedures, and a sizeable majority would not honor student DNAROs under any condition. The study also noted that potentially problematic discrepancies existed between school board policies and state laws [39]. These incongruities highlight the potential conflict between school system concerns and parental and student rights [36].

Only a few states explicitly authorize EMS providers to apply advance directives to children [40]. Although lacking explicit authorization, existing statutes generally do not prohibit extension of DNARO for children to out-of-hospital situations [38]. This lack of clarity invites misinterpretation and failure to act according to the wishes of the child and family. It is the practitioner's responsibility to initiate conversations about advance care planning with families to clarify decisions about medical treatment and nontreatment. Until statutes are clear, the challenge is to be able to communicate. The challenge is to communicate the caregivers' wishes for their children in an organized, succinct document available to the local EMS system and schools.

Honoring an out-of-hospital DNARO does not mean doing nothing for the child. During the discussion about out-of-hospital DNAROs with families and other involved parties, caregivers should avoid the phrase, "There is nothing more that can be done for your child." This language erects a barrier to children getting appropriate care and comfort measures near the end of life. Conversations with families about their wishes should focus on what can and should be done rather that what will not be done. Caregivers may not want their children to receive cardiopulmonary resuscitation or intubation, but they may want less invasive but equally important interventions such as the provision of oxygen, relief of pain, and aggressive symptom management. The orders containing the DNARO should provide clear guidance regarding how to proceed in the event of a medical decompensation or cardiopulmonary arrest [35]. A clearly defined out-of-hospital DNARO document would assure that the child will receive appropriate care in an emergency situation. The collaborative efforts of general practitioners, parents, school officials, community health care providers, and EMS personnel are essential to provide a document that invokes comfort care as opposed to life-sustaining measures for the complex chronic or terminally ill child in the community.

Reimbursement issues

Community medical practitioners who refer patients for hospice and palliative care services outside the hospital setting do encounter barriers to providing and receiving adequate reimbursement for services that meet the minimum standards indicated for appropriate pediatric palliative care [14,41–44]. The Institute of Medicine (IOM) report recommends that the hospice benefit be restructured to better meet the needs of children [26]. Their recommendations include eliminating eligibility restrictions related to life expectancy, eliminating the requirement to discontinue all curative treatment, and adding an outlier payment category for children whose care is unusually costly. The report also cautions in strong language that the current hospice health care delivery model for adults and children alike can create "incentives for undertreatment, overtreatment, inappropriate transitions between settings of care, inadequate coordination of care, and poor overall quality of care" [26].

In response to the existing referral and reimbursement barriers to providing and funding the care of children with life-threatening conditions, Children's Hospice International developed the Program for All-Inclusive Care for Children (PACC) and their Families [45]. The PACC model provides access to care for all children diagnosed with life-threatening conditions. It also provides for reimbursement by all payers including private insurance, workplace coverage, managed care, and Medicaid. Initial pilot programs in Colorado, Florida, Kentucky, New York, New England, Utah, and Virginia were funded by Congressional appropriations through the Centers for Medicare and Medicaid Services (CMS). Following the pilot programs, Florida and Colorado were approved for CMS waivers. Florida received approval of its CMS waiver in July 2005 for a 5-year, statewide demonstration project of the PACC program [46,47]. Colorado received approval in January 2007 for its request for a CMS waiver and will be implementing a 3-year renewable demonstration project for pediatric palliative care [48]. Utah is in the process of submitting a waiver and California is in the process of writing a waiver request to be submitted no later than

January 1, 2008, as mandated by legislation passed in the fall of 2006 [49,50]. Several other states and the District of Columbia are in the early phases of data gathering to prepare for waiver development.

Other barriers to receiving care at home

In addition to reimbursement issues related to home hospice services, some other barriers that may influence a family's decision to take their sick child home to die are

- Concern for other siblings living in the home
- Concern about the house itself forever being associated with the loss of a beloved child
- Inadequate family support
- Unsafe conditions in the home
- Lack of skilled hospice home care providers
- Cultural or religious beliefs/influences

The general practitioner should consider the desires of the family as well as their ability to manage their children's care at home regardless of issues like reimbursement. Parents need to be presented with the various options of care (ie, hospital, home setting, or in-patient skilled nursing facility) and the attendant financial and physical obligations. Home care scenarios assume that parents will provide a substantial amount of the care themselves, which can include mechanical ventilation, feeding tubes, and central intravenous lines. Parents may incur financial obligations for copayments and deductibles for home hospice services that are not reimbursable. Despite a willingness to care for their children at home, not all families are able to provide the care. Even for families who can bear the financial cost, caring for their dying children at home may be too great a burden. To achieve the goal of quality end-of-life care for dying children whose families are unable to care for them at home, the pediatric skilled nursing facilities can provide another option for care for children with complex, chronic conditions.

Summary

JR was successfully reintegrated into the home and school settings with these revised plans in place. He died peacefully at home after the completion of his school year without any further hospitalizations.

When children die of complex, chronic, or life-limiting conditions, death is a journey that belongs to the child and family. Those of us who care for these children and their families are the honored guests. Our role as medical practitioners must become one of advocate, communicator, and facilitator to support the wishes of the child and family on this journey. The goals of care should always focus on the family's needs and desires, removing the barriers that hinder the journey, and optimizing quality of life and relief of suffering along the way.

Although evidence exists that appropriate care and services for children with complex, chronic, or life-limiting conditions and their families can help to assuage their physical, emotional, and spiritual suffering, services for them are still inadequate. To address this dilemma and its related issues, all health care providers, not just the medical practitioner, must first recognize that the problems exist and then join the effort to make critical and lasting improvements in services and care delivery through research, education, funding, and innovative programs.

Acknowledgment

The authors would like to thank the following individuals for their assistance in reviewing this article: Betty Davies, RN, PhD, FAAN, Department of Family Health Care Nursing, N411Y, University of California, San Francisco School of Nursing and Betty R. Ferrell, PhD, FAAN, Department of Nursing Education and Research, City of Hope National Medical Center.

References

[1] Hill L. The history and development of children's hospices. Nurs Times 1998;94(33):58–60.
[2] Worswick J. A house called Helen: the development of hospice care for children. 2nd edition. Oxford (UK): Oxfod University Press; 2000.
[3] Association of Children's Hospices. Available at: www.childhospice.org.uk. Accessed January 8, 2006.
[4] Association for Children's Palliative Care. Available at: www.act.org.uk. Accessed December 8, 2006.
[5] Armstrong-Dailey A, Zarbock S. A history of children's hospice and palliative care. 2001. Available at: http://www.chionline.org/resources/history.php. Accessed February, 2007.
[6] Levetown M, Barnard M, Hellston M, et al. A call for change: recommendations to improve the care of children living withlife-threatening conditions. A white paper produced by the Children's International Project on Palliative/Hospice Services (ChIPPS) Administrative/ Policy workgroup of the National Hospice and Palliative Care Organization. Alexandria (VA): NHPCO; 2001.
[7] Mallinson J, Jones PD. A 7-year review of deaths on the general paediatric wards at John Hunter Children's Hospital, 1991–97. J Paediatr Child Health 2000;36(3):252–5.
[8] Feudtner C, Christakis D, Zimmerman F, et al. Characteristics of deaths occurring in children's hospitals: implications for supportive care. Pediatrics 2002;109(5):887–93.
[9] Feudtner C, Hays R, Haynes G, et al. Deaths attributed to pediatric complex chronic conditions: national trends and implications for supportive services. Pediatrics 2001;107(6):E99.
[10] National Consensus Project for Quality Palliative Care. Clinical practice guidelines for quality palliative care, 2004. Available at: www.nationalconsensusproject.org. Accessed January 27, 2007.
[11] American academy of pediatrics. Committee on bioethics and committee on hospital care. Palliative care for children. Pediatrics 2000;106(2 Pt 1):351–7.
[12] Armstrong-Daily A, Zarbock S, editors. Hospice care for children. New York: Oxford University Press; 2001.

[13] Feudtner C, DiGiuseppe DL, Neff JM. Hospital care for children and young adults in the last year of life: a population-based study. BMC Med 2003;1:3.

[14] Simpson L, Owens PL, Zodet MW, et al. Health care for children and youth in the United States: annual report on patterns of coverage, utilization, quality, and expenditures by income. Ambul Pediatr 2005;5(1):6–44.

[15] AAP. Palliative care for children. Pediatrics 2000;106(2):351–7.

[16] A national framework and preferred practices for palliative and hospice care quality: a consensus report. 2006.

[17] Lieberman L, Hilliard RI. How well do paediatric residency programmes prepare residents for clinical practice and their future careers? Med Educ 2006;40(6):539–46.

[18] Himelstein BP, Hilden JM, Boldt AM, et al. Pediatric palliative care. N Engl J Med 2004; 350(17):1752–62.

[19] Fowler K, Poehling K, Billheimer D, et al. Hospice referral practices for children with cancer: a survey of pediatric oncologists. J Clin Oncol 2006;24(4):1099–104.

[20] Baker J, Torkildson C, Baillargeon J, et al. A national survey of pediatric residency program directors and residents regarding education in palliative medicine and end-of-life care. In press.

[21] National Center for Health Statistics. Available at: http://www.cdc.gov/nchs/datawh/statab/unpubd/mortabs/gmwk307.htm. Accessed January 8, 2006.

[22] Contro NA, Larson J, Scofield S, et al. Hospital staff and family perspectives regarding quality of pediatric palliative care. Pediatrics 2004;114(5):1248–52.

[23] Drake R, Frost J, Collins JJ. The symptoms of dying children. J Pain Symptom Manage 2003;26(1):594–603.

[24] Wolfe J, Grier HE, Klar N, et al. Symptoms and suffering at the end of life in children with cancer. N Engl J Med 2000;342(5):326–33.

[25] National data set - NHPCO's facts and figures 2005 findings. NHPCO, 2006.

[26] Behrman RE, Field MJ, editors. When children die: improving palliative and end-of-life care for children and their families. Washington, DC: The National Academy of Sciences; 2003. Institute of Medicine of the National Academies.

[27] FY2006 Hospice wage index and rates: Center for Medicare and Medicaid Services, 2006.

[28] Hilden J, Tobin D. Shelter from the storm: caring for a child with a life-threatening condition. Cambridge (UK): Perseus; 2003. p. 164.

[29] Sumner L. Pediatric care: the hospice perspective. In: Ferrell B, Coyle N, editors. Textbook of palliative nursing. 2nd edition. New York: Oxford University Press; 2006. p. 916.

[30] Maxwell T, Reifsnyder J, Davis C, et al. Our littlest patients: a national description of pediatric hospice patients. Paper presented at the American academy of hospice and palliative medicine annual assembly. Nashville (TN), 2006.

[31] Kang T, Hoehn S, Licht D, et al. Pediatric palliative, end-of-life and bereavement care. Pediatr Clin North Am 2005;(52):1029–46.

[32] Tan GH, Totapally BR, Torbati D, et al. End-of-life decisions and palliative care in a children's hospital. J Palliat Med 2006;9(2):332–42.

[33] Jonsen A, Siegler M, Winslade W. Clinical ethics: a practical approach to ethical decisions in clinical medicine. 5th edition. New York: McGraw-Hill; 2002.

[34] Prince v Massachusetts In: US, ed. vol. 321 US 158, 166–167;1994.

[35] Rushton C, Will J, Murray M. To honor and obey - DNR orders and the school. Pediatr Nurs 1994;20(6):581–5.

[36] Rehm R, Bradley J. The search for social safety and comfort in families raising children with complex chronic conditions. J Fam Nurs 2005;11(1):59–78.

[37] Individuals with Disabilities Education Act. vol 94-142 Title 20 United States code section 1400; 1975.

[38] AAP. Do not resuscitate orders in schools. Pediatrics 2000;105(4):878–9.

[39] Kimberly MB, Forte AL, Carroll JM, et al. Pediatric do-not-attempt-resuscitation orders and public schools: a national assessment of policies and laws. Am J Bioeth 2005;5(1):59–65.

[40] AAP. Guidelines on forgoing life-sustaining medical treatment. Pediatrics 1997;93(3):532–6.
[41] Mentro AM. Health care policy for medically fragile children. Journal of Pediatric Nursing 2003;18(4):225–32.
[42] Perrin JM. EPSDT (Early and periodic screening, diagnosis, and treatment): a primer in time of change. Ambul Pediatr 2006;6(2):63–4.
[43] Rowse V. Palliative care for children: a public health initiative. Paediatr Nurs 2006;18(4): 41–5.
[44] Sardell A, Johnson B. The politics of EPSDT policy in the 1990s: policy entrepreneurs, political streams, and children's health benefits. The Milbank Quarterly 1998;76(2):175–205.
[45] Children's Hospice International program for all-inclusive care for children and their families (CHI PACC). Available at: http://www.chionline.org/programs/. Accessed January 15, 2007.
[46] CHI. CHI PACC model: The Kentucky, Colorado, Florida, Kentucky, Utah and New York experience. Children's Hospice International. Available at: http://www.chionline.org/ programs/. Accessed December, 2006.
[47] The Florida CHI PACC model: partners in care, together for kids. Available at: http://www. chionline.org/states/fl.php. Accessed January 15, 2007.
[48] The butterfly program: a Children's Hospice International program for all-inclusive care for children and their families (CHI PACC). Available at: http://www.chionline.org/states/co. php. Accessed January 15, 2007.
[49]] CHI PACC Utah: promoting hospice and optimal palliative efforts. Available at: http:// www.chionline.org/states/ut.php. Accessed January 15, 2007.
[50] The Nick Snow Children's Hospice & Palliative Care Act of 2006-Assembly Bill 1745. Available at: http://childrenshospice.org/news/index.php?itemid=21. Accessed January 15, 2007.

**ELSEVIER
SAUNDERS**

Pediatr Clin N Am 54 (2007) 829–836

PEDIATRIC CLINICS

OF NORTH AMERICA

Index

Note: Page numbers of article titles are in **boldface** type.

0031-3955/07/$ - see front matter © 2007 Elsevier Inc. All rights reserved.
doi:10.1016/S0031-3955(07)00130-7

United States Postal Service

Statement of Ownership, Management, and Circulation
(All Periodicals Publications Except Requestor Publications)

1. Publication Title	2. Publication Number	3. Filing Date
Pediatric Clinics of North America	4 2 4 - 6 6 0	9/14/07

4. Issue Frequency	5. Number of Issues Published Annually	6. Annual Subscription Price
Feb, Apr, Jun, Aug, Oct, Dec	6	$138.00

7. Complete Mailing Address of Known Office of Publication (Not printer) (Street, city, county, state, and ZIP+4)

Elsevier Inc.
360 Park Avenue South
New York, NY 10010-1710

Contact Person
Stephen Bushing
Telephone (Include area code)
215-239-3688

8. Complete Mailing Address of Headquarters or General Business Office of Publisher (Not printer)

Elsevier Inc., 360 Park Avenue South, New York, NY 10010-1710

9. Full Names and Complete Mailing Addresses of Publisher, Editor, and Managing Editor (Do not leave blank)

Publisher (Name and complete mailing address)

John Schrefer, Elsevier, Inc., 1600 John F. Kennedy Blvd. Suite 1800, Philadelphia, PA 19103-2899

Editor (Name and complete mailing address)

Carla Holloway, Elsevier, Inc., 1600 John F. Kennedy Blvd. Suite 1800, Philadelphia, PA 19103-2899

Managing Editor (Name and complete mailing address)

Catherine Bewick, Elsevier, Inc., 1600 John F. Kennedy Blvd. Suite 1800, Philadelphia, PA 19103-2899

10. Owner (Do not leave blank. If the publication is owned by a corporation, give the name and address of the corporation immediately followed by the names and addresses of all stockholders owning or holding 1 percent or more of the total amount of stock. If not owned by a corporation, give the names and addresses of the individual owners. If owned by a partnership or other unincorporated firm, give its name and address as well as those of each individual owner. If the publication is published by a nonprofit organization, give its name and address.)

Full Name	Complete Mailing Address
Wholly owned subsidiary of	4520 East-West Highway
Reed/Elsevier, US holdings	Bethesda, MD 20814

11. Known Bondholders, Mortgagees, and Other Security Holders Owning or Holding 1 Percent or More of Total Amount of Bonds, Mortgages, or Other Securities. If none, check box ☑ None

Full Name	Complete Mailing Address
N/A	

12. Tax Status (For completion by nonprofit organizations authorized to mail at nonprofit rates) (Check one)
The purpose, function, and nonprofit status of this organization and the exempt status for federal income tax purposes:
☑ Has Not Changed During Preceding 12 Months
☐ Has Changed During Preceding 12 Months (Publisher must submit explanation of change with this statement)

PS Form 3526, September 2006 (Page 1 of 3 (Instructions Page 3)) PSN 7530-01-000-9931 PRIVACY NOTICE: See our Privacy policy in www.usps.com

---

13. Publication Title	14. Issue Date for Circulation Data Below
Pediatric Clinics of North America	June 2007

15. Extent and Nature of Circulation			Average No. Copies Each Issue During Preceding 12 Months	No. Copies of Single Issue Published Nearest to Filing Date
a. Total Number of Copies (Net press run)			7150	7200
b. Paid Circulation (By Mail and Outside the Mail)	(1)	Mailed Outside-County Paid Subscriptions Stated on PS Form 3541 (Include paid distribution above nominal rate, advertiser's proof copies, and exchange copies)	3463	3220
	(2)	Mailed In-County Paid Subscriptions Stated on PS Form 3541 (Include paid distribution above nominal rate, advertiser's proof copies, and exchange copies)		
	(3)	Paid Distribution Outside the Mails Including Sales Through Dealers and Carriers, Street Vendors, Counter Sales, and Other Paid Distribution Outside USPS®	2230	1951
	(4)	Paid Distribution by Other Classes Mailed Through the USPS (e.g. First-Class Mail®)		
c. Total Paid Distribution (Sum of 15b (1), (2), (3), and (4))		▲	5693	5171
d. Free or Nominal Rate Distribution (By Mail and Outside the Mail)	(1)	Free or Nominal Rate Outside-County Copies Included on PS Form 3541	155	142
	(2)	Free or Nominal Rate In-County Copies Included on PS Form 3541		
	(3)	Free or Nominal Rate Copies Mailed at Other Classes Mailed Through the USPS (e.g. First-Class Mail)		
	(4)	Free or Nominal Rate Distribution Outside the Mail (Carriers or other means)		
e. Total Free or Nominal Rate Distribution (Sum of 15d (1), (2), (3) and (4))		▲	155	142
f. Total Distribution (Sum of 15c and 15e)		▲	5848	5313
g. Copies not Distributed (See instructions to publishers #4 (page #3))		▲	1302	1887
h. Total (Sum of 15f and g)		▲	7150	7200
i. Percent Paid (15c divided by 15f times 100)			97.35%	97.33%

16. Publication of Statement of Ownership
If the publication is a general publication, publication of this statement is required. Will be printed ☑ Publication not required
in the October 2007 issue of this publication.

17. Signature and Title of Editor, Publisher, Business Manager, or Owner	Date
Stephen Bushing – Executive Director of Subscription Services	September 14, 2007

I certify that all information furnished on this form is true and complete. I understand that anyone who furnishes false or misleading information on this form or who omits material or information requested on the form may be subject to criminal sanctions (including fines and imprisonment) and/or civil sanctions (including civil penalties).

PS Form 3526, September 2006 (Page 2 of 3)